PROTEIN packed

125 Low-Carb, High-Protein Recipes to Build Strength, Health, and Longevity

ANNIE LAMPELLA

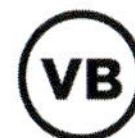

VICTORY BELT PUBLISHING INC.
LAS VEGAS

First published in 2025 by Victory Belt Publishing Inc.

ISBN-13: 978-1-628605-64-8

The information included in this book is for educational purposes only. It is not intended or implied to be a substitute for professional medical advice. The reader should always consult their healthcare provider to determine the appropriateness of the information for their own situation or if they have any questions regarding a medical condition or treatment plan. Reading the information in this book does not constitute a physician-patient relationship.

Cover design by Kat Lannom

Interior design by Crizalie Olimpo

Author photos on pages 4, 6, 8, 42, and 52 by Miranda Kelton

Recipe photos by Eva Riazati and Annie Lampella

Illustrations by Elita San Juan and Alyanna Alcira

Printed in Canada

TC 0125

TABLE OF CONTENTS

INTRODUCTION

If you haven't met me yet, I'm Annie, the creator of the KetoFocus YouTube channel and website. Over the past twelve years, I've been dedicated to creating meals that not only fit into a keto or low-carb lifestyle but also are delicious and family friendly. I'm a mom to picky eaters with a husband who doesn't hold back his critiques (in a loving, constructive way), so I've had plenty of practice perfecting recipes that pass the ultimate taste test. If it's in this book, you can trust that it's been thoroughly tested in my home kitchen.

My keto journey started in 2012, when my husband told me about a way of eating that is supposed to help you lose weight, give you tons of energy, and help you think clearly. After giving birth to my second son, I had a whole lot of extra baby weight to lose. Plus, I was set to go back to work full-time as a pharmacist while balancing two kids under the age of two. I needed as much energy and mental clarity as I could get.

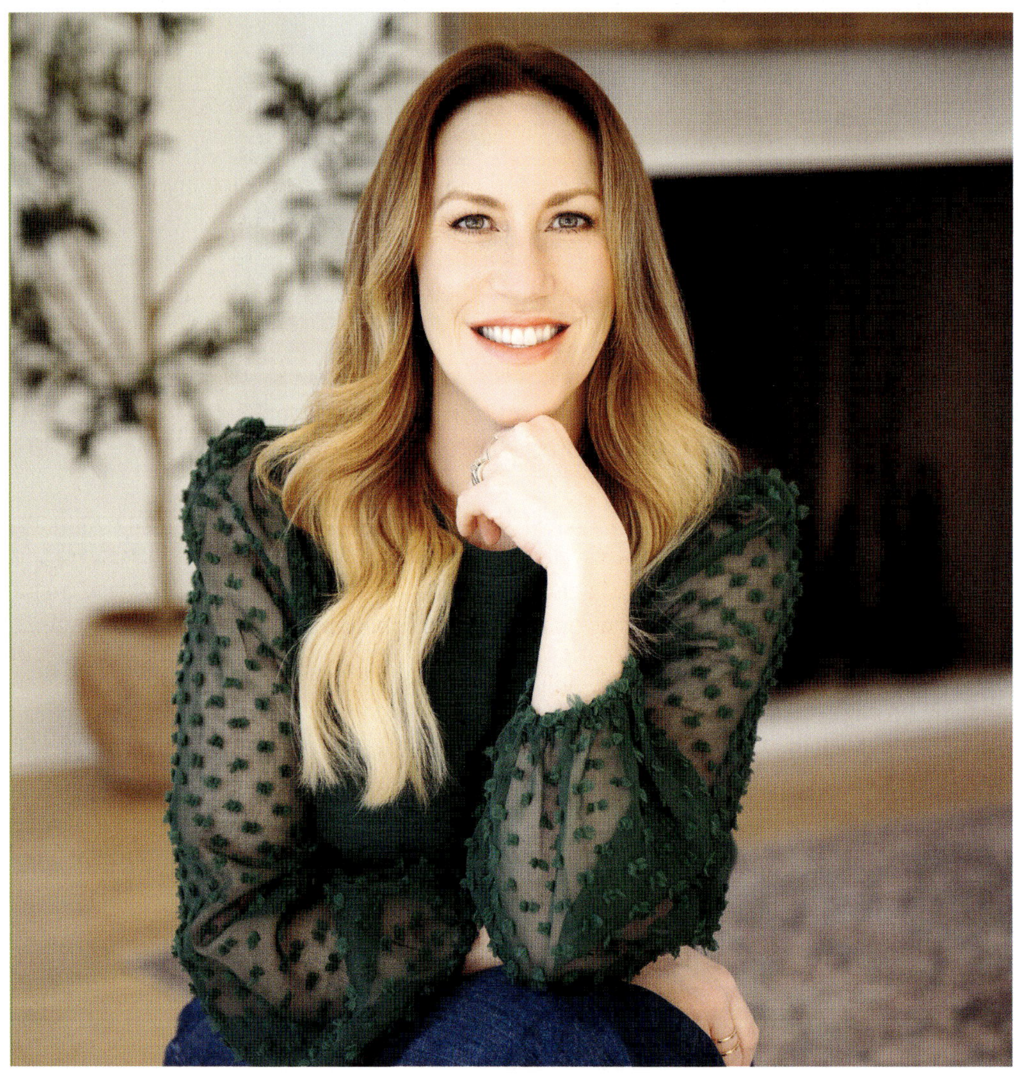

Given my background in science and medicine, I was a little hesitant to eat all the fat involved in the keto diet. But my years of taking biochemistry classes that focused on human metabolism at UC Davis and University of the Pacific while pursuing my doctorate degree also helped me understand why eating keto made sense for the outcomes I wanted to achieve.

What clicked for me was how keto supports the body on a metabolic level. When you lower your carbohydrate intake, your insulin levels drop, and the body shifts into a state called ketosis—where it starts breaking down fat into ketones to use as fuel instead. With high amounts of insulin no longer present, the body switches to using stored fat for energy. You're no longer stuck in a cycle of constant blood sugar spikes and crashes. Your energy is stable, and your cravings are reduced. Plus, the higher fat intake keeps you full, so you're not thinking about food all day. Once I understood that, I felt more confident about leaning into the process.

The results were remarkable. I lost close to 70 pounds and felt better than ever—sharp, energetic, and clear-headed. Keto became a lifestyle, not just a diet, although the path wasn't always completely smooth. Like any journey, there were bumps along the way. As I launched my KetoFocus YouTube channel and website, self-care took a backseat. Trying to balance working, being a parent to two active boys, and starting my side hustle meant that I woke up at 3:30 a.m. to edit videos. Sleep deprivation, fatigue, stress, and the dreaded carb creep disrupted my progress. My hormones were out of balance, and I knew I needed a change.

A few years ago, I decided to take a new approach. I returned to keto with a renewed focus, but I adjusted it to suit my evolving needs. When I first started keto, I kept total carbs under 20 grams per day, but I found myself missing the vibrant vegetables and fruits that I loved. Eventually, I transitioned to a low-carb approach that included more nonstarchy vegetables and low-sugar fruits, keeping my daily intake to around 50 grams of carbs. At the same time, I increased my protein intake after learning about its role in weight loss, muscle building, and overall health. Even though I had been working out with resistance training five times a week, I was having a hard time putting on muscle and hoped the extra protein would help.

This way of eating has completely reshaped my health and lifestyle. By prioritizing protein and embracing a more balanced approach to low-carb eating, I've found long-term sustainability and rebalanced my hormones. I feel stronger, more satisfied, and no longer restricted.

You've picked up this book because you want to make changes in your life. You want to learn more about eating a high-protein, low-carb diet, or perhaps you're a fan of my YouTube channel who's eager for more recipes to add to your collection. In this book, I share the recipes that have helped me hit my protein goals and find balance. These meals are simple, satisfying, and designed for busy lives. From breakfasts to desserts, every dish is crafted to help you succeed in your low-carb, high-protein journey—just as they've helped me and my family. Let's dig in and fuel your best self!

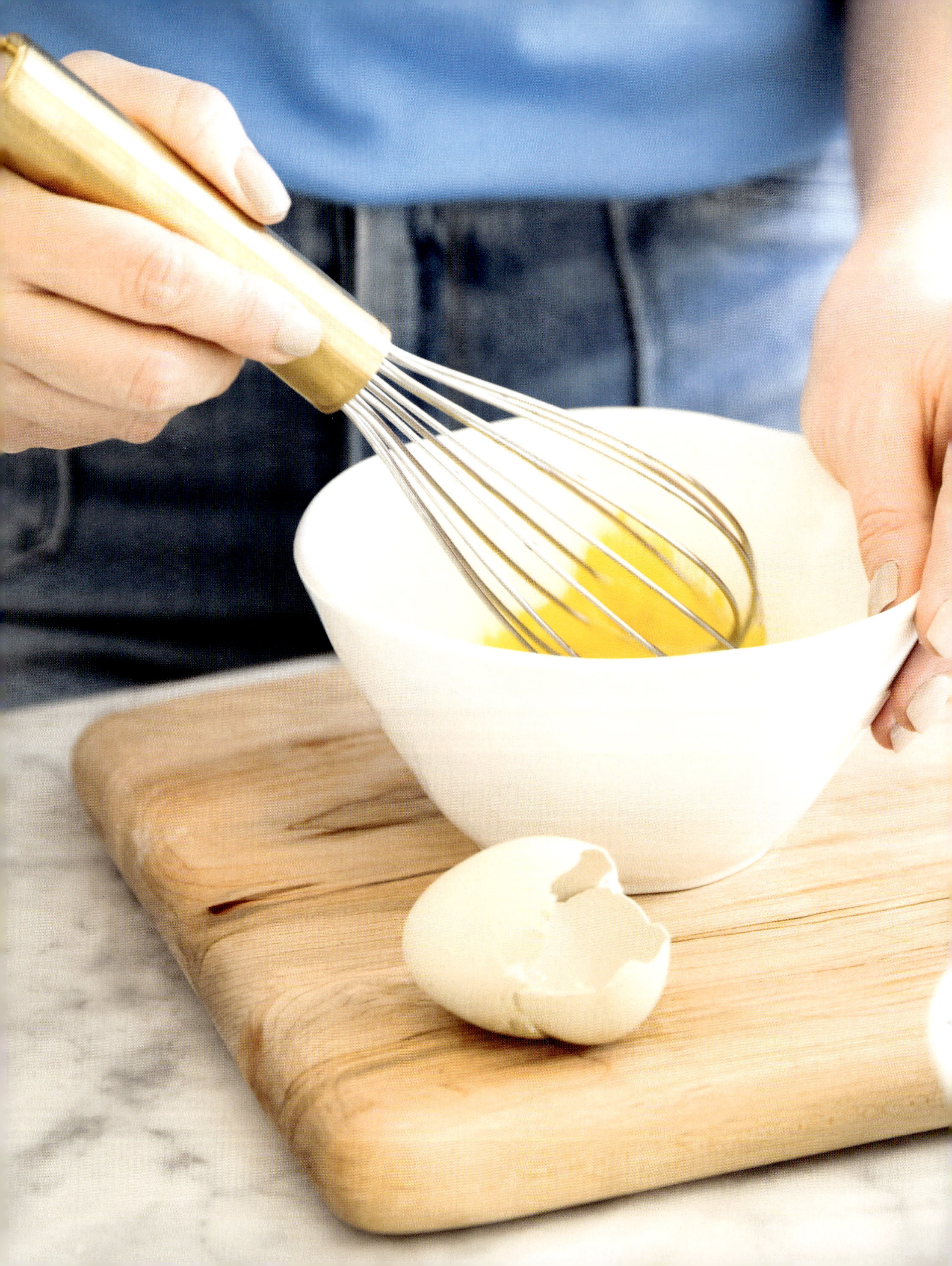

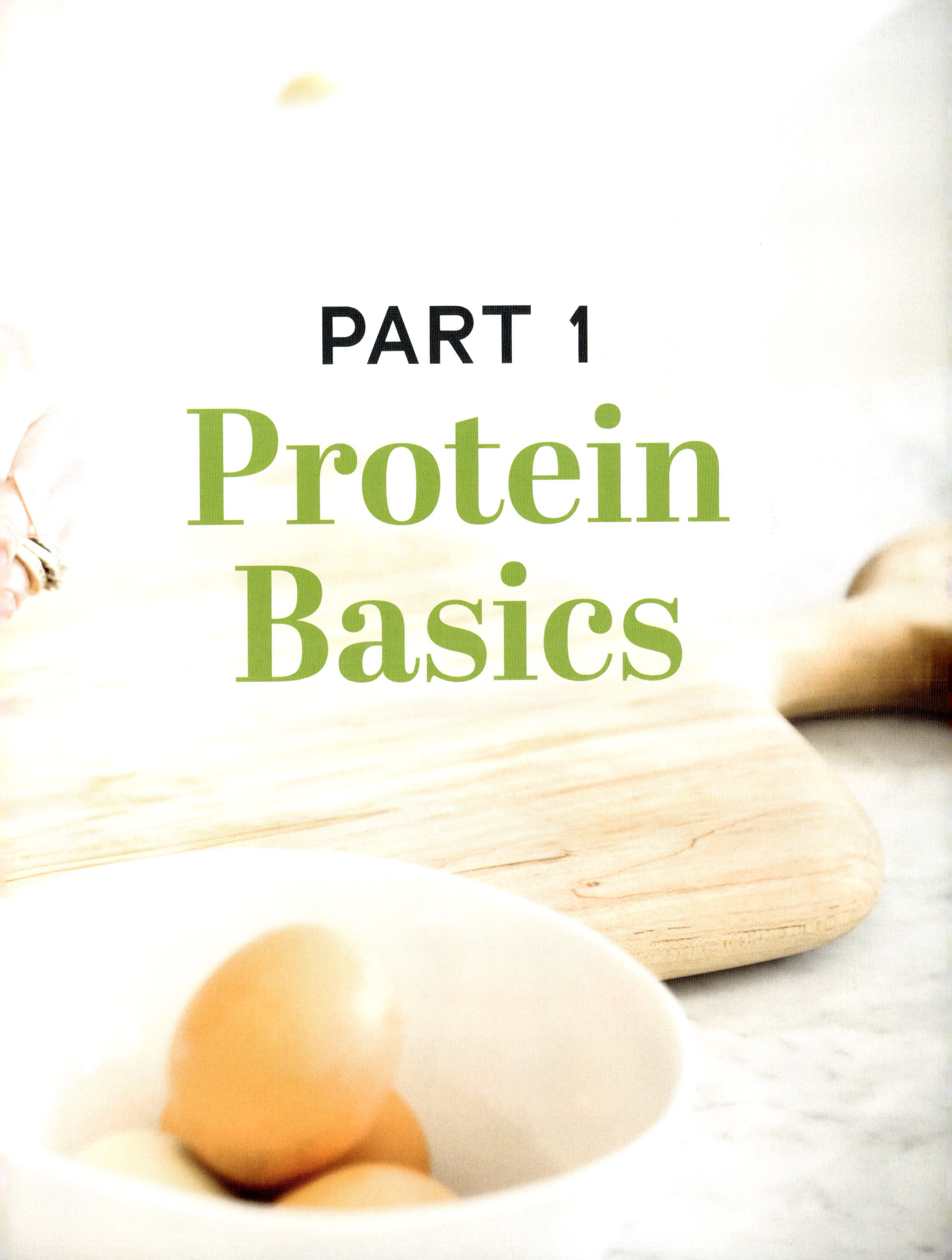

PART 1
Protein Basics

CHAPTER 1

WHAT IS PROTEIN?

To get things started, I want to explain what protein is, what it's made of, why it's essential, and how your body metabolizes it. Understanding these basics is key to appreciating just how important protein is for your health.

Protein is a macronutrient that plays vital roles in the body. Protein is unlike fat and carbohydrates because it's the only macronutrient that contains nitrogen, an essential building block for DNA and RNA. Cell and tissue repair requires nitrogen. Simply put, without nitrogen, your body can't function or survive.

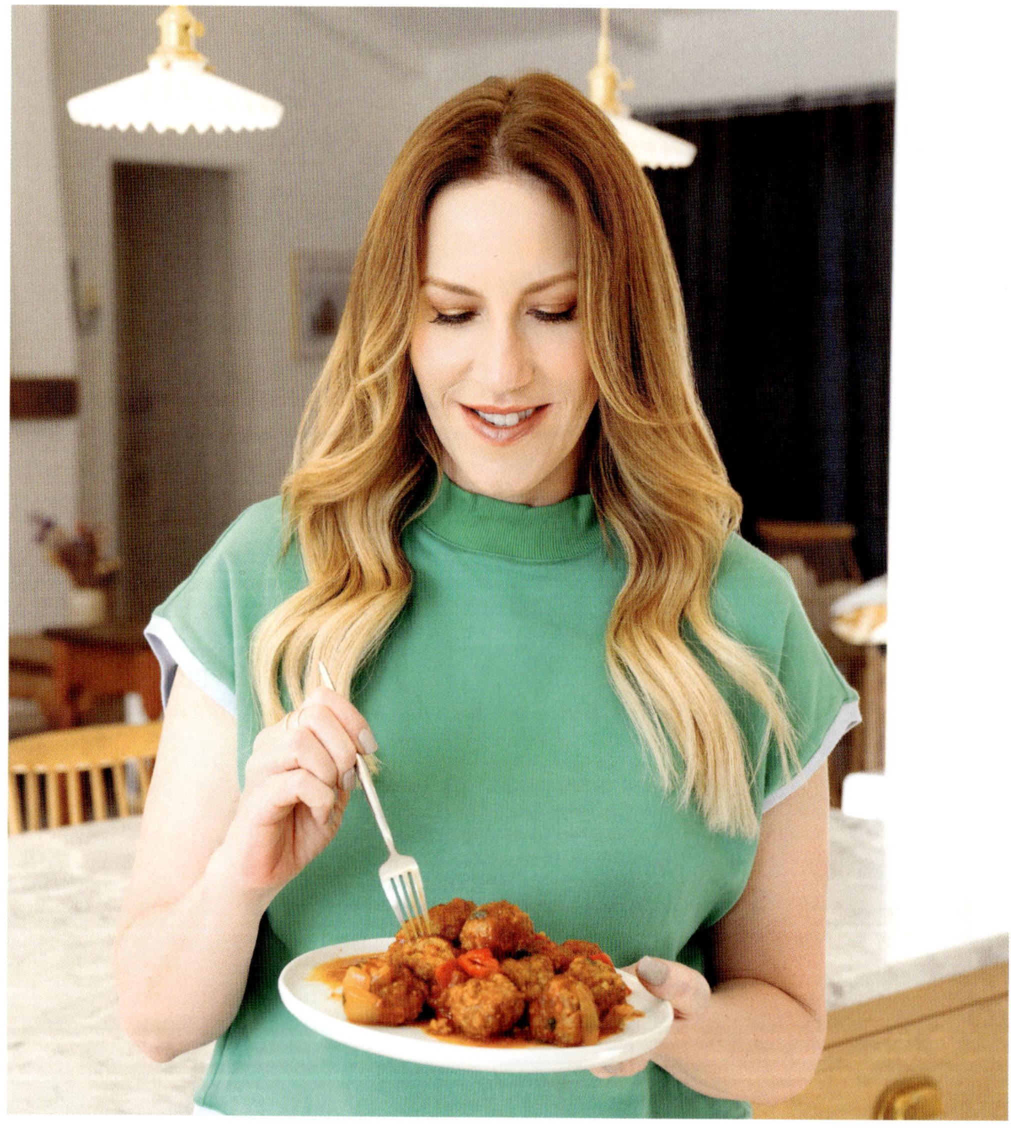

AMINO ACIDS

Protein is made up of smaller units called amino acids, which are linked together in specific sequences. This precise arrangement gives each protein its specific function.

The human body needs twenty different amino acids to work properly, but only nine of them are considered essential. These essential amino acids—histidine, isoleucine, leucine, lysine, methionine, phenylalanine, threonine, tryptophan, and valine[1]—must come from your diet because your body can't make them on its own. There's also a third category called semi-essential amino acids, which are made by the body, but not in sufficient quantities during periods of stress or growth (for example, during sickness, pregnancy, and lactation and in children).

ESSENTIAL AMINO ACIDS	NONESSENTIAL AMINO ACIDS
Histidine	Alanine
Isoleucine	Arginine
Leucine	Asparagine
Lysine	Aspartate
Methionine	Cysteine
Phenylalanine	Glutamate
Threonine	Glutamine
Tryptophan	Glycine
Valine	Proline
	Serine
	Tyrosine

Without the essential amino acids, you would eventually experience impaired growth as well as clinical symptoms such as vomiting, low appetite, depression, anxiety, insomnia, fatigue, and weakness.[2] Sufficient amino acids are essential for producing neurotransmitters and hormones, supporting muscle growth, and carrying out various cellular functions.

However, the fact that the body can make these nonessential amino acids doesn't mean you don't need to consume them in your diet. For optimal growth and cellular function, these nonessential amino acids are required. They play roles in blood flow, hormone secretion, gene expression, cell signaling, immune responses, antioxidative defense, and other vital functions.[3]

THE ROLE OF PROTEIN

Protein is often celebrated for its role in muscle growth and repair. However, its importance goes far beyond strong muscles. It's a crucial component of every cell in the body, playing critical parts in numerous functions that keep us alive and thriving.

Muscle Growth and Repair

Protein plays a vital role in both the growth and repair of muscles, which is why it's essential for maintaining and building a strong, healthy body. The human body has three types of muscle: skeletal, cardiac, and smooth. Most people think of skeletal muscle first because it is the muscle type responsible for voluntary movement. However, cardiac muscle (in the heart) and smooth muscle (surrounding blood vessels and organs) are also vital and made primarily of protein.

When you exercise, your muscles get damaged. The body uses protein to repair damaged muscle fibers, increasing the thickness and number of those fibers to create muscle hypertrophy, or growth.

Immune Function

Your body needs protein and amino acids to stay healthy, repair damage, and fight off sickness. If you don't get enough protein in your diet, your immune system can weaken, making it difficult to fight off infection or delaying wound healing.

Certain amino acids help the immune system by supporting cells like T cells and B cells, helping make antibodies, and keeping the body's defense system strong. Here are some things amino acids do:

- **Alanine** helps the liver make glucose to be used as energy for the immune cells.
- **Arginine** helps the body release important hormones like insulin and growth hormone, which regulate the metabolism of glucose and other amino acids to supply energy for immune cells and help make more T cells to fight infections.
- **Glutamine** helps the body produce glutathione, which protects cells from damage and repairs them. It's also a key ingredient that helps create lymphocytes, the immune cells that fight infection.[4]

Proteins aid in healing wounds and injuries. For example, if you get a cut, your body sends proteins called bradykinins to dilate the blood vessels so repair molecules can quickly get to the injured area. Another protein called fibrin helps form a clot to stop the bleeding. A third protein, collagen, acts as a scaffold and helps fill in the wound and strengthen the tissue.[5]

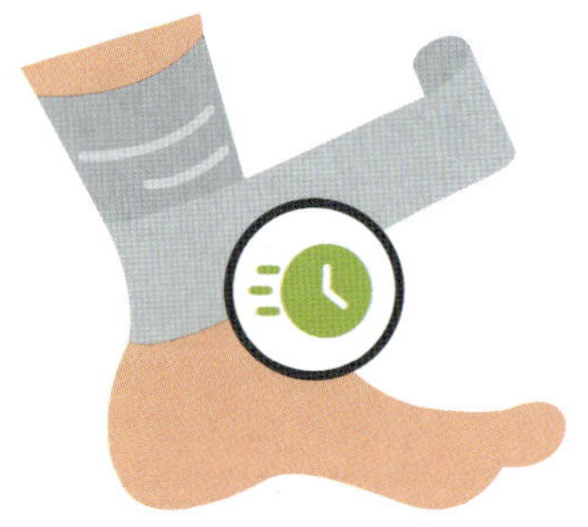

For certain groups, such as those who are malnourished, battling infections, or dealing with serious health conditions, getting enough protein is crucial. Eating more protein can help the body repair itself faster.

Hormone Production

Another job of proteins is to participate in hormone production. Hormones are special messenger molecules that communicate with various parts of the body. They help control and regulate specific processes, such as growth, metabolism, and reproduction. For example, insulin is a protein hormone that aids in blood sugar regulation.[5]

Some proteins act like sensors, called receptors, that detect changes in the body and send signals for cells to be fixed. The protein receptors can attach to specific signaling molecules to trigger a response. For example, dopamine is a neurotransmitter that plays important roles in how you feel, think, and move. It helps with motivation, feelings of pleasure, learning, memory, and fine motor movements.[6] The protein receptors for dopamine help manage all these processes, making it a key player in how your brain and body function together.

> **note**
>
> Not all hormones are made from proteins. Some, like estrogen and testosterone, are made from fats.

Structural Support

Four main types of proteins are essential for structure and support: collagen, keratin, elastin, and fibrin. They act as scaffolding, holding tissues together and helping them stay strong and flexible.

- **Collagen**, the most common structural protein in the body, makes up about 6 percent of your total body weight and is a key component in bones, skin, muscles, tendons, and ligaments. It is made up of three long protein strands that are twisted together like a rope, which makes it incredibly strong.[7] Collagen does a lot of important jobs. In combination with a mineral called calcium phosphate, it makes bones strong, but it's flexible enough to handle pressure.[8] In your skin, collagen provides structure, while **elastin** makes it stretchy. When you pinch your skin, collagen and elastin work together to bounce it back into its original shape. Blood vessels also have collagen and elastin, which give them structure and let them stretch as blood pumps through them.
- **Keratin** is found in skin, hair, and nails. It makes these parts of the body structurally tough to serve as a barrier from wounds and infection.[9]
- **Fibrin** is a strong, thread-like protein that helps stop the bleeding when you get a cut or injury. When bleeding occurs, fibrin is produced and forms a weblike structure, or clot, that traps blood cells and blocks the flow of blood. These fibrin clots are also stretchy and can be squished without breaking, which means they can handle a lot of movement or pressure while still holding together to protect the wound.[10]

Together, these structural proteins keep the body strong, flexible, and able to move. Without them, your bones, skin, and muscles wouldn't be able to function the way they should.

CHAPTER 2
PROTEIN CONSIDERATIONS & REQUIREMENTS

The amount of protein each person needs depends on factors like age, activity level, health status, and gender, making it far from a one-size-fits-all recommendation. An active athlete, an elderly person, and someone recovering from surgery all have different requirements to support their bodies' needs. Despite these differences, many current guidelines fail to consider how these factors impact protein intake. This chapter examines how protein needs vary across different populations and reveals how the current recommendations might fall short of helping people achieve optimal health.

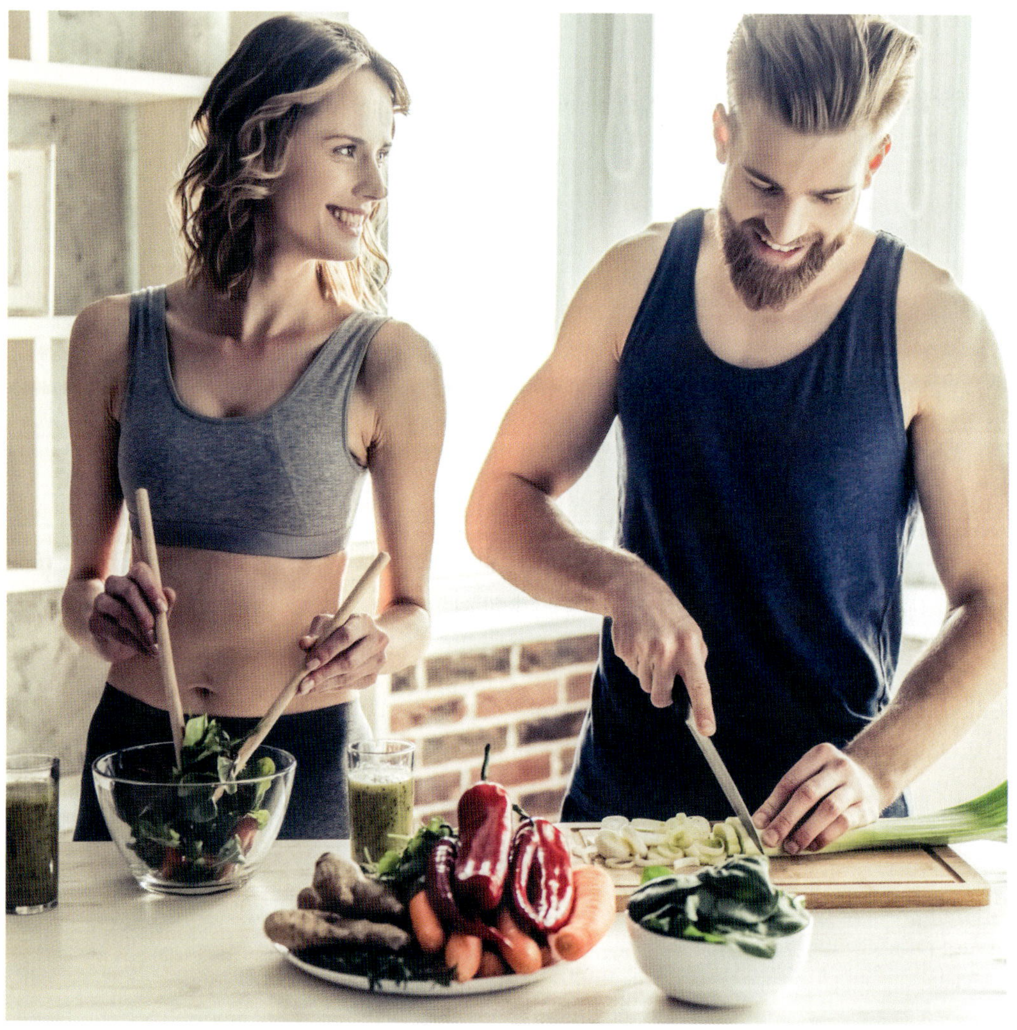

THE CURRENT GUIDELINES

To guide individuals in planning a nutritionally adequate diet, United States government-related groups developed the recommended daily allowances (RDAs) in 1941. The RDA outlines how much of a specific nutrient, like protein, calcium, or fiber, most people need to eat every day to meet their nutritional needs.[1]

The US began transitioning from RDAs to dietary reference intakes (DRIs) in the mid-nineties. Whereas the RDA focused on preventing nutrient deficiencies by providing a single value to meet the needs of most individuals, the DRI provides a more comprehensive framework. It includes not only the RDA but also the estimated average requirement (EAR), estimated energy requirement (EER), adequate intake (AI), and tolerable upper intake level (UL). This structure addresses deficiency prevention as well as optimal nutrient intakes for reducing chronic disease risks.[2]

Despite transitioning to the DRI, the RDA is still used as a guideline to determine protein requirements for all individuals. The following table outlines the current RDA and EAR for protein from the National Institutes of Health in grams of protein per kilogram of body weight per day.[3]

POPULATION	RDA	EAR
Men		
Age 4–13	0.95 g/kg/day	0.76 g/kg/day
Age 14–18	0.85 g/kg/day	0.73 g/kg/day
Age 19–70+	0.8 g/kg/day	0.66 g/kg/day
Women		
Age 4–13	0.95 g/kg/day	0.76 g/kg/day
Age 14–18	0.85 g/kg/day	0.71 g/kg/day
Age 19–70+	0.8 g/kg/day	0.66 g/kg/day
Pregnant people	1.1 g/kg/day	0.88 g/kg/day
Lactating people	1.3 g/kg/day	1.05 g/kg/day

The EAR represents the minimum protein intake needed to meet the essential amino acid requirements of 50 percent of that particular population in the US. The RDA, on the other hand, indicates the minimum protein intake needed to meet the essential amino acid requirements, maintain nitrogen balance, and prevent muscle loss for nearly 97.5 percent of that population.

The current guidelines don't recommend any additional dietary protein for healthy adults engaging in resistance or endurance exercise, citing the lack of compelling evidence. The evidence cited is from two studies published in the 1990s.

SHORTFALLS OF PROTEIN RDA

The current RDA for protein represents the minimum intake needed to prevent the loss of lean body mass and prevent diseases associated with nutritional deficiency, but it's often incorrectly presented as the optimal level for consumption.

The protein RDA is based on the concept of nitrogen balance, a method that evaluates the difference between nitrogen intake (protein in food) and nitrogen loss (mostly via urine, but also from stool, sweat, skin, hair, and breath). While it's easy to measure nitrogen intake because you can easily track the nitrogen coming in from protein in food, accurately measuring nitrogen loss is challenging. The methods for capturing all sources of nitrogen excretion—beyond urine and stool—are imprecise. For this reason, the derived RDA values are more of a baseline to avoid deficiency than an optimal target for health.[4]

Modern research methods that use isotopes to trace nitrogen specifically from amino acids reveal that the body's actual protein requirements likely exceed the RDA. Emerging evidence suggests that the current protein RDA is insufficient for older adults in particular because it doesn't address age-related decline in muscle mass, known as sarcopenia. Protein metabolism becomes less efficient with age, increasing the need for higher protein intakes. Studies and observational data indicate that higher protein intakes are linked to improved muscle mass and function with age.[5]

THE CASE FOR HIGHER PROTEIN RECOMMENDATIONS

Across all age groups, higher protein intake supports greater strength and muscle growth when combined with resistance training.[6] It also helps preserve muscle mass during periods of caloric restriction,[7] reduces muscle loss associated with aging,[8] and enhances muscle protein synthesis when spread evenly across meals.

Recent research, which reexamined nitrogen balance studies and incorporated amino acid oxidation-based requirements, suggests that the minimum protein needs for adults are closer to 0.93 to 1.2 g/kg/day—much higher than the previously established range of 0.66 to 0.8 g/kg/day.[9]

Furthermore, internationally recognized professional organizations advocate for higher protein intakes than the current RDA for physically active individuals. For instance, the Academy of Nutrition and Dietetics, Dietitians of Canada, and the American College of Sports Medicine jointly recommend consuming 1.2 to 2.0 g/kg/day of protein,[10] while the International Society for Sports Nutrition suggests a similar range of 1.4 to 2.0 g/kg/day.[11] These recommendations address the needs of active individuals whose protein requirements surpass the baseline.

Protein requirements vary across different life stages and health conditions. From children to active adults and athletes, elderly individuals, pregnant and lactating people, and those in special circumstances—such as people recovering from surgery, people who have undergone bariatric surgery, and GLP-1 users—higher protein intakes are often recommended to meet unique metabolic needs. The following sections explore the recent evidence and highlight how tailored recommendations can better support overall health across these groups.

Recommendations for Active Adults

The RDA for protein is designed to represent the minimum amount needed to prevent malnutrition but doesn't necessarily reflect the ideal intake for optimal health. For active adults who engage in some form of daily movement—whether it's walking, resistance training, yoga, or even light housework—a higher protein intake is more appropriate. As mentioned earlier, taking another look at nitrogen balance studies and amino acid oxidation studies has shown that the current RDA of 0.8 g/kg/day may be insufficient. Updated research suggests that a better baseline is at least 1.0 g/kg/day.

One study highlighted this greater need by placing sedentary adults on diets with varying protein levels—0.7, 1.8, or 3.0 g/kg/day—while providing 40 percent more calories than required for weight maintenance. Participants in the low-protein group (0.7 g/kg/day) experienced a slight decrease in lean body mass (muscle, bones, organs, water). This suggests that even with excess calories, protein intake plays a vital role in maintaining muscle.[12]

Dr. Peter Attia, author of the *New York Times* best-selling book *Outlive* and a leading voice in health and longevity, recommends a daily intake of at least 1.6 g/kg/day for his patients.[13] Combining this with findings from recent studies, an optimal range for healthy, active adults is likely around 1.2 to 1.8 g/kg/day. Here's how this recommendation calculates for a 150-pound adult:

150 lb / 2.2 = 68.1 kg

Grams of protein per day = 1.2 g/kg/day x 68.1 kg = 82 g

Grams of protein per day = 1.8 g/kg/day x 68.1 kg = 122 g

So, a 150-pound adult should be eating somewhere between 82 and 122 grams of protein per day. This level supports not only muscle maintenance but also overall health and well-being, emphasizing the importance of protein as a cornerstone of a balanced, active lifestyle.

Recommendations for Athletes

Multiple professional sports nutrition organizations are advocating for high protein intake in athletes, recommending at least 1.2 to 2.0 g/kg/day. Recent evidence suggests that athletes, especially those with demanding training regimens, may benefit from protein consumption at the higher end of or even beyond this range.[14]

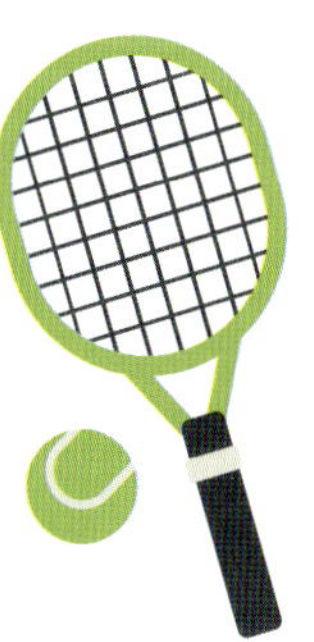

Protein needs vary based on an athlete's goals. Strength and power athletes often aim to maximize muscle mass, whereas endurance athletes focus on reducing fat mass while preserving muscle. Both need sufficient protein in their diets to achieve their goals—often triple the RDA.

A 2018 meta-analysis found that an average intake of 1.6 g/kg/day maximized muscle gains from resistance training, with some individuals benefiting from amounts up to 2.2 g/kg/day.[15] When athletes are restricting calories, they may require even more protein, with some studies suggesting intakes of 2.4 to 2.7 g/kg/day to preserve muscle while losing fat.[16]

Overall, athletes aiming for muscle gain or fat loss while preserving or increasing muscle should aim for between 1.6 to 2.7 g/kg/day depending on training intensity, body composition goals, and individual response.

Recommendations for Older Adults

Sarcopenia is the natural loss of muscle mass and strength that occurs with age and reduced physical activity. It begins at around age 30 and continues after, with muscle decreasing by about 3 to 5 percent with each decade. Over a lifetime, most men will lose about 30 percent of their muscle mass. This decline leads to reduced strength and mobility, increasing the risk of falls and fractures.

Researchers estimate that 5 to 13 percent of people over age 60 and up to 50 percent of those over age 80 experience sarcopenia.[17] A 2015 report by the American Society for Bone and Mineral Research found that individuals with sarcopenia are 2.3 times more likely to suffer fractures in bones, such as hips, arms, or wrists, from falls.[18]

As we age, muscle mass and strength decline due to several changes happening at the cellular level. The number of muscle cells decreases, and the remaining cells become less efficient. Inside the muscle, there's less energy-storing material, and the parts of the cells that produce energy, called mitochondria, don't work as well. These changes slow down how muscles use energy and recover.[19] On top of that, factors like lower hormone levels, reduced physical activity, and poor nutrition can worsen the process.

Testosterone naturally decreases with age. By age 65, about 60 percent of men have levels below the normal range for younger men.[20] Since testosterone is essential for building and maintaining muscle, its decline can reduce muscle protein production, leading to muscle loss and weakness. Studies on testosterone replacement therapy in men with low testosterone levels have shown that bringing testosterone back to normal levels can greatly improve muscle mass, strength, protein synthesis, and bone density.[21]

In women, estrogen levels drop quickly during menopause. There is growing evidence that loss of estrogen contributes to muscle loss and weakness. This hormone plays a role in protecting muscle cells from dying and supports muscle quality by supporting proteins and cells that help muscles repair and generate force.[22]

As people get older, getting enough protein becomes increasingly important to maintain muscle mass and overall health. However, many older adults don't consume enough protein for several reasons. Appetite often decreases with age, and some eat less due to lower energy needs. Others do not get enough protein because they face financial challenges or because they live alone. These factors can lead to diets that don't meet their nutritional needs, including protein.

One study looking at protein intakes in adults age 51 and older showed that protein intake decreased significantly in older age groups, with nearly half of the oldest adults not reaching the RDA of 0.8 g/kg/day.[23] Those who consumed less than the recommended amount of protein were more likely to face physical limitations, such as difficulty stooping, standing, or walking long distances. Ensuring adequate protein intake in older adults is essential for maintaining mobility, strength, and overall quality of life.[24]

Research also suggests that older adults process protein less effectively than younger individuals. This phenomenon is called anabolic resistance.[25] If someone young and someone older were to consume the same 20 grams of protein, the younger person's body would produce more muscle protein than the older person's.

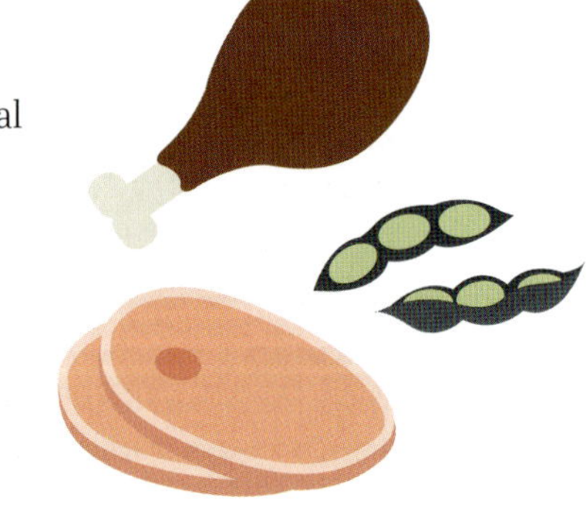

For these reasons, it's important for older individuals to prioritize protein intake. Recent research suggests a minimum of 1.2 g/kg/day,[17] or more if they're physically active. One study found that adults aged 65 and older saw significant improvements in muscle mass when they ate 1.2 to 1.59 g/kg/day while doing resistance exercise.[26]

I firmly believe that daily physical activity is essential for everyone, but it's especially important for older adults. Staying active helps maintain strength, bone health, and muscle mass, which are not only key indicators of longevity but also vital for staying independent and mobile as you age. Regular movement supports the ability to walk, drive, and perform everyday tasks, like cooking and getting dressed, without assistance. Whether you walk or do things like resistance training, yoga, or even light housework, making physical activity and consuming sufficient protein part of your daily life can significantly enhance your quality of life and ensure you remain independently capable in your later years.

Recommendations During Pregnancy and Lactation

Protein is essential during pregnancy because the body undergoes many changes that increase the demand for it. During pregnancy, the body is building tissues and storing nutrients to support the growing fetus. Protein is also needed to build the placenta and expand the blood supply so all the nutrients can get to the womb.

The current protein RDA during pregnancy is 1.1 g/kg/day. This baseline was established by taking the RDA for an adult and accounting for the extra protein needed to support changes in the body and the fetus. However, research using the new amino acid methods suggests that this amount might not be enough. One study looking at protein requirements for a healthy pregnancy indicates that at least 1.22 g/kg/day and maybe as much as 1.66 g/kg/day is appropriate; by late pregnancy, the amount would increase to 1.52 to 1.77 g/kg/day.[27] Of course, these numbers are based on individual needs and may vary based on activity level and for supporting multiple pregnancy.

Lactation also increases protein requirements to support production of high-quality milk. While the RDA during lactation is set at 1.3 g/kg/day, newer research suggests that this recommendation may underestimate actual needs. Research in one study showed that some participants consuming up to 1.5 g/kg/day were still in a negative nitrogen balance, meaning they weren't getting enough protein to meet their needs.[28] Other findings indicate supporting babies who exclusively breastfeed, particularly three to six months postpartum, might require 1.7 to 1.9 g/kg/day.[29]

Recommendations for Children

It makes sense that children have a higher RDA for protein when compared to adults because they are still growing and need extra protein to support that growth. However, research suggests that the recommendation of 0.95 g/kg/day for children ages 4 to 13 years may underestimate their true requirements. Studies using the indicator amino acid oxidation method in children aged 6 to 10 indicate that 1.55 g/kg/day would be a more accurate protein target to support growth and development.[30] Protein needs are likely even higher for children who participate in sports and athletic activities.

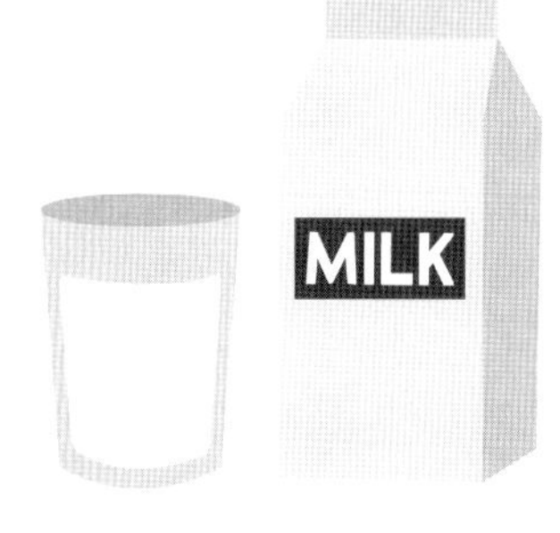

Considerations for Special Populations

Protein should be a top priority for individuals in certain groups, such as those recovering from bariatric surgery; healing after other surgeries; living with cancer; and recovering from infections, burns, or other injuries. These situations place unique demands on the body, making protein essential for supporting healing while maintaining muscle mass. For these situations, it's important to work side by side with your doctor or a nutritionist to ensure you are getting all the nutrients vital to aid in healing.

A newer group to consider is individuals using GLP-1 medications for weight management. These medications work by suppressing appetite, which can make it challenging to consume enough protein. As a result, some of the weight lost during treatment may come from lean body mass, including muscle, rather than just fat. Ensuring adequate protein intake is essential for preserving lean body mass and supporting overall health while on a GLP-1 journey.

WHO SHOULD AVOID HIGH-PROTEIN DIETS?

Research suggests that healthy individuals can handle higher protein intakes without harm, but individuals with decreased kidney function or high risk of kidney disease should be cautious when considering a high-protein diet, or perhaps should avoid it altogether.[31] Although protein is an essential nutrient, consuming large amounts can place too much stress on unhealthy kidneys by increasing their processing workload. This increased strain, called intraglomerular hypertension, can potentially speed up damage to compromised kidneys.[32]

Given the potential for harm, anyone with known or suspected kidney issues should speak with a healthcare professional before significantly raising their protein intake.

SETTING YOUR PROTEIN GOAL

To determine the amount of protein you need daily, use the recommendations and research I presented earlier in this chapter. You'll need to determine your weight in kilograms, so remember there are 2.2 kilograms in 1 pound. You'll need to divide your body weight in pounds by 2.2 to get your weight in kilograms. For example, if you weigh 175 pounds, divide that number by 2.2 to calculate that your weight in kilograms is about 79.

There are two different weights you can use to determine your protein goal. The first is your lean body mass, which is the weight of your muscles, bones, organs, and water—basically everything except fat. It makes sense to use this number to determine your protein needs because protein primarily supports muscle tissue. However, lean body mass is difficult to accurately determine without doing a DEXA scan, using skinfold calipers or a Bod Pod, or tracking down other costly methods that require specialized equipment. Fortunately, there are several calculators online that you can use to estimate your lean body mass.

Since determining lean body mass can be challenging, some experts recommend using total body weight as a simpler and more practical method for estimating protein requirements. Unless you are morbidly obese, you could take this approach or consult with your healthcare practitioner to determine your lean body mass.

Once you know your daily protein requirement, determine how many meals you want to consume a day. I find it easiest to divide my protein requirements evenly over my meals. That way, when I'm making breakfast, lunch, or dinner, I know I should be including enough protein to hit that target.

For example, if your daily protein goal is 100 grams, I suggest aiming to consume around 30 grams of protein for breakfast, lunch, and dinner, leaving around 10 grams of protein for a snack, dessert, or protein coffee.

Keep in mind that your individual protein needs may vary depending on your age, activity level, muscle mass, health goals, and any medical conditions you may have. It's always a good idea to check in with your healthcare practitioner or a registered dietitian for help determining the amount of protein that's right for you. They can take into account your overall health and help tailor a plan that supports your personal goals.

PROTEIN TIMING

If you've ever wondered whether the timing of when you eat protein makes a difference in building muscle, improving strength, or maintaining overall health, this section is for you. Here, I break down whether it's more effective to spread protein evenly throughout the day or consume it all at once. I also dive into the best time to consume protein relative to when you exercise and explain how protein fits into intermittent fasting patterns.

Nutrient timing is the strategy of eating specific foods (specifically, carbohydrates and protein) at certain times around exercise to improve performance and help your body recover and adapt better. Studies have shown that consuming high-quality, fast-digesting protein combined with carbohydrates after exercise not only aids in muscle recovery but also helps reduce muscle breakdown. When it comes to building muscle, researchers are particularly interested in the anabolic window, a period after exercise when the body is especially primed to use nutrients for muscle repair and protein synthesis, making it an ideal time to consume protein for optimal recovery.[33]

For years, the anabolic window was believed to be a strict thirty- to sixty-minute period after exercise.[34] However, recent research suggests that this window may be much larger and lasts several hours. Muscle protein synthesis—building of new skeletal muscle—can remain elevated for at least twenty-four hours after resistance exercise.[35] So eating soon after a workout is beneficial, but it's not absolutely necessary as long as you're meeting your total daily protein and other nutrient needs.[36] In other words, it appears that spreading your protein intake across meals matters more than rushing to slam a protein shake immediately after a workout.

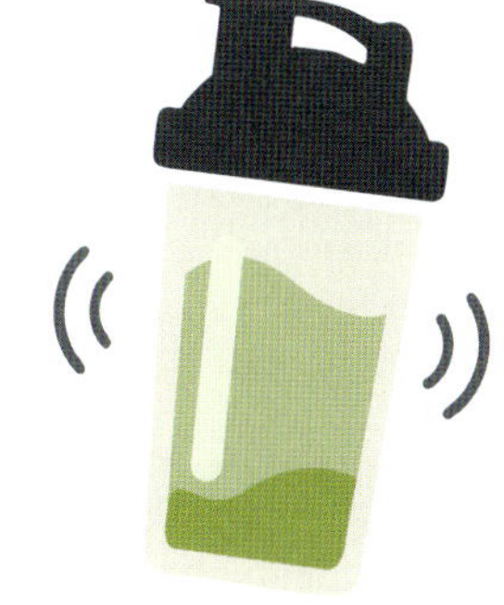

Eating protein soon after a workout can still help you meet your daily protein goal, so if you love that post-workout protein shake or meal, then go ahead and have it!

PROTEIN PACING

Feeding consistently throughout the day has been shown to be more beneficial in building muscle and having overall positive health outcomes than consuming the bulk of your protein in one meal. Protein pacing, when you consistently and evenly distribute protein throughout the day, has been studied across both overweight and healthy, fit populations. This approach aims to maximize muscle protein synthesis, enhance recovery, and improve performance.

For example, one study compared balanced protein consumption (30 grams per meal) to uneven patterns (10 grams at breakfast, 15 grams at lunch, and 65 grams at dinner). The results showed that evenly distributed protein intake led to greater muscle protein synthesis.[37] Other research suggests that consuming protein evenly across six meals daily significantly improved metabolic health markers, increased lean mass, and reduced body fat, all without changes in body weight.[38]

PROTEIN AMOUNT PER MEAL

One study that looked at protein intake (using whey protein) among men showed that for young adults, consuming 0.24 gram of protein per kilogram of body weight per meal maximized muscle protein synthesis. The optimal intake for an adult male in the study was 0.4 g/kg/meal.[39] This effect has been observed in other studies as well. Older males needed higher amounts to achieve max muscle protein synthesis (0.4 to 0.6 g/kg/meal).[40]

PROTEIN LIMITS

The maximum amount of protein the body can absorb and use in a single meal has been the subject of debate. Some studies suggest that the maximum is between 20 and 25 grams. Beyond that, it is believed that excess protein would be used for energy or excreted as waste. However, there are limitations to these studies. These findings were specific to fast-digesting proteins (that is, whey protein), and those proteins were consumed without other macronutrients (fats and/or carbs). When most people eat, they combine protein with fats and carbohydrates, which slows absorption, allowing the body to use the amino acids more effectively.[41]

A 2023 study highlights this point by examining muscle protein synthesis over a twelve-hour period post exercise. The researchers found that having 100 grams of protein led to a 40 percent higher muscle protein synthesis rate between hours 4 and 12 than having only 25 grams of protein (although there was no difference in the synthesis rate in hours 1 to 4).[42]

These findings go against the idea that too much protein in a single meal gets wasted or even completely oxidized for energy. The body uses it over time to repair muscles.

INTERMITTENT FASTING

Intermittent fasting can be a powerful tool for weight management and overall health, but it requires careful planning to ensure adequate protein intake. Prioritizing protein in the feeding window is crucial for maintaining muscle mass.

Time-restricted eating often involves fewer than the typical three meals per day, which can negatively impact muscle protein turnover if you consume too little protein. To mitigate this effect, there are a couple of recommendations you can follow.

A review looking at the vast research around fasting and protein suggests that you consume at least 1.6 grams of protein/kg/day. It should be distributed as evenly as possible across the meals within the feeding window, spaced three to five hours apart.[43]

Consuming protein-rich meals frequently and evenly throughout the day is beneficial to maintaining muscle mass while losing weight. A 2024 study highlighted the benefits of combining intermittent fasting with protein pacing. In the study, participants who followed intermittent fasting while consuming four protein-rich meals (25 to 50 grams of protein each) saw greater weight loss, reduced abdominal and visceral fat, and increased fat-free mass compared to those who simply restricted calories. Additionally, the participants who focused on protein intake saw improvements in gut health, indicating potential benefits beyond weight loss.[44]

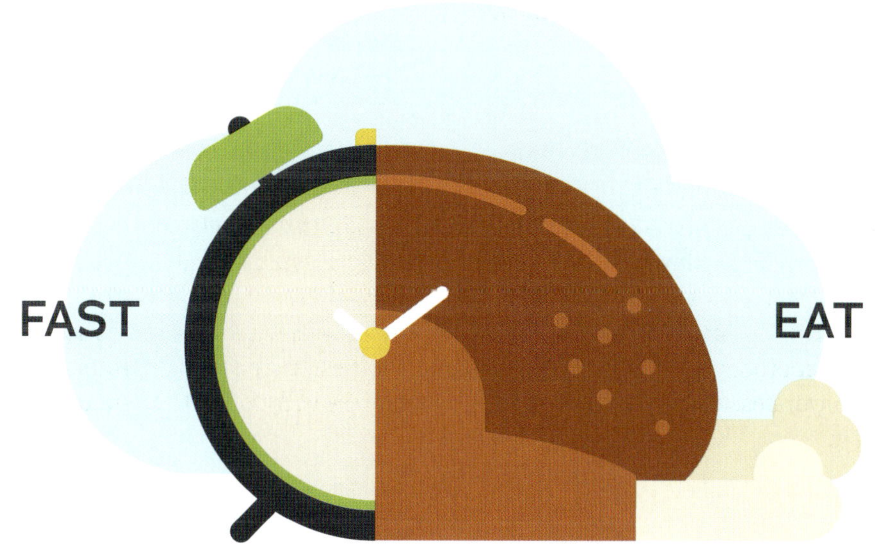

CHAPTER 3
PROTEIN SOURCES

Protein comes from a variety of sources, each with its own benefits and nutritional profile. From meats like chicken, beef, and fish to dairy products like yogurt and cheese, animal proteins are often rich in essential amino acids that support muscle growth and repair. But for vegetarians and vegans, plant-based protein options are available and often supply additional nutrients like fiber and healthy fats. If you're looking for convenience or supplementation, protein powders are a quick and easy solution to meeting your daily protein needs. Let's explore the different sources of protein, their nutritional value, and how they can fit into a balanced high-protein diet.

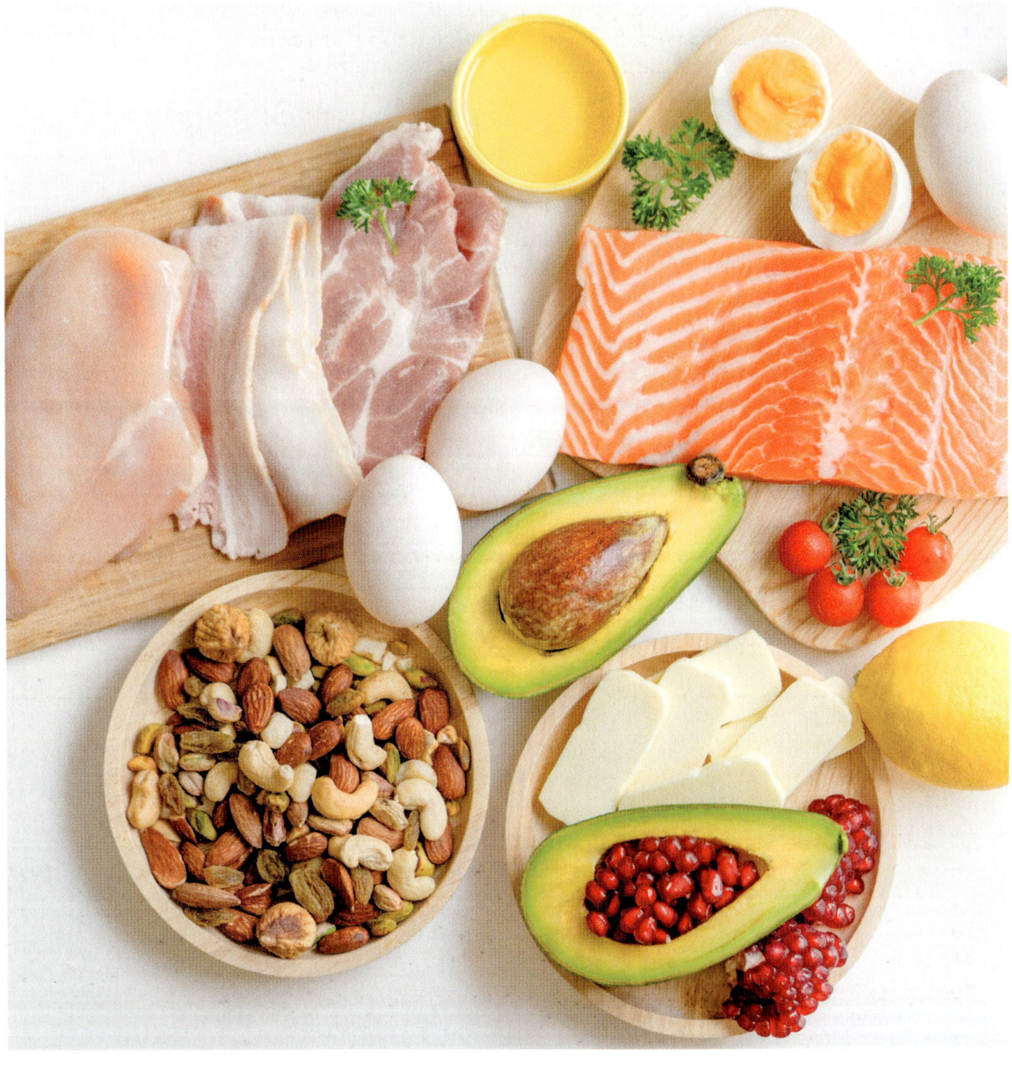

POULTRY

Poultry, which includes chicken, turkey, duck, goose, and other types of fowl, is a high-quality protein that provides many of the essential amino acids needed for muscle growth and repair. Like all animal proteins, the protein in poultry is highly bioavailable, meaning the body can readily digest and use it. Poultry is also rich in nutrients such as B vitamins, iron, and zinc, which support energy production and immunity.[1]

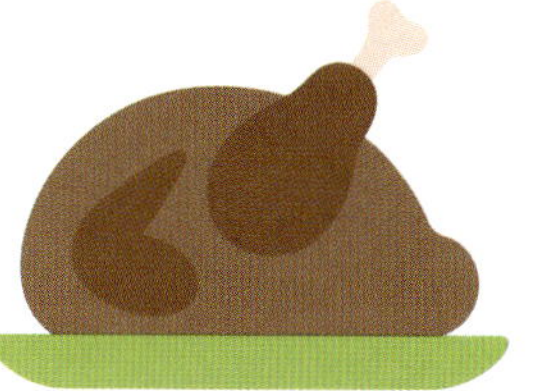

note

Zinc might not get as much attention as some other nutrients, but it plays a huge role in keeping your body running smoothly. It supports your immune system, helps with wound healing, boosts brain function, and even plays a role in hormone health and fertility. Zinc is also crucial for growth and development, which is why it's especially important during pregnancy and adolescence.[2]

The body doesn't store zinc long term, so you need to get enough regularly—especially if you eat a mostly plant-based diet, since compounds like phytic acid in grains and legumes can block its absorption.

The fat content in poultry varies depending on the type of meat. Dark meat, such as thighs and legs, tends to be higher in fat, while white meat, such as chicken breast, is leaner. Breast meat without skin is nearly fat-free, making it a popular lean protein source.

BEEF AND LAMB

Beef and lamb are considered red meat and are high-quality protein sources that provide essential nutrients for health and performance. Like all animal proteins, they contain all the essential amino acids needed for muscle growth and repair. Beef and lamb are also rich in zinc, iron, B vitamins, creatine, and conjugated linoleic acid (CLA).

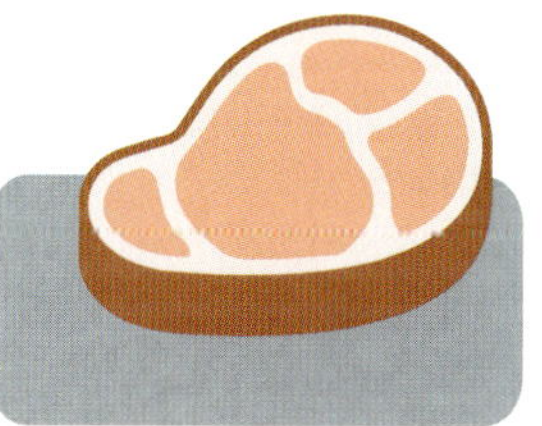

note

Creatine isn't just for bodybuilders. New research reveals that the benefits of creatine go way beyond muscle growth and recovery. It also supports brain health, bone strength, and even your metabolism. Studies show creatine can improve memory during stressful times[3] and support better sleep after training.[4]

For older adults, creatine has the potential to support healthy aging when paired with resistance training. Research shows it can help increase lean muscle mass, boost strength, and improve physical performance in daily activities like climbing stairs. Creatine may also help slow bone loss, particularly in areas prone to fractures, like the hip.[5]

note

Naturally found in beef and dairy, CLA is a unique type of fatty acid that's been shown in animal and cell studies to support fat loss, improve lean body mass, enhance immune function, and even reduce inflammation.[6] Grass-fed beef contains significantly higher levels of CLA than conventionally raised beef, making it a better source of this beneficial fatty acid.

Female athletes, who are prone to iron deficiency due to menstrual blood loss, can benefit from the highly bioavailable heme iron found in red meat. Heme iron is absorbed up to ten times more efficiently than the non-heme iron in plant-based foods.[7]

The fat content of beef and lamb varies widely depending on the cut of meat. Lean cuts include eye of round roast and steak, top and bottom round roast and steak, and top sirloin steak. Fattier cuts like rib eye, skirt steak, and short ribs contain around 20 grams of fat for a 3-ounce portion.[8] Lean cuts of lamb typically come from the leg, loin, and rack. For the leanest options, look for leg (especially sirloin or shank half), loin chops with visible fat trimmed, and trimmed rib chops.

PORK

Another high-quality animal protein is pork, which includes bacon, ham, pork tenderloin, pork chops, and more. While pork provides all the essential amino acids needed for muscle growth and repair, the fat content is higher in many cuts, such as bacon and pork belly. Lean cuts like loin and tenderloin are good options for those looking for lower-fat protein sources.

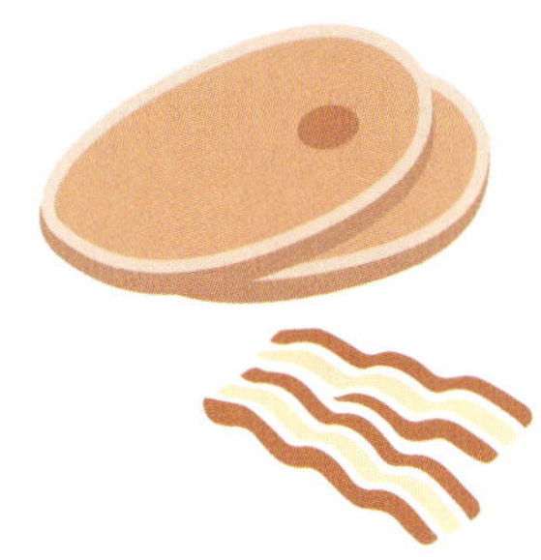

Processed pork products, such as hot dogs, Spam, and deli meat, often come with some concerns. These items are generally higher in sodium and may contain added ingredients, like nitrates, nitrites, fillers, and preservatives, which may negatively impact health if consumed in excess.

FISH AND SEAFOOD

Like other animal proteins, fish and seafood provide all the essential amino acids. Many types of fish—such as cod, tilapia, and mahi mahi—are naturally low in fat, making them good options if you want a leaner fish. But higher-fat fish, like salmon and sardines, provide healthy omega-3 fatty acids. These fats are known for their health benefits, including reducing inflammation and improving heart health and mood.

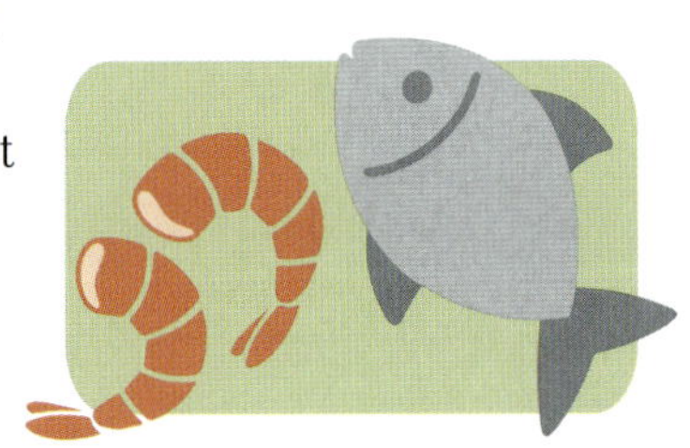

EGGS

Eggs are often considered the perfect protein source because they provide all nine essential amino acids in a highly digestible form. Eggs have long served as a standard against which other protein sources are compared.[9]

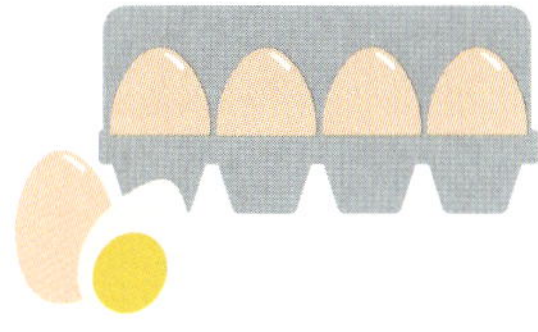

Each large egg contains about 6.3 grams of protein, distributed between the white and the yolk. The egg white is more protein rich—providing 3.6 grams of protein—than the yolk, which contains around 2.7 grams. The yolk contains other necessary nutrients, like healthy fat, vitamin D, B vitamins, and iron.[10]

WILD GAME

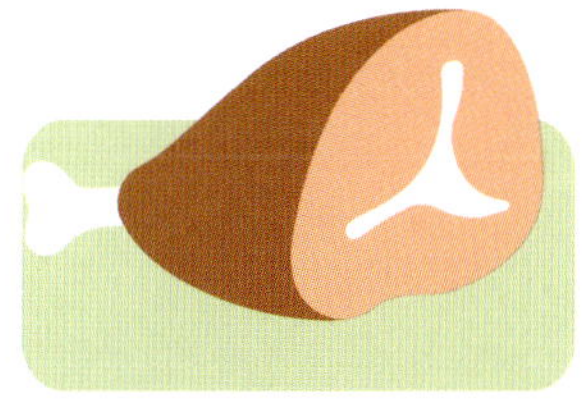

Wild game, including elk, venison (deer), bison (buffalo), and antelope, is an excellent source of lean protein. It contains all the essential amino acids and is rich in B vitamins, iron, and zinc. Wild game is naturally low in saturated fat, making it a good alternative to beef.

Wild game is versatile and can easily replace other meats in a variety of dishes, from casseroles to hearty stews. Its unique flavor and nutrient profile make it a popular choice among people looking to diversify their protein intake.

DAIRY

Dairy foods, including milk, yogurt, cheese, cottage cheese, sour cream, and ice cream, are another source of protein. Most dairy products are made from cow's milk, though alternatives from goats and sheep are sometimes used. About 80 percent of the protein in milk is casein. The other 20 percent is whey protein. Casein is digested much slower than other proteins, so it provides a steady and prolonged release of amino acids into the muscles. In contrast, whey protein is digested very quickly, making it a readily available source of amino acids.[11]

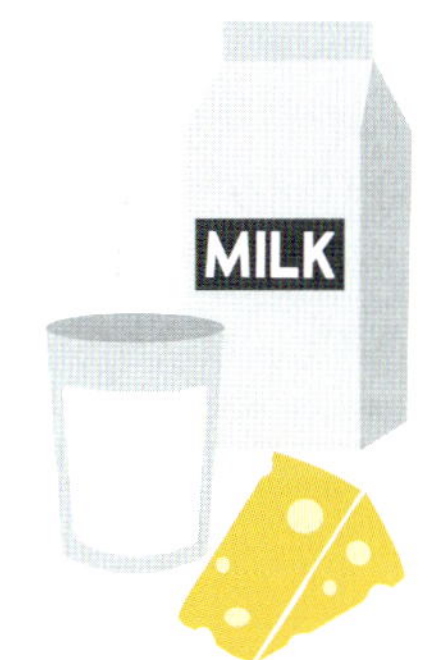

Dairy can be added to meals and snacks to boost the protein and flavor. For example, sprinkling cheese on chili or mixing protein powder into cottage cheese can bump up your protein intake and make your dish more delicious.

PLANT-BASED PROTEIN OPTIONS

Plant-based protein sources include legumes, nuts, seeds, grains, and soy products. They generally contain less protein per serving compared to animal foods, which means you need to eat larger portions of them to meet your protein needs. Most plant foods do not individually contain all twenty amino acids. However, by consuming a variety of plant-based protein sources, you should be able to obtain all the essential amino acids you need.

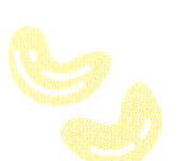

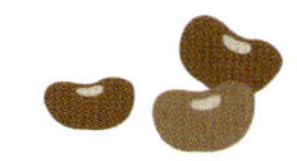

Another drawback of plant proteins is that their digestibility is lower compared to animal proteins.[12]

Legumes, such as kidney beans, pinto beans, lentils, chickpeas, peanuts, and lupini beans, are popular among both vegetarians and meat-eaters. However, most legumes are higher in carbohydrates than meats, with the exception of lupini beans and peanuts. The carbohydrate content in lupini beans is mostly from fiber, so they're an excellent source of protein on a plant-based low-carb diet.

Soy products, including tofu, tempeh, edamame, soy milk, and texturized vegetable protein, are other popular sources of plant-based protein. Soy is one of the few plant foods that contains all the amino acids.

Grains and vegetables can also contribute to protein intake, although their protein content varies. Vegetables like broccoli, asparagus, Brussels sprouts, and kale contain small amounts of protein. Grains can provide up to 10 grams of protein per serving, but they're also higher in carbohydrates.

For those seeking lower-carb plant protein options, foods like hemp seeds, chia seeds, edamame, lupini beans, tofu, tempeh, nuts, and peanuts are excellent choices.

Plant-based protein sources offer a wide range of nutritional benefits beyond protein. While they may not match the digestibility or amino acid content of animal proteins, they can still support muscle growth, recovery, and overall health when consumed in the right combinations.

PROTEIN POWDERS

Protein powders are a popular choice for athletes because of their convenience and effectiveness as a protein source. While whole-food sources of protein should make up the bulk of your protein intake, protein powders offer several advantages.

They are often more cost-effective per gram of protein compared to whole foods. They have a long shelf life and allow for precise control over nutrient intake. They're easy to use, making them an ideal option for post-workout nutrition.

Most protein powders contain 20 to 40 grams of protein per serving and can be mixed with water, milk, cottage cheese, or yogurt, or you can use them in baking. This convenience is ideal for anyone with a busy schedule or who struggles to get enough protein.

Protein powders are available in three primary forms:

- **Protein concentrates** contain about 80 percent protein with 5 to 6 percent carbohydrates and are generally the least expensive option.
- **Protein isolates** contain around 90 percent protein and minimal carbohydrates, making them a favorite protein for those on a low-carb diet.
- **Hydrolysates** are proteins created by adding digestive enzymes, which can make them faster to absorb; however, they are usually the most expensive.

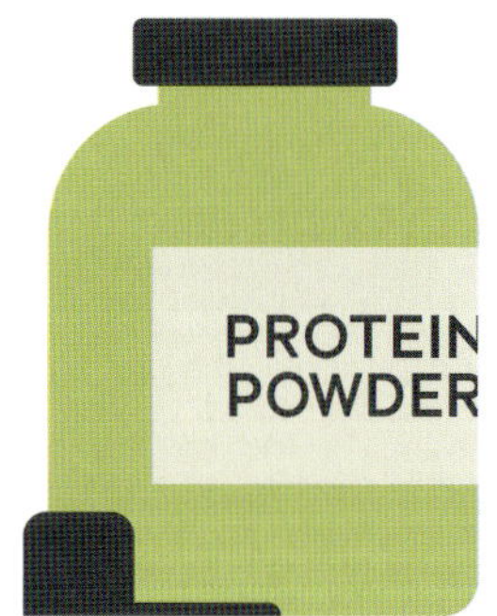

QUICK PROTEIN REFERENCE

The following tables are a quick reference guide of popular foods that provide approximately 30 grams of protein. You can use them to easily identify options to meet your protein needs. All foods listed are uncooked.[13,14,15]

BEEF	QUANTITY	PROTEIN (GRAMS)
Ground beef, 90/10	6 ounces	33
Ground beef, 85/15	6 ounces	31
Ground beef, 80/20	6 ounces	29
Chuck eye steak	4 ounces	28
Flank steak	5 ounces	30
New York strip steak	4 ounces	29
Rib-eye steak	6 ounces	30
Sirloin steak	5 ounces	29
Skirt steak	4 ounces	29
T-bone steak	4 ounces	28
Tenderloin steak	6 ounces	30
Tri-tip	5 ounces	30
Short ribs	6 ounces	30
Chuck roast	6 ounces	31
Rib roast	5 ounces	31

POULTRY	QUANTITY	PROTEIN (GRAMS)
Ground chicken	6 ounces	30
Chicken breast	5 ounces	32
Chicken drumstick	5 ounces	28
Chicken thighs	6 ounces	31
Chicken wings	6 ounces	31
Ground turkey, 93/7	6 ounces	33
Ground turkey, 99/1	4 ounces	28
Turkey breast	5 ounces	33

PORK	QUANTITY	PROTEIN (GRAMS)
Bacon	12 slices	30
Ground pork	6 ounces	30
Ham	1 cup diced	30
Pork chop	5 ounces	32
Pork loin	5 ounces	30
Pork belly	11 ounces	29
Pork ribs	6 ounces	30
Pork tenderloin	5 ounces	30

FISH & SEAFOOD	QUANTITY	PROTEIN (GRAMS)
Cod	7 ounces	32
Halibut	6 ounces	32
Mahi mahi	6 ounces	31
Salmon	5 ounces	29
Sardines (canned)	6 ounces	33
Tilapia	7 ounces	30
Tuna, albacore (canned)	5 ounces	30
Tuna, yellowfin	5 ounces	33
Tuna, ahi	4 ounces	27
Catfish	7 ounces	33
Trout	5 ounces	29
Clams	8 ounces	29
Crab	6 ounces	31
Lobster	6 ounces	28
Mussels	9 ounces	30
Oysters	11 ounces	29
Shrimp	6 ounces	31
Scallops	7 ounces	30

LAMB	QUANTITY	PROTEIN (GRAMS)
Ground lamb, 85/15	6 ounces	33
Leg	5 ounces	29
Shoulder	5 ounces	29

WILD GAME	QUANTITY	PROTEIN (GRAMS)
Ground bison, 90/10	5 ounces	28
Ground elk	4 ounces	30
Ground venison	4 ounces	29
Elk steak	4 ounces	34
Venison steak	3 ounces	27

PLANT-BASED SOURCES	QUANTITY	PROTEIN (GRAMS)
Black soybeans	1½ cups	33
Edamame (shelled)	2 cups	30
Black beans (canned)*	2 cups	29
Chickpeas (canned)*	1½ cups	30
Kidney beans (canned)*	2 cups	27
Tempeh	5 ounces	28
Tofu, extra firm	10 ounces	30
Lupini beans (aka lupin beans), jarred	2½ cups	30
Chia seeds	15 tablespoons	30
Hemp hearts	9 tablespoons	30
Peanuts, dry roasted	1 cup	28
Peanut butter, creamy	½ cup	32
Almonds	5 ounces	30
Almond milk	30 cups	30
Hemp seed milk	10 cups	30
Flaxmilk + protein (Good Karma brand)	6 cups	30

*Higher-carb sources

EGGS	QUANTITY	PROTEIN (GRAMS)
Chicken egg, large	5	30
Duck egg, 70g	3	27
Quail egg	25	30

DAIRY	QUANTITY	PROTEIN (GRAMS)
Cheddar cheese	5 ounces	30
Monterey Jack cheese	5 ounces	30
Mozzarella cheese	5 ounces	30
Parmesan cheese	3 ounces	27
Pepper Jack cheese	5 ounces	30
Cottage cheese, 4% milkfat	1 cup	28
Greek yogurt	1½ cups	34
Milk, whole	3 cups	27

PROTEIN QUALITY

Protein quality is a factor to consider when comparing sources of protein. It refers to how effectively the body can use a protein based on its essential amino acid profile, how well the body can digest it, and how easily and efficiently the body can absorb and use the amino acids.[16]

Not all proteins are created equal, and their quality can vary significantly depending on the source. This section explores the various aspects of protein quality and compares incomplete proteins with complete ones, animal proteins with plant-based options, and whole-food proteins with synthetic protein powders. Examining these differences can help you make more informed choices about protein sources to support optimal health and performance.

Complete Versus Incomplete Proteins

Proteins are categorized as complete or incomplete based on their amino acid profile. A food is considered a complete protein if it contains adequate levels of all nine essential amino acids: histidine, isoleucine, leucine, lysine, methionine, phenylalanine, threonine, tryptophan, and valine. Remember, these are the amino acids your body can't make on its own, so you must obtain them from food.

Incomplete proteins lack one or more of these essential amino acids or provide very small amounts.

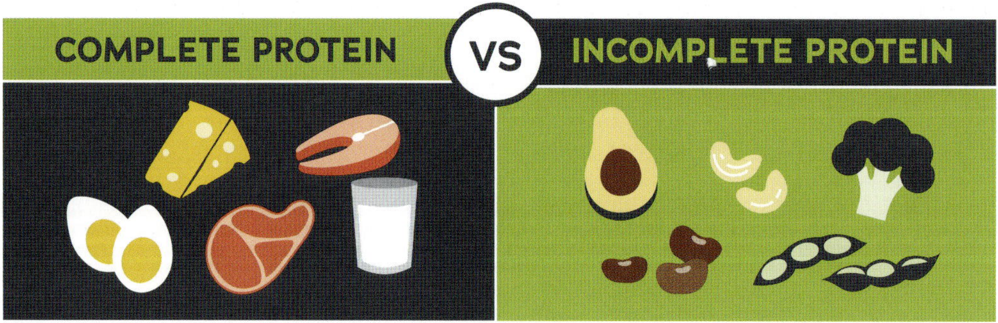

Animal Versus Plant-Based Proteins

Animal foods like meat, fish, eggs, and dairy are typically complete proteins. Some plant foods, such as soy, are also considered complete proteins because they provide all nine essential amino acids in sufficient quantities.

Many plant-based proteins, such as legumes, whole grains, nuts, and seeds, are incomplete proteins. Some plant foods like quinoa, hemp, chia, and spirulina can be labeled as "nearly complete" because they have low levels of certain essential amino acids.

If you follow a plant-based diet, it's important that you eat a variety of protein sources throughout the day. You can combine different plant-based foods, such as nuts, soy, lupini beans, vegetables, and seeds, to ensure you consume all the essential amino acids your body needs.

The process by which your body repairs and builds muscle is largely triggered by the rise in essential amino acids after you eat.[17] Plant-based proteins are often considered less effective for building muscle than animal proteins because they contain lower amounts of the essential amino acids, specifically leucine, lysine, and methionine.[18] Since all amino acids are needed for muscle synthesis to occur, being short of one or more can limit your body's ability to build and repair muscle.

Studies comparing plant-based and animal proteins have shown that, gram for gram, plant proteins are less effective at stimulating muscle protein synthesis.[19] Additionally, plant proteins are less digestible than animal proteins because they contain compounds like phytates and tannins, which can interfere with your body's ability to absorb protein.[20]

One study showed that 85 to 95 percent of protein from sources like egg whites, whole eggs, and chicken is absorbed by the body, compared to only 50 to 75 percent of the protein from plant sources like chickpeas, mung beans, and yellow peas.[21,22] However, when plant-based proteins are processed to remove antinutritional factors and are turned into protein isolates or concentrates (such as pea protein powder), their absorbability becomes comparable to that of traditional animal proteins.[23]

Whole-Food-Sourced Versus Synthetic Proteins

Although some protein powders are readily absorbed and used to build and repair tissues, whole-food protein sources may offer a unique advantage. Recent research suggests that the food matrix, which includes protein and other vitamins, minerals, and fats, from a whole-food source (such as a rib-eye steak or shrimp) can enhance the body's ability to use amino acids for muscle repair. All these nutrients working together in whole foods may make them more effective at supporting muscle protein synthesis than isolated protein sources. Additionally, the interaction of proteins and other nutrients contained in a whole food could play a significant role in recovery, especially after exercise when the gut is able to absorb more nutrients to reach the muscles.[24]

Adopting a food-first approach to protein intake not only supports muscle recovery but also helps with overall diet quality. Whole foods provide a variety of essential nutrients that protein isolates may lack. However, there is a case for using protein powders—especially when traveling, immediately after training, or when you need a convenient way to get extra protein to meet your daily needs.

CHAPTER 4

PROTEIN MYTHS & CONTROVERSIES

High-protein diets are often the subject of misunderstanding, with many myths surrounding their effects on health. From claims that high protein intake damages the kidneys or weakens bones to fears that consuming too much protein will age you prematurely, these misconceptions can create confusion about the role of protein in a balanced lifestyle. Here, I explore some common misconceptions about high-protein diets and clarify what the research actually says.

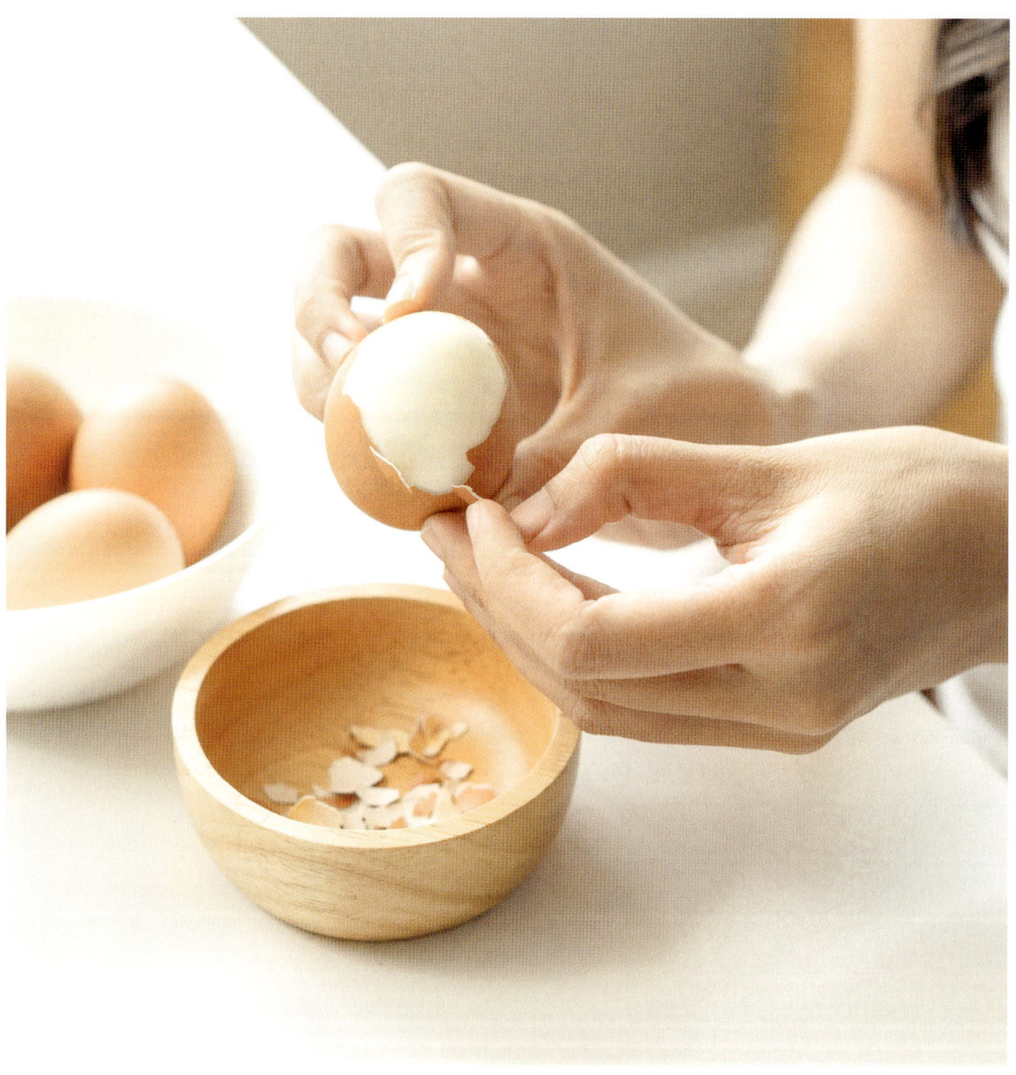

MYTH #1: COLLAGEN IS A GOOD SUBSTITUTE FOR WHEY PROTEIN POWDER

Collagen supplements have become increasingly popular due to their health benefits, particularly for improving skin elasticity, reducing wrinkles,[1] and supporting joint health. As noted in Chapter 1, collagen is a type of protein that is especially prevalent in connective tissues like skin, bones, cartilage, ligaments, and joints. It has high concentrations of three amino acids, glycine, proline, and hydroxyproline, which play a role in maintaining cell and tissue integrity. This is why collagen supplements are primarily used for skin and joint health.

Although collagen is a protein, it's not a complete protein source like whey protein. It lacks sufficient levels of tryptophan, one of the nine essential amino acids.[2] Consequently, it can't fully replace protein powders when it comes to building or repairing muscle. But it does contribute to your total daily protein intake, and its joint and skin benefits make it a complementary addition to your protein routine.

> **note**
>
> Collagen powder doesn't substitute well for protein powder in baking. The texture of the resulting baked good can vary quite a bit.

MYTH #2: EGG WHITES ARE A GOOD SOURCE OF PROTEIN

Maybe this isn't a total myth, because egg whites are often praised for being a complete source of protein. They do contain all the essential amino acids, but using only the whites means you're missing out on much of the nutritional value of a whole egg.

Although egg whites do contain a small amount of B vitamins, other important fat-soluble vitamins and minerals like vitamin D, zinc, and selenium are concentrated in the yolk.[3] Additionally, eating the whole egg provides a few extra grams of protein, which can be helpful if you struggle to meet your daily protein intake.

MYTH #3: HIGH-PROTEIN DIETS CAUSE KIDNEY FAILURE

There's a common misconception that high-protein diets can damage the kidneys, but this idea is not supported by evidence when it comes to people with healthy kidneys. I already discussed that those with underlying kidney disease should use caution and consult their healthcare providers when eating high amounts of protein. However, this is not the case for healthy individuals with fully functioning kidneys.

For those without kidney problems, research shows that healthy kidneys can adapt well to higher protein intake.[4] Eating more protein increases the kidneys' workload because they process extra nitrogen from the amino acids, but it doesn't seem to correlate to any harm or risk of kidney failure.

In fact, research has found no connection between high protein intake and markers of compromised kidney function, like blood urea nitrogen (BUN)[5] or glomerular filtration rate (GFR). A meta-analysis of trials even suggested that higher protein intake slightly improved GFR, indicating the kidneys' ability to adapt.[6]

MYTH #4: HIGH-PROTEIN DIETS DECREASE LONGEVITY AND INCREASE CANCER RISK

In recent news, it's been suggested that high-protein diets may decrease longevity and increase cancer risk because they raise mTOR (mammalian target of rapamycin), which is a key component in cell growth, metabolism, and survival.[7] mTOR is like the body's "growth switch," helping cells decide when to grow and when to clean up based on nutrient availability. It responds to amino acids, glucose, and insulin to stimulate muscle growth and repair. When food is plentiful, mTOR activates and promotes cell growth and reproduction. However, when nutrients are scarce, mTOR is suppressed and cells switch to "recycling mode," when they break down old parts to conserve energy and clean themselves.[8] The balance of growth and repair is essential for maintaining good health.

While it's true that protein can briefly activate mTOR, this response is short-lived and localized mainly to muscle tissue, where it supports repair and growth—essential processes for maintaining strength and health, especially as you age. In contrast, chronic and widespread mTOR activation, often caused by insulin resistance, can contribute to aging and disease.[9] However, the temporary increase in mTOR from protein intake has not been shown to raise cancer risk. In fact, studies show that people who engage in resistance training tend to have lower cancer rates,[10,11] and that population also tends to eat more than the RDA for protein.

Additionally, there is little evidence to support the idea that mTOR activation from protein intake leads to early death.[12] Both cell growth (stimulated by mTOR during a fed state) and cellular repair (which occurs when mTOR is not active) are valuable processes that work together to keep your body healthy and balanced. The mTOR pathway is not inherently harmful, and it's absolutely necessary for growth and survival.

MYTH #5: TOO MUCH PROTEIN WILL INCREASE BLOOD GLUCOSE

If you have dabbled in the keto diet, you know the fear that eating too much protein will kick you out of ketosis. This happens through a process called gluconeogenesis, where glucose is made from noncarbohydrate sources like amino acids. The rate at which protein intake triggers this process can vary among individuals and the type of diet they regularly consume.[13] So, while there's some truth to the idea that too much protein messes with ketosis, I don't believe you have to worry about it too much as long as you stick to no more than 50 to 60 grams of protein per meal.

When you start a keto diet, your body has to adjust to having fewer carbs and using fat for fuel. During this time, gluconeogenesis increases to convert protein to glucose to help maintain blood glucose levels and feed those cells that require glucose for energy (for example, red blood cells). While this is happening, your blood glucose and ketone levels can temporarily fluctuate. Eating too much protein during this time can tip the scales toward creating too much glucose, potentially disrupting ketosis. Over time, the body becomes better at using fat and ketones for energy, and gluconeogenesis decreases.[13]

How much protein needs to be consumed to stimulate gluconeogenesis? There is no exact number. There have been studies showing that the amount of glucose made from around 20 grams of protein (the amount in four eggs) is fairly small.[14]

Some experts, like Dr. Don Layman, professor of Food Science and Human Nutrition at the University of Illinois Urbana-Champaign, believe that the body can handle anywhere between 25 and 60 grams of protein at a time to maximize muscle-building.[15]

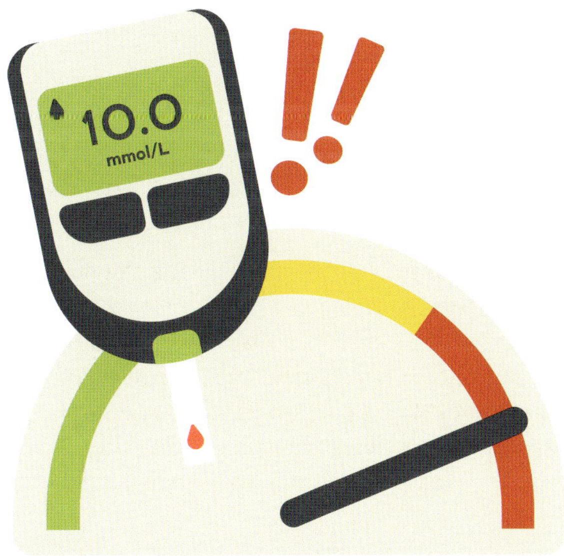

CHAPTER 5
LOW-CARB, HIGH-PROTEIN BASICS

Low-carb eating and the keto diet have been all the rage for the last ten years, although both have been around for much longer. People have flocked to this way of eating for many reasons—weight loss and better health outcomes being the most popular. This chapter helps you better understand what it means to eat low carb and what kind of benefits come from eating this way.

WHAT IS A LOW-CARB DIET?

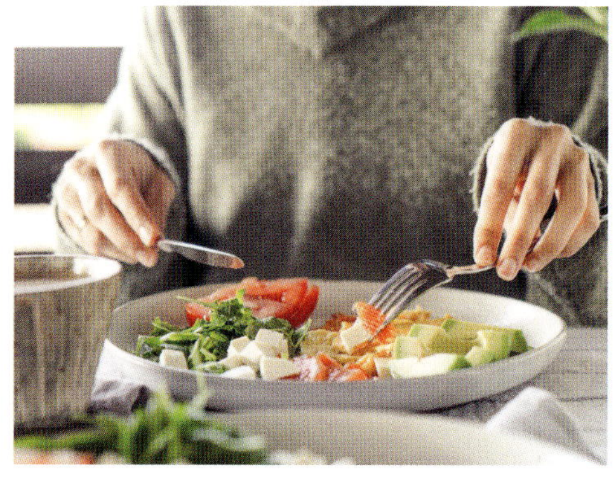

A low-carb diet limits the amount of carbohydrates you consume, typically by reducing or omitting foods like bread, pasta, sugar, rice, and starchy vegetables. Instead, you eat more protein, healthy fats, green leafy vegetables, and fruit. The goal is to lower carb intake to stabilize blood sugar, support weight loss, and improve overall health. Typically, the carbohydrate intake on a low-carb diet is 50 to 100 grams per day, depending on an individual's goals and needs. I personally like to keep that number closer to 50 grams.

A keto diet is one type of low-carb diet. It's stricter than some other options because it drastically reduces carbohydrate intake—typically keeping it to less than 20 grams per day. The main goal of a keto diet is to get the body into ketosis, where it burns fat for fuel instead of burning carbohydrates.

YOUR METABOLISM ON HIGH-CARB AND LOW-CARB DIETS

When you consume a lot of sugar and processed carbohydrates, your body rapidly breaks them down into glucose that enters your bloodstream, causing a spike in blood sugar levels. This signals the pancreas to release insulin to move that glucose into the cells. This glucose is either used as energy, stored as glycogen in the liver and muscles, or converted to fat for long-term storage of energy.

Over time, frequent spikes in blood sugar and insulin can negatively impact your metabolism. Constant release of insulin can lead to insulin resistance, making it harder for your body to respond to insulin's signals. This will eventually lead to diabetes.

In addition, eating too many sugary and processed carbs (such as chips, crackers, breakfast cereals, pastries, and white bread) can leave you feeling less than your best. These types of carbs are converted to glucose quickly and produce an immediate and pronounced release of insulin. Often, you experience the following issues:

- **Fatigue:** Sugary and high-carb processed foods can cause a quick spike in blood sugar that gives you a boost of energy, but it's followed by a crash that leaves you feeling tired and sluggish.
- **Brain fog:** Following the sugar crash, you may find it difficult to concentrate and think clearly.
- **Bloating:** Sugary foods can feed gut bacteria and cause gas buildup.
- **Addictive tendencies:** The more you eat sugar, the more you crave it. Sugar activates the brain's reward systems, creating a cycle that makes it hard to stop.
- **Low blood sugar:** Ironically, too much sugar can eventually cause low blood sugar. This usually happens with insulin resistance and leaves you feeling jittery, shaky, dizzy, irritable, and hungry again.

Chronic consumption of too much sugar and processed carbohydrates may lead to a variety of serious health issues. Here are just a few of the well-known ones, but there is a growing list of other health conditions linked to eating too much sugar:

- **High blood pressure and heart disease:** You can't feel that you have high blood pressure. It's often called the "silent killer" because you don't have any symptoms you can feel, but over time it can cause serious damage and/or lead to death. High blood sugar causes your body to retain more water. When insulin is released in response to high blood sugar, it also triggers the reabsorption of sodium in the kidneys. The body holds on to sodium instead of excreting it in the urine. This sodium retention in turn causes water retention, which results in elevated blood pressure.[1] This is why people with insulin resistance start to have high blood pressure. The high blood pressure and increased water retention puts added strain on the blood vessels, which increases the risk of heart disease.
- **Type 2 diabetes:** Over time, continuously consuming an excess of sugar can lead to diabetes. Consistent elevated blood sugar levels force the body to produce more insulin. Eventually, this can lead to insulin resistance and then diabetes.
- **Obesity:** Evidence suggests that diets high in sugar promote the development of obesity.[2] Foods and drinks high in added sugars, like candy, pastries, and soda, are calorie-dense but often lack fiber, protein, and other nutrients to keep you feeling full. This can lead to overeating because sugary foods are digested quickly, causing a rapid rise and fall in blood sugar levels. This triggers hunger signals sooner than if a balance of protein, fat, and slower-digested carbs was consumed. Excess sugar is also stored as fat after the body's energy requirements are met and glycogen stores are filled.

When you eat a low-carb diet, your body doesn't experience frequent and pronounced blood sugar and insulin spikes like it does on a high-carb diet. In combination with eating a balanced diet of protein and healthy fats, this helps stabilize energy levels and suppress appetite. Without frequent insulin release from eating carbs, the body no longer constantly receives signals to store fat.

WEIGHT LOSS WITH LOW-CARB DIETS

Low-carb diets can be highly effective for weight loss. Studies show that eating this way often leads to two to three times more weight loss compared to traditional low-fat diets.[3] One of the major reasons is that low-carb diets significantly reduce insulin levels in the body. Remember, insulin is released in response to consuming carbohydrates. It's a hormone that promotes fat storage and inhibits fat burning. By restricting carbs, the body lowers insulin, making it easier to break down stored fat.

Another significant advantage of low-carb diets is their effect on reducing appetite. Low-carb meals tend to be more satiating, so they help you feel full longer because they're usually higher in fat and protein. Not only does this help reduce hunger throughout the day, but your overall calorie intake on a low-carb diet can be lower. Often, people can get away with reducing calories without the strict calorie counting that may be required for success on a low-fat diet.

GENERAL GUIDELINES FOR EATING LOW CARB

Here are some of the general guidelines that I recommend (and follow) for living a low-carb lifestyle:

- **Limit carb intake.** Depending on what type of low-carb diet you do (keto, Atkins, South Beach, or general low carb), deciding on your daily carb limit is the first step. Typically, this ranges from 10 to 100 grams of carbohydrates per day. Setting this limit depends on your goals (for example, weight loss, maintenance, or specific health conditions) and your tolerance to carbs. My goal is to maintain my weight, and I feel my best when I eat 50 to 60 grams of carbohydrates per day.

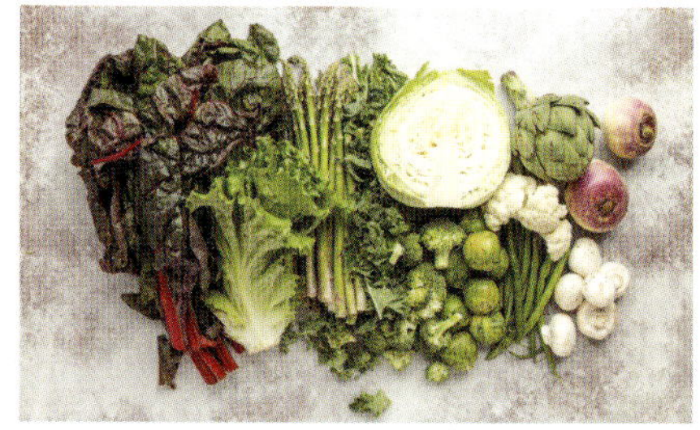

Nonstarchy Vegetables

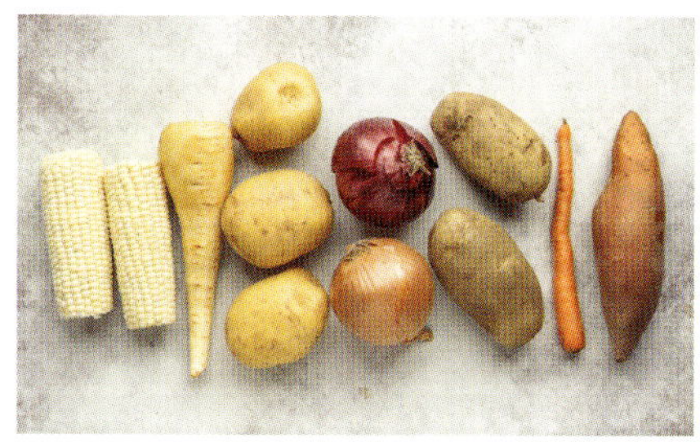

Starchy Vegetables

- **Prioritize nonstarchy vegetables.** All vegetables contain carbohydrates. The carbs primarily come from natural sugars, starches, and fiber. The natural sugars are small amounts of glucose, fructose, and sucrose, which are all simple carbohydrates that are readily absorbed in the body. The starches are complex carbs that aren't absorbed as quickly as sugars because they have to be broken down before they're converted to glucose. Potatoes and corn are examples of starchy vegetables. Fiber is a type of carbohydrate that the body can't fully digest, so high-fiber, nonstarchy vegetables like broccoli, spinach, zucchini, and lettuce don't produce a pronounced insulin response.

  Although vegetables contribute to the daily carbohydrate count, I don't limit the amount of nonstarchy vegetables I eat. They are filled with fiber, and they're excellent sources of vital minerals and vitamins, too.

- **Limit or avoid sugary and processed foods.** Cut out as much sugary food—like candy, baked goods, and sugary sodas or other drinks—as possible. You should also limit processed foods like crackers, chips, and cookies because they can spike blood sugar and trigger a pronounced insulin response.
- **Reduce grains and starchy foods.** Minimize or eliminate traditional breads, pastas, and rice because they're high in carbohydrates. You can easily replace them with low-carb breads, noodles, and cauliflower rice.
- **Eat fruits in moderation.** Fruits contain fiber and natural sugars. Some are higher in natural sugars than others. Bananas, grapes, cherries, mangoes, apples, pears, pineapple, and dried fruits have a higher sugar content than fruits like berries, lemons, and limes. All fruit contains other important nutrients like vitamins and antioxidants, so I believe they have a place in a low-carb diet. You should limit high-sugar fruits, but don't completely skip them unless you're following a very low-carb diet like a ketogenic diet.

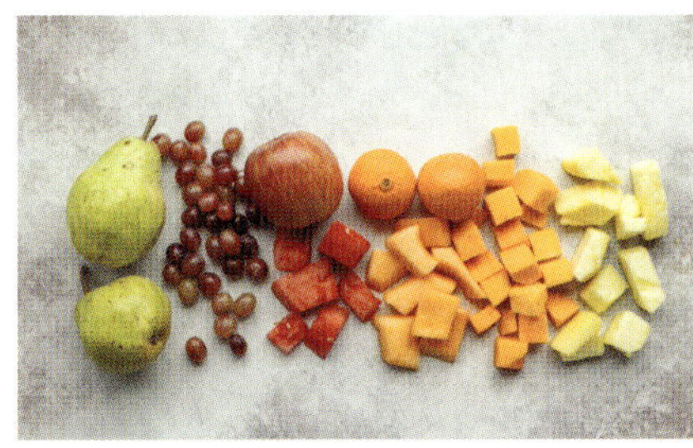

High-Sugar Fruits

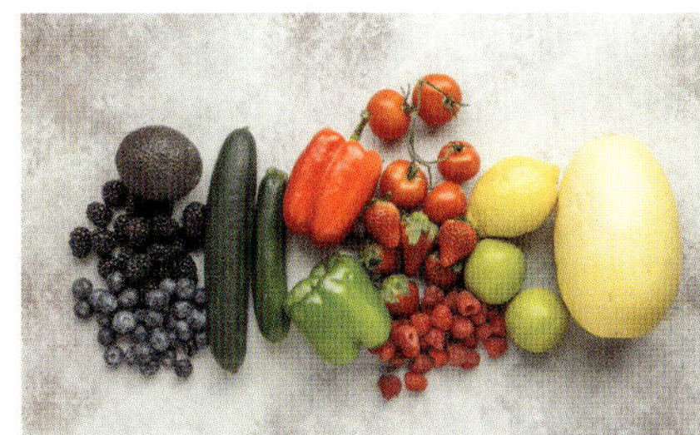

Low-Sugar Fruits

- **Focus on healthy fats and more protein.** Incorporate sources of healthy fats like avocados, nuts, seeds, olive oil, avocado oil, and tallow. Include more proteins like eggs, fish, poultry, beef, pork, wild game, and/or plant-based protein sources.
- **Don't forget your electrolytes.** Remember how I talked about insulin's effect on the kidneys? It plays a role in electrolyte balance, too. A low-carb diet diminishes your insulin response. Insulin is what tells the kidneys to reabsorb sodium into the body. If you have little insulin, it's not there to tell your kidneys to pull back sodium, so the sodium gets flushed out. Other electrolytes like potassium and magnesium can follow. Low electrolytes can cause you to be fatigued, dizzy, and unable to think and perform properly since electrolytes are needed for proper nerve firing, cell signaling, and muscle contractions.

THE KEY THING TO REMEMBER

Eating low carb and high protein is a lifestyle. I don't look at it as a temporary fix. I take a long-term, sustainable approach to eating; it's part of my daily life.

I also realize no one is perfect, and no diet is one size fits all. For a way of eating to be sustainable in the long run, you have to leave room for flexibility, balance, and forgiveness. I don't subscribe to the idea that you can never have a slice of bread again or never enjoy a candy bar on a low-carb diet.

By allowing yourself the occasional treat, you can avoid feeling restricted or guilty, which can often lead to frustration and giving up altogether. Life is meant to be enjoyed, and food is part of that enjoyment, especially if you're a foodie like me. The goal isn't perfection but overall consistency.

Most of the time, I focus on nutrient-dense, low-carb, high-protein meals, but when there's a special occasion or I just feel like indulging, I don't deny myself. That's what makes this a lifestyle. Be adaptable and realistic, and you'll find that you can stick with eating the way that makes you feel good for the long haul.

EATING HIGH PROTEIN FOR WEIGHT LOSS

Incorporating more protein into your diet can be a powerful tool for weight loss. More and more evidence supports how it helps control appetite, regulate hormones, and increase metabolism, all while preventing muscle loss.

Evidence from multiple studies shows that high-protein diets are effective for weight loss and improving body composition. A meta-analysis by Wycherley et al. analyzed 24 randomized controlled trials and found that participants following a high-protein diet (consuming 1.07 to 1.60 grams of protein/kg/day) experienced greater reductions in body weight and fat mass compared to those on a standard-protein diet (consuming the RDA for an adult). Even with similar calorie restrictions, the high-protein group lost an average of 0.79 kg more body weight and 0.87 kg more fat mass than the standard group over a 12-week period.[4]

Similarly, a meta-analysis by Santesso et al. reviewed 74 randomized controlled trials and concluded that high-protein diet participants consuming protein as 16 to 45 percent of their daily energy intake experienced significant reductions in weight, BMI, and waist circumference compared to standard-protein diet participants.[5]

Additional evidence from studies where participants can eat freely without calorie restriction supports how effective a high-protein diet is even without calorie intake being tightly controlled. In a six-month trial, participants consuming 25 percent of their energy intake from protein lost significantly more weight (3.7 kg on average) and fat mass (3.3 kg on average) compared to those on a high-carbohydrate diet.[6] This suggests that the satiety-inducing effects of protein may reduce overall calorie consumption, leading to weight loss.

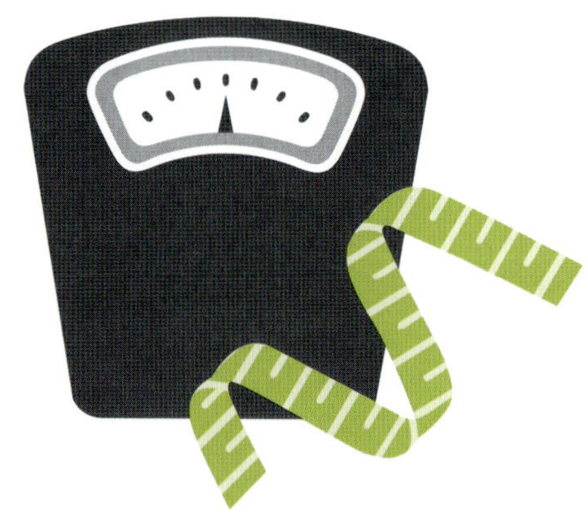

Not only have high-protein diets been shown to be effective for weight loss, but studies have suggested they're effective for maintaining that weight loss in the long term, even in the absence of strict caloric control.[7]

High-Protein Diets Reduce Appetite

High-protein diets are effective for weight loss largely because they help reduce appetite, making it easier to consume fewer calories. Satiety studies have shown that protein is the most satiating macronutrient, meaning that consuming protein helps you feel full and satisfied longer compared to fat and carbs.[8]

Protein helps reduce hunger by influencing hunger hormones. Protein intake decreases the hunger hormone, ghrelin, and increases levels of hormones that signal fullness—peptide YY, glucagon-like peptide (GLP-1), and cholecystokinin.[9,10] These hormones are secreted in the gut when protein is present, stimulating the vagus nerve to enhance feelings of fullness.[11]

High-Protein Diets Increase Metabolic Rate

Another way that eating a diet high in protein helps with weight loss is by boosting your metabolism through a process called the thermic effect of food (TEF), which describes the energy it takes for your body to digest, absorb, and metabolize food.[12] Protein has the highest TEF of the three macronutrients, with 15 to 20 percent of the calories from protein being burned during digestion compared to 5 to 10 percent for carbs and 0 to 3 percent for fats.[13,14] Basically, you burn calories just by eating! This calorie burn may seem small on a daily basis, but it adds up over time.

Gluconeogenesis

If you have any experience with the keto diet, you may think gluconeogenesis is a bad word. In a diet where the goal is to keep carbs and blood glucose to a minimum, having the liver make glucose from excess noncarbohydrate sources like amino acids seems counterproductive when it comes to weight loss, but let me explain how it might be helpful.

Gluconeogenesis increases the expenditure contributing to an overall increase in calorie burn, which supports weight loss efforts.[15] On top of that, the glucose produced during this process and the increased production of glycogen in the liver from that production of glucose sends signals to the brain that tell the body it is full.[16]

CHAPTER 6

THE HIGH-PROTEIN KITCHEN

Now that you know why eating higher protein and low carb is recommended, the rest of this book helps you put it all together and make a plan to fit it into your life. In this chapter, I explain how to use the special features of the recipes and prepare your kitchen to pack your meals with protein.

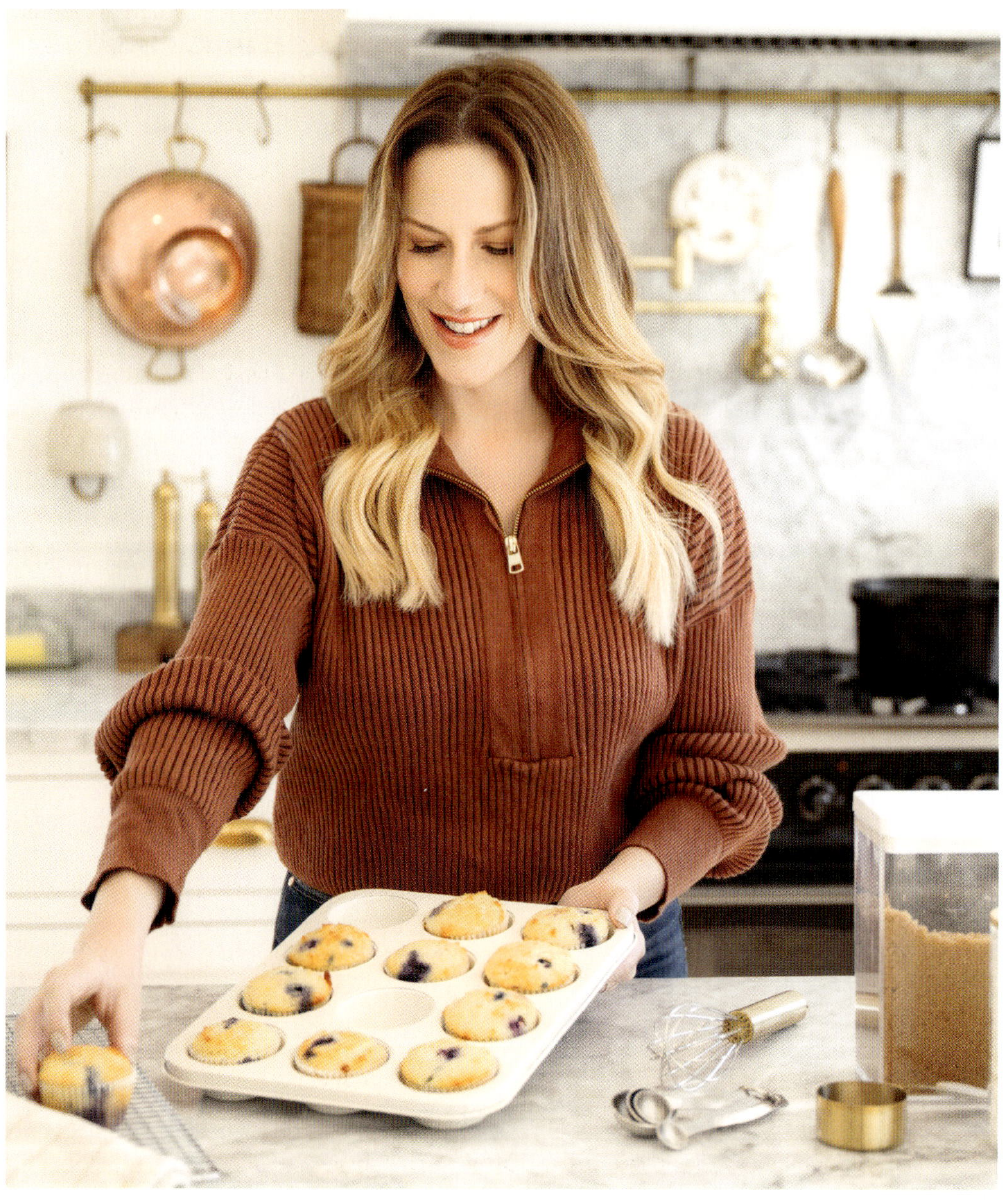

USING THE RECIPES

I designed these recipes to use ingredients that should be familiar to most people who already follow a low-carb diet. If you're new to low-carb eating, some of these ingredients may be unfamiliar to you. I've included notes in the "Ingredients I Keep in My Kitchen" section about ingredients that may not be staples in your refrigerator or pantry yet. Additionally, check out the "Must-Have Tools" section to find a list of kitchen equipment that may be helpful in cooking and baking some of these recipes.

Understanding the Icons

I've included icons at the top of each recipe to help you with your meal planning. The icons indicate allergens you may need or want to avoid, meal prep friendliness, and compatible cooking equipment. Use the following icons to assist with your meal planning:

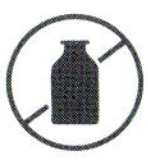

Dairy free: Recipes labeled as dairy free do not call for any dairy products. In those recipes that do include dairy, I've suggested dairy-free alternatives when possible, although I haven't necessarily tested these substitutions.

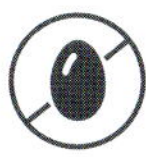

Egg free: For those with egg sensitivities or allergies, this icon highlights recipes that are egg free.

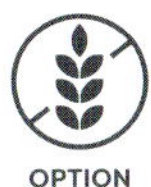

Gluten-free option: Almost all of my recipes are gluten free, but I occasionally call for soy sauce and for keto breads, tortillas, and chips that do contain gluten. In those cases, I have marked the recipe with this icon and noted what modifications are needed to make the recipe gluten free. If you have celiac disease or a true gluten allergy, I strongly encourage you to check all ingredient labels carefully, because some products may contain hidden sources of gluten.

Nut free: For those with nut sensitivities or allergies, this icon highlights recipes that are nut free. Although some recipes use nut flours or include nuts, I have provided nut-free substitutions where possible. For this allergen icon, coconut is not classified as a nut, despite "nut" being in the name. Most individuals with nut allergies can tolerate coconut. Recipes using pine nuts will not have the nut-free icon since some people with tree nut allergies cannot tolerate pine nuts either.

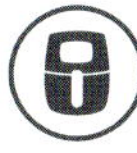

Air fryer: Recipes marked with this icon can be prepared in an air fryer. Air fryers offer a healthier alternative to traditional frying by using less oil while still delivering crispy results in a fraction of the time compared to baking in the oven.

Instant Pot: Recipes marked with this icon are suitable for an Instant Pot or other type of pressure cooker. Using a pressure cooker significantly reduces cooking time while retaining flavors, making it a convenient tool for busy days.

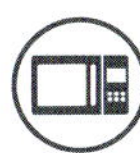

Microwave: This icon marks recipes that can be cooked (not just reheated) in a microwave—quick and easy dishes that come together in a flash.

Slow cooker: This icon highlights recipes that you can make in a slow cooker, which makes meal prep easier by allowing you to start your meal earlier in the day so it cooks gradually with minimal supervision. You can set a timer, focus on your day, and come back to a meal that's nearly ready to serve.

Freezer safe: This icon indicates recipes that freeze well, making them perfect for storing leftovers or preparing meals in advance to enjoy later.

Meal prep friendly: Meal prepping is essential for maintaining your new eating habits. Recipes that you can prepare in advance can ease the burden of cooking during hectic times and busy schedules. This icon highlights dishes that can be made ahead and stored for several days while retaining their taste and quality.

Using the Nutritional Information

(per serving)
CALORIES: **401** | PROTEIN: **42.7g** | FAT: **19.8g** | TOTAL CARBS: **12.6g** | NET CARBS: **7.9g** | FIBER: **4.7g**

Every recipe includes the following nutritional information per serving: calories, protein, fat, total carbohydrates, net carbohydrates, fiber, and sugar alcohols (where applicable). All the nutritional information was calculated using MyFitnessPal. I make every effort to ensure accuracy when calculating macros; however, these figures are estimates based on the average size of ingredients. I recommend calculating your own nutritional information.

Additionally, the sweeteners used in this book technically include carbohydrates from fiber and sugar alcohols. However, they typically have little to no impact on blood sugar for most individuals. While I include them in the total carb counts, fiber and sugar alcohols are subtracted to determine net carbs.

If an ingredient is listed as optional, a topping, or a garnish, it is not included in the given macronutrient calculations.

MAKING SUBSTITUTIONS

Some of the recipes in this book use ingredients that might be new to you. If you're just starting to cook or bake with low-carb ingredients, it's best to follow the recipes exactly as written until you gain confidence experimenting with substitutions and low-carb cooking.

Keep in mind that some ingredients cannot be swapped one for one. For instance, a cup of coconut flour is not equivalent to a cup of almond flour because its high absorbency dramatically alters the moisture balance and texture of a recipe, often requiring additional eggs or liquid to compensate. If you need to make a substitution, it's a good idea to look up the conversion online to help figure out how much you need of the item you're substituting. However, know that the substituted item may not yield the same results as the item in the ingredient list.

Where possible, I've suggested substitutions, but the nutritional information provided is based on the original ingredients listed in the recipe. The following table shows some suggested substitutes.

Easy Substitution Guide

INSTEAD OF	TRY
Soy sauce or tamari	Coconut aminos or liquid aminos
Cow's milk	Almond milk, flax milk, macadamia nut milk, hemp seed milk, or coconut milk
Heavy cream	Coconut cream
Sour cream	Greek yogurt
Honey or maple syrup	Sugar-free honey or sugar-free maple syrup
Rice	Cauliflower rice, Kaizen rice, or heart of palm rice
Pasta	Heart of palm noodles, Kaizen noodles, lupini pasta, or Miracle Noodle egg white spaghetti
Breadcrumbs	Pork panko, almond flour, or grated Parmesan cheese

STORING LEFTOVERS

Unless otherwise stated, you can use the following recommendations for storing leftovers or dishes made ahead of time:

- **Baked goods:** Because most low-carb baked goods are made with sugar alternatives, they tend to dry out faster than those made with real sugar. Store low-carb baked goods at room temperature for up to 3 days. Or store them in an airtight container in the refrigerator for up to a week. You can also freeze most low-carb baked goods—just wrap them tightly in plastic wrap or foil and store in a freezer-safe bag or container for up to 2 months. Thaw at room temperature or reheat gently in the microwave or oven before serving.
- **Casseroles:** Leftover casseroles can be stored in the refrigerator for up to 4 days or frozen for longer storage, typically 1 to 3 months. To reheat, cover the casserole with foil to retain moisture. Most casseroles can be heated in the oven at 350°F until heated through. You can also use a microwave for smaller portions.
- **Chips:** Store homemade chips in a paper bag at room temperature for up to 10 days. Make sure they're completely cool before storing to prevent steam from softening them.
- **Cooked egg dishes:** Leftover egg dishes can be stored in an airtight container in the refrigerator for 3 to 4 days. To reheat, use a microwave at a low setting or warm in the oven at 300°F until warmed.
- **Cooked meats:** Store leftover cooked meats in an airtight container in the refrigerator and use within 3 to 4 days. For longer storage, freeze for up to 3 months. To maintain the best texture and flavor, let the meat cool completely before refrigerating or freezing.
- **Cooked vegetables:** Store leftover cooked vegetables in an airtight container in the refrigerator for up to 4 days. Let them cool completely before storing.
- **Pasta dishes:** Store leftover pasta dishes in an airtight container in the refrigerator for up to 4 days. If you plan to freeze them, transfer to a freezer-safe container or bag and store for up to 2 months. Keep in mind that egg-based sauces like carbonara (see page 128) don't freeze well, as they can become grainy or separate when reheated.
- **Pizza:** Leftover pizza can be stored in an airtight container, or slices can be wrapped in foil or plastic wrap, and refrigerated for up to 4 days. To freeze, place slices in a single layer on a plate and freeze until solid. Then transfer to a freezer-safe bag or container and freeze for up to 2 months. Reheat refrigerated pizza in a 375°F oven for 5 to 8 minutes. Frozen pizza slices can go straight into the oven but will require a few extra minutes to bake.
- **Salads/salad dressings:** Store salads and salad dressings separately to keep everything fresh and the salad crisp. Place undressed salad in an airtight container with a paper towel to absorb moisture and refrigerate for 3 to 5 days. Store homemade dressings in a sealed jar or container in the refrigerator for 1 to 2 weeks. Add dressing just before serving to prevent the salad from becoming soggy.

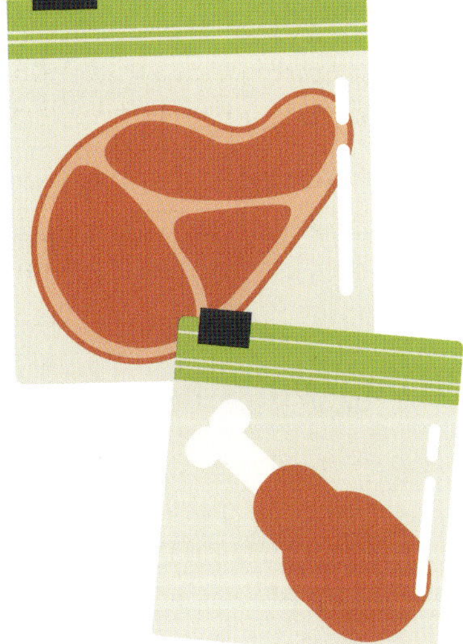

- **Soups:** Leftover soup can be stored in the refrigerator for 3 to 4 days, but it will last at least a month in the freezer. Be sure to let it cool completely before freezing it. Store in resealable freezer bags or freezer-safe containers.
- **Wraps:** To store sandwich wraps, wrap them in plastic wrap and place in an airtight container or plastic bag in the refrigerator for up to 3 days. If the wrap contains ingredients that release moisture (like tomatoes or cucumbers), consider storing those separately and adding them just before eating to prevent sogginess.

INGREDIENTS I KEEP IN MY KITCHEN

Stocking your kitchen with the right ingredients is essential for maintaining healthy eating habits. Keep these pantry staples on hand to support your journey toward a healthier lifestyle.

Eating low carb often means filling your kitchen with new and different foods that align with this lifestyle. In this section, I share the items I always keep on hand and my go-to choices for staying successful with a high-protein, low-carb way of eating.

Dairy and Eggs

Butter: I always keep butter on hand for cooking and baking, and I prefer to use butter from grass-fed cows. Grass-fed butter is richer in omega-3 fatty acids, vitamin K2, and conjugated linoleic acid (CLA). In this book, I use both salted and unsalted butter, so the type is always specified.

Cheese: I always keep a variety of cheeses on hand: cheddar, feta, Parmesan, cream cheese, and string cheese. Feta cheese, in particular, is a great choice for adding extra protein to salads or other dishes, with 6 grams of protein per 1-ounce serving. I use two types of Parmesan: pregrated and preshredded.

Cottage cheese: I buy whole-milk cottage cheese with at least 4% milkfat. I prefer it over low-fat or fat-free cottage cheese because it is creamier and has a better flavor due to the higher fat content. Good Culture is a popular brand because it has less carbohydrates than other brands. It's the kind I used to create the recipes in this book and calculate the macros.

Eggs: My fridge is well stocked with fresh eggs and hard-boiled eggs, perfect for whipping up a protein-packed breakfast, enjoying as a quick snack, or adding extra protein to any meal.

Milk: Most of the recipes in this book are versatile enough to work with the milk of your choice. Cow's milk is higher in carbs than other alternatives, so if you don't strongly prefer it, you may want to try unsweetened and unflavored almond milk, coconut milk, cashew milk, flax milk, hemp seed milk, or macadamia nut milk. I developed all the recipes for this book using Good Karma Flaxmilk + Protein, an unsweetened flax milk with 5 grams of protein per 1-cup serving.

Yogurt: I always keep plain Greek or low-carb yogurt in my refrigerator, with my go-to brands being Fage 5% Greek yogurt and Two Good. I particularly like Two Good for its very low carb content: just 3 grams per ¾ cup, plus 14 grams of protein. This is the type I used to calculate the macros for the recipes in this book.

Oils and Fats

Avocado oil: This is my go-to cooking oil for nearly everything because of its high smoke point and neutral flavor. It's also rich in heart-healthy monounsaturated fats and antioxidants.

Olive oil: I love using olive oil for cold applications like making dressings because its rich flavor enhances salads and marinades. It has a lower smoke point than avocado oil, but it's packed with monounsaturated fats and antioxidants.

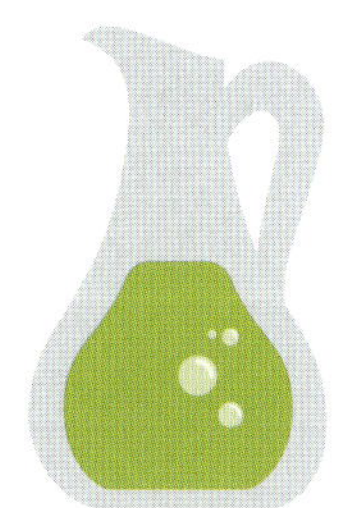

Tallow: Tallow is a nutrient-dense cooking fat that's rich in healthy fats like CLA and fat-soluble vitamins, making it a great option for high-heat cooking while giving health benefits. I love using tallow for cooking eggs and searing meats like steak, pork chops, and chicken because it creates the perfect crust and adds incredible flavor. Store it in the refrigerator after opening.

Produce

Lemons and limes: I always keep lemons and limes in the fridge because their juice and zest add a fresh, bright flavor to meals. They're also a great source of vitamin C and can enhance the taste of dishes without adding extra carbs.

Parsley: Flat-leaf (Italian) parsley and curly parsley differ in both flavor and texture. Flat-leaf parsley has a more robust, slightly peppery taste, making it better suited for cooking, while curly parsley is milder. For this cookbook, I use flat-leaf parsley because it brings more flavor to the recipes.

Broths and Sauces

Beef and chicken bone broth: I love making bone broth from scratch (see pages 284 to 287 for my recipes) and always keep some in the fridge to use in recipes. Its rich nutrients and collagen make it a healthy and incredibly flavorful addition to meals. However, I also keep my pantry stocked with cartons of store-bought beef and chicken broth as a backup in case I run out of my homemade batches. For vegetarian dishes, vegetable broth is an easy alternative.

Chili garlic sauce: This is a must-have in my kitchen for enhancing the flavor of savory dishes like stir-fries and marinades. Huy Fong brand is my favorite.

Marinara sauce: I always keep marinara sauce in my pantry because it's perfect for making quick Italian dishes. When choosing marinara, look for brands with no added sugar to keep carbs low. One of my favorites is Yo Mama's marinara sauce. Sometimes I find it at my local grocery store, but it's also available on Amazon.

Soy sauce, tamari, liquid aminos, and/or coconut aminos: These umami-packed sauces are used in many Asian-style dishes. My husband doesn't eat gluten, so I keep gluten-free tamari in the house as a soy sauce substitute, but I also use liquid aminos, which has a savory flavor similar to soy sauce while being gluten free and lower in sodium. Coconut aminos is a soy-free option.

Sriracha: This sauce is always in my fridge, and I usually keep a backup in the pantry, too. Sriracha adds a spicy kick to dishes and sauces. When it's mixed with mayo, it's perfect for dipping steak or chicken. Be sure to check out my Sriracha Egg Salad recipe on page 232!

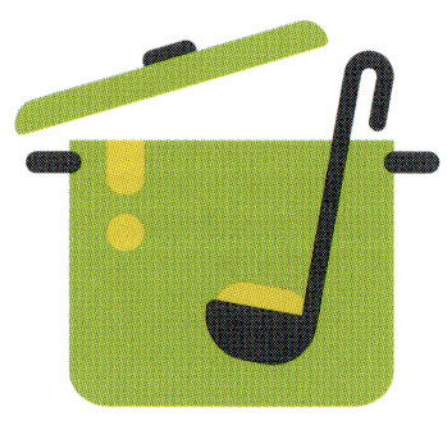

Sweet chili sauce: A few recipes in this book call for sweet chili sauce. Look for the brands that have the least sugar.

Flours and Thickeners

Almond flour: Almond flour is made from finely ground almonds. I prefer finely milled, blanched almond flour because it has a smoother texture and excludes the almond skins found in coarser almond meal. This finer texture creates baked goods with a more delicate crumb. My go-to brands are Kirkland (from Costco) and Bob's Red Mill.

Arrowroot powder: This is my preferred gluten-free thickener. Cup for cup, arrowroot powder is a stronger thickening agent than all-purpose flour, so you don't need to add much of it to thicken a sauce or soup. This keeps it low carb, too.

Coconut flour: Coconut flour is a popular low-carb option, but it's higher in carbs than almond flour. It also has a strong flavor and does not measure cup for cup with all-purpose flour because of how absorptive it is. The conversion I tend to follow is 1 cup of all-purpose flour equaling ¼ cup of coconut flour.

Lupin flour: This flour is derived from lupini beans, a type of legume that is high in protein and fiber while being low in carbs. It has a unique flavor that, in my opinion, resembles the taste of corn, so it's a perfect choice for my tortilla recipe on page 249.

Oat fiber: Don't confuse oat fiber with oat flour. Oat fiber is an insoluble fiber from the outer husk of the oat. Because it can't be digested or absorbed, it has zero net carbs. Adding a few tablespoons to baked goods gives them a better breadlike texture and a hint of oat flavor.

Xanthan gum: I use xanthan gum in some recipes in this book. It helps hold doughs together and provides structure. Although some people use it as a thickener, it's not my preferred thickener because it can make a dish slimy.

Protein Powders

Egg white protein powder: This can be used in protein shakes and smoothies, and I love to bake with it as well. You can make the perfect meringue just by adding water. In fact, it's a great shelf-stable alternative to fresh egg whites.

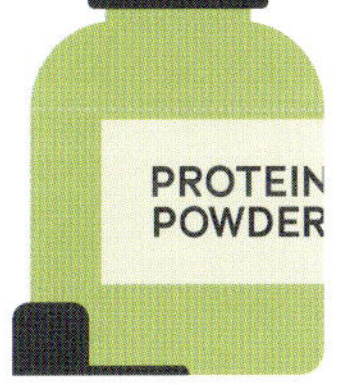

Whey protein powder: A few recipes in this book call for protein powder. The protein powder I prefer for baking and cooking is a whey isolate protein from Isopure. The Isopure Zero Carb Unflavored Protein Powder has 25 grams of protein and zero carbohydrates per scoop. Another protein powder I use in protein shakes is from 1 UP Nutrition—it's a fast-absorbing, low-carb whey protein isolate that comes in delicious flavors like Peanut Butter Cookie. I haven't experimented with other types or brands of protein powder in these recipes.

Sweeteners

Sugar-free chocolate chips: When a recipe calls for chocolate chips, I use Lily's sugar-free chocolate chips.

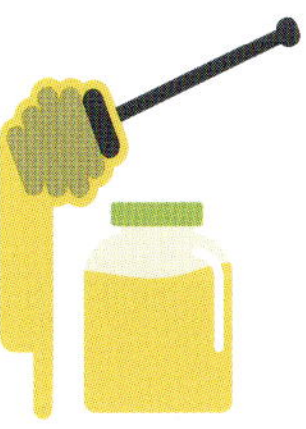

Sugar-free honey: Some of my recipes call for sugar-free honey. Luckily, you can find sugar-free honey that tastes and performs like regular honey from brands like Wholesome Yum Foods.

Sugar-free maple syrup: In place of maple syrup, you can use a sugar-free option like Lakanto Maple Syrup or the Wholesome Yum Foods Zero Sugar Maple Syrup.

Sugar-free sweeteners: There are many sugar-free sweeteners available, which makes it easy to find options that fit your needs. These sweeteners don't tend to raise blood sugar levels in most people because they're typically made from sugar alcohols and/or nondigestible fibers, resulting in zero net carbs. I prefer to use brands that measure cup for cup with sugar. For a granulated sugar substitute, I use Lakanto Classic. For a brown sugar alternative, I rely on Swerve Brown. And for powdered sweeteners, I alternate between powdered allulose from Wholesome Yum Foods and Swerve Confectioners, which is erythritol based.

Miscellaneous Pantry Items

Black soybeans: Black soybeans have a similar appearance and flavor to black beans, but they're lower in carbs. They're high in protein and fiber with 5 grams of net carbs and 11 grams of protein per ½-cup serving. Eden makes canned organic black soybeans, and you can find them on Amazon.

Lupini beans: Lupini beans are a fantastic high-protein, low-carb snack thanks to their fiber content. They make a great replacement for beans in soups and stews because they offer a similar texture and flavor while keeping the carb count low. Since lupini beans are legumes with a flavor similar to chickpeas, I've used them to create my low-carb hummus recipe, which you can find on page 310.

Low-carb chips: I like to keep a variety of low-carb chips in my pantry for quick snacks or to pair with dips and meals. Some of my favorite brands are Quest Chips, Hilo, Beyond Chipz, and Mr. Tortilla, which makes delicious tortilla chips. These options are perfect for satisfying crunchy cravings.

Low-carb pastas: There are a variety of low-carb pastas available to suit different recipes and tastes. Options include heart of palm, wheat, shirataki (made from konjac root), and lupini bean. Many of these are gluten free, too. Kaizen is one of my go-to brands for low-carb, high-protein (20 grams per serving!) pasta. I also love heart of palm noodles, especially the ones from Natural Heaven; they're great for lighter dishes. Miracle Noodle, famous for shirataki noodles, now offers a noodle made from egg whites. They're perfect for replacing traditional spaghetti and have 10 grams of protein per serving.

Low-carb tortillas: If you don't want to make your own tortillas (see page 249), there are plenty of low-carb options available at most grocery stores. Mission makes both Zero Carb and Carb Balance tortillas, but keep in mind that they do contain gluten. If you're looking for a gluten-free alternative, brands like Unbun and Maria & Ricardo's offer low-carb tortillas that fit the bill.

Pork panko: My go-to substitute for breadcrumbs is pork panko, which is just ground-up pork rinds. You can make your own by pulverizing them in a food processor, but it's more convenient to buy them preground. The brand I used for this cookbook is Bacon's Heir. I find it on Amazon.

Salt: For these recipes, I used fine grain Redmond Real Salt, a mineral-rich, unrefined sea salt that adds clean, natural flavor to each dish.

MUST-HAVE TOOLS

These kitchen tools simplify prep work and cooking, and I rely on them weekly, if not almost daily.

Air fryer: An air fryer is a fantastic tool for quick cooking and for reheating leftovers. It gives you crispy, golden results without using excess oil. It makes the best fried chicken tenders and crispy roasted vegetables in less time than using an oven.

Instant Pot: This versatile kitchen tool combines the functions of a pressure cooker and slow cooker, plus newer models offer other functions like sous vide and steaming. It significantly reduces cooking time for meals like soups, stews, and even roasts but still delivers flavorful results. I also use it to meal-prep shredded chicken for the week, which is perfect for adding to high-protein meals like salads, wraps, or casseroles.

Slow cooker: A slow cooker is an incredibly useful tool for effortless cooking when you don't have time to cook dinner in the evenings but do have a few minutes to pull ingredients together in the morning. It allows you to prepare a meal in advance by putting in ingredients and letting them cook slowly throughout the day. This hands-off approach to dinner saves me time and the stress of putting something healthy on the table when we come home late.

Sous vide cooker: This is one of my favorite tools for cooking proteins to perfection. It cooks meats, fish, or poultry in a temperature-controlled water bath, which ensures even doneness while preserving tenderness and juiciness. This method is especially helpful for meal prep because you can batch-cook proteins and store them for quick high-protein meals throughout the week. Plus, it eliminates the guesswork. Your steak or chicken turns out flawlessly every time! One of my favorite time-saving tips is to season a bunch of meats ahead of time, vacuum seal them, and freeze them. When you're ready to cook, just pull out what you need and drop it straight into the sous vide from frozen.

Traeger or pellet grill: A Traeger grill is my go-to grill for cooking proteins. Its wood pellet system adds delicious flavor to chicken, steak, and fish while maintaining juiciness.

Parchment paper: Parchment paper is excellent for lining baking sheets to prevent sticking and make cleanup easier. It's also available in precut circles that perfectly fit tortilla presses and cake pans.

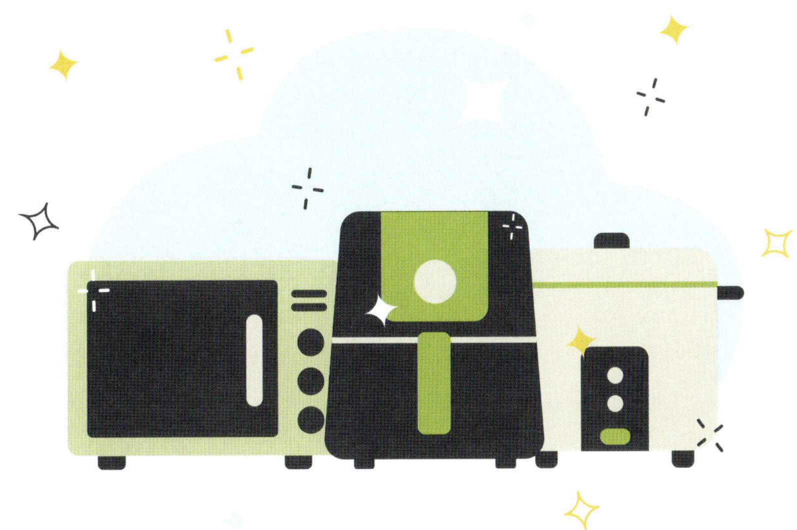

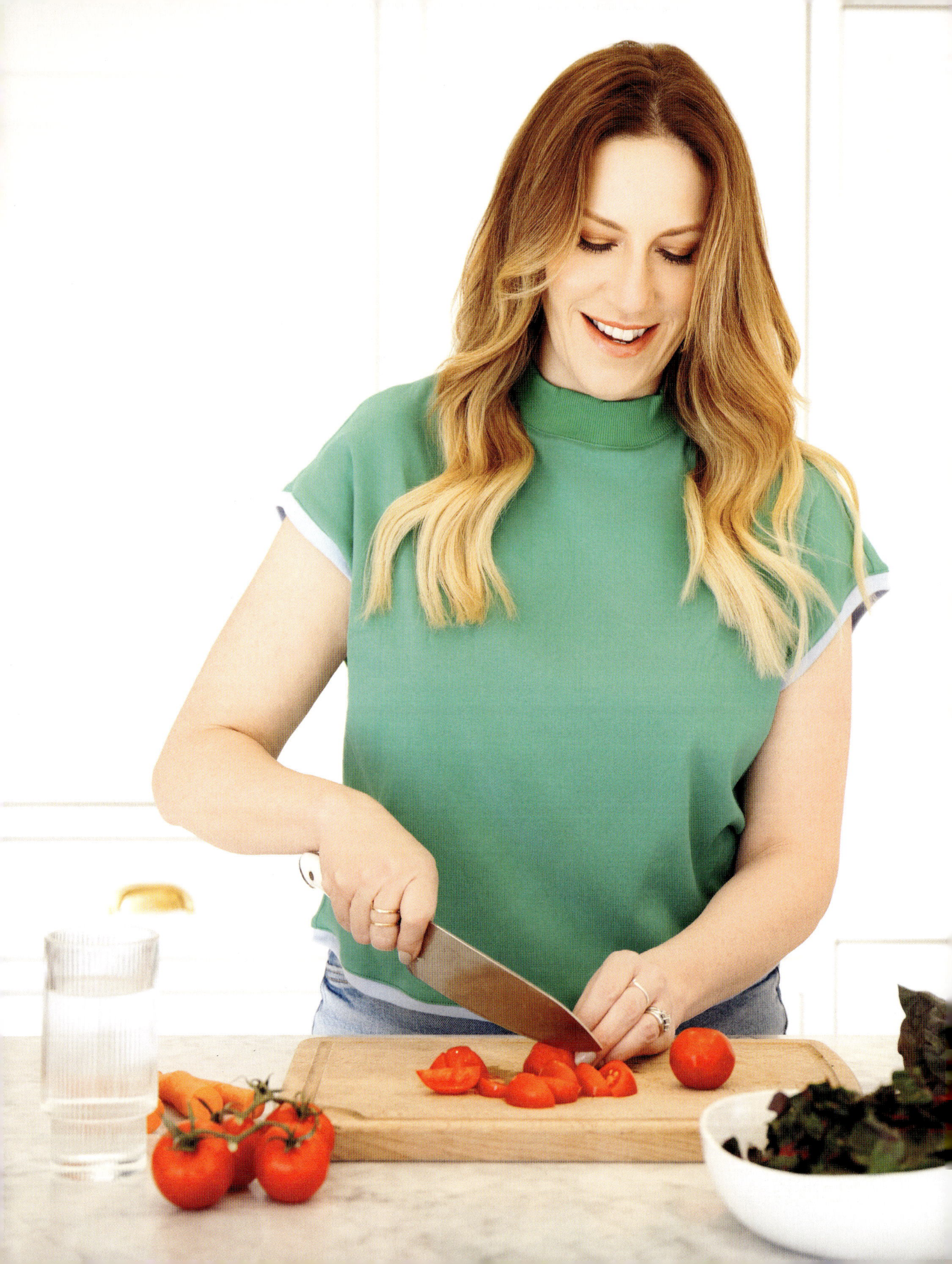

PART 2
Recipes

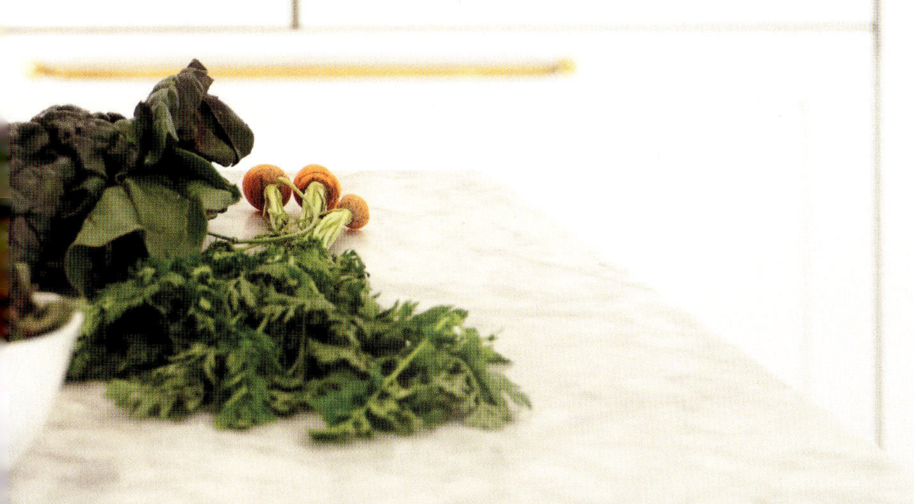

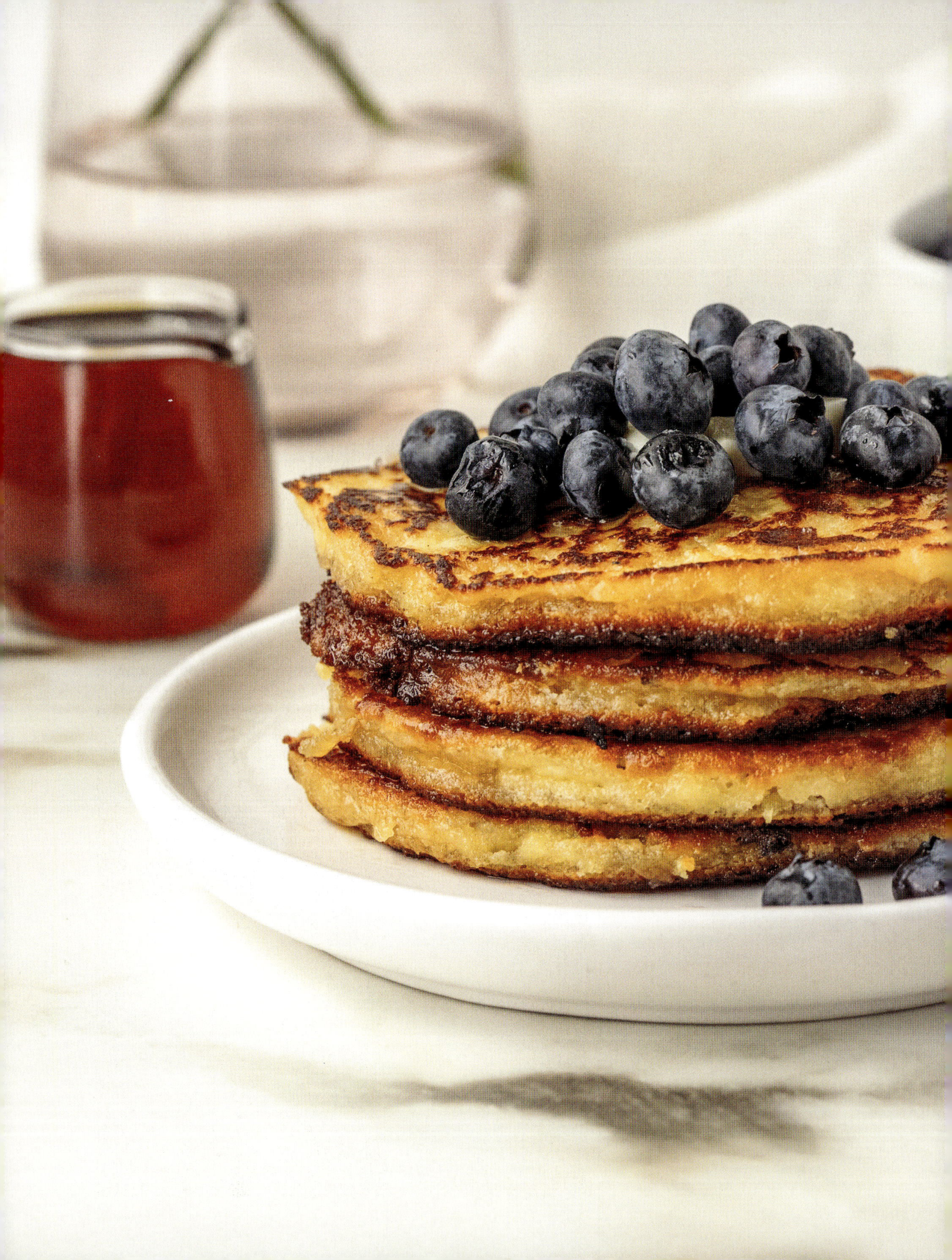

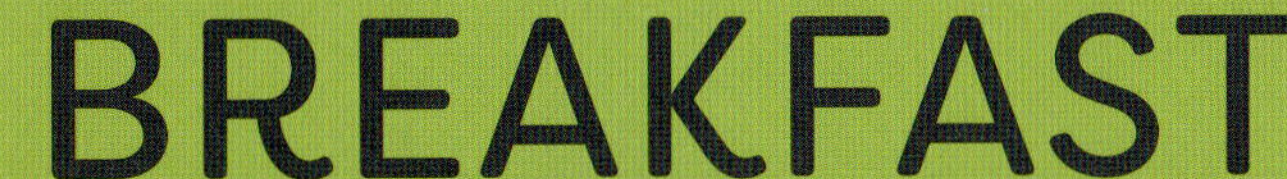

BREAKFAST

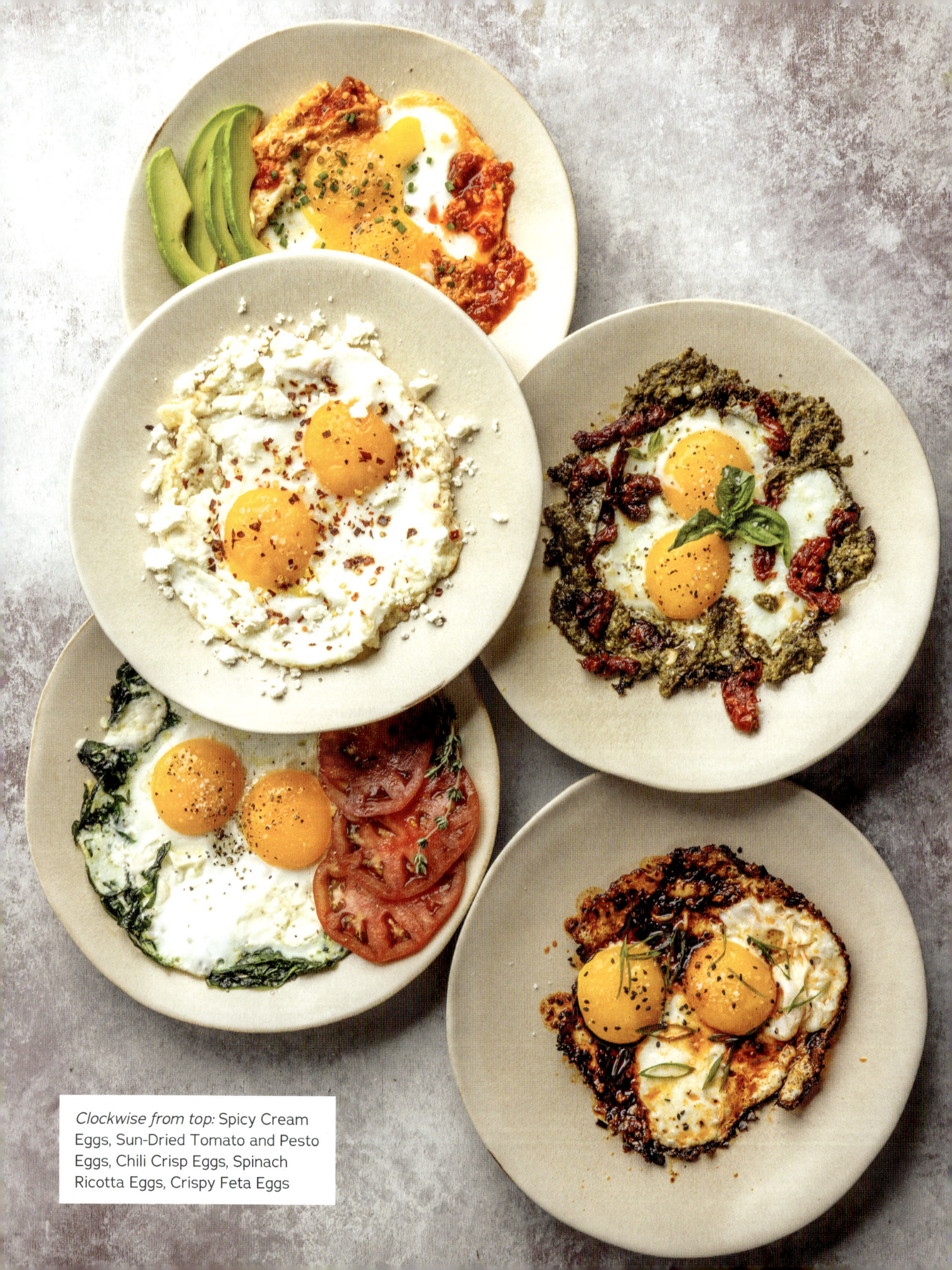

Clockwise from top: Spicy Cream Eggs, Sun-Dried Tomato and Pesto Eggs, Chili Crisp Eggs, Spinach Ricotta Eggs, Crispy Feta Eggs

LEVELED-UP FRIED EGGS—5 WAYS

Eggs don't have to be boring. With just a few additions, you can have bougie eggs with next-level flavor without taking a lot of effort or time. These recipes allow you to cook the eggs to your preference. Don't like your eggs sunny side up? Flip and fry them over easy or change them up completely and scramble them. Enjoy these egg preparations as is or serve them atop your favorite low-carb toast.

SPICY CREAM EGGS

SERVES 1

PREP TIME: 2 minutes

COOK TIME: 4 minutes

2 tablespoons heavy cream

1½ teaspoons chili paste or chili garlic sauce (see notes)

2 large eggs

Salt and pepper

FOR SERVING (OPTIONAL)

¼ avocado, sliced

2 fresh chives, thinly sliced

1. Preheat a small nonstick skillet over high heat for 2 minutes.
2. Pour in the cream, then add the chili paste and stir to combine. Lower the heat to medium and simmer for 1 minute to caramelize and thicken the cream. It should become slightly golden in color and the bubbles on the surface will have increased in size.
3. Crack in the eggs, season with a pinch of salt, and cover. Cook the eggs until the whites are set and the yolks are still runny, 2 to 3 minutes. If you like very firm whites with a set yolk, cook for an additional 30 to 90 seconds.
4. Season to taste with pepper. If desired, serve with avocado slices and garnish with sliced chives.

notes

Pouring the cream into a hot pan helps caramelize the cream, giving it a hint of sweetness to complement the spicy chili paste.

I recommend either Huy Fong Sambal Oelek Chili Paste or Chili Garlic Sauce.

CALORIES: **263** | PROTEIN: **13.2g** | FAT: **21.5g** | TOTAL CARBS: **1.3g** | NET CARBS: **1.3g** | FIBER: **0g**

SUN-DRIED TOMATO & PESTO EGGS

SERVES 1

PREP TIME: 2 minutes

COOK TIME: 3 minutes

---

2 tablespoons basil pesto

1 tablespoon roughly chopped sun-dried tomatoes (packed in oil)

2 large eggs

Salt and pepper

Fresh basil leaves, for garnish (optional)

1. Preheat a small nonstick skillet over medium heat.
2. Put the pesto and sun-dried tomatoes in the pan and stir to combine.
3. Crack the eggs into the skillet, season with a pinch of salt, and cover. Cook the eggs until the whites are set and the yolks are runny, 2 to 3 minutes. If you like very firm whites with set yolks, cook for an additional 30 to 90 seconds.
4. Season to taste with pepper. Garnish with fresh basil leaves, if desired.

CALORIES: **313** | PROTEIN: **14.8g** | FAT: **26g** | TOTAL CARBS: **3.1g** | NET CARBS: **1.8g** | FIBER: **1.3g**

SPINACH RICOTTA EGGS

SERVES 1

PREP TIME: 3 minutes

COOK TIME: 4 minutes

---

1 tablespoon salted butter

½ cup baby spinach, chopped

2 tablespoons ricotta cheese

2 large eggs

Salt and pepper

3 tomato slices

Fresh herb(s) of choice, for garnish (optional)

1. Preheat a small nonstick skillet over medium heat.
2. Melt the butter in the skillet. Add the spinach and cook until almost wilted, about 1 minute.
3. Stir in the ricotta cheese. Crack the eggs into the pan, season with a pinch of salt, and cover. Cook the eggs until the whites are set and the yolks are runny, 2 to 3 minutes. If you like very firm whites with set yolks, cook for an additional 30 to 90 seconds.
4. Season to taste with pepper. Serve with sliced tomatoes. Garnish with fresh herbs, if desired.

CALORIES: **308** | PROTEIN: **15.4g** | FAT: **24.3g** | TOTAL CARBS: **5.4g** | NET CARBS: **4.5g** | FIBER: **0.9g**

CRISPY FETA EGGS

SERVES 1

PREP TIME: 2 minutes

COOK TIME: 4 minutes

Aside from serving these eggs over low-carb toast, you might also try them wrapped in a tortilla (see page 249) with mashed avocado, arugula, and pickled onion. They are particularly good that way.

¼ cup crumbled feta cheese

2 large eggs

Salt and pepper

Sprinkle of red pepper flakes (optional)

1. Preheat a small nonstick skillet over medium heat. Spray the skillet with cooking oil.
2. Sprinkle the crumbled feta into a wide ring in the skillet, leaving the center open for the eggs. Let the feta melt for 1 minute.
3. Crack the eggs into the center of the feta ring. Season with a pinch each of salt and pepper and red pepper flakes, if using. Cook until the edges of the eggs are crispy and the yolks are runny, 2 to 3 minutes. If you like very firm whites with set yolks, cover the eggs and cook for an additional 30 to 90 seconds.

CALORIES: **213** | PROTEIN: **16.6g** | FAT: **15.5g** | TOTAL CARBS: **1.7g** | NET CARBS: **1.7g** | FIBER: **0g**

CHILI CRISP EGGS

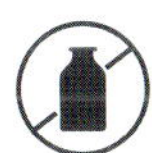

SERVES 1

PREP TIME: 1 minute

COOK TIME: 3 minutes

1 tablespoon chili crisp (see note)

2 large eggs

Salt

Sliced green onions, for garnish (optional)

1. Preheat a small nonstick skillet over medium heat.
2. Using a rubber spatula, evenly spread the chili crisp across the bottom of the pan.
3. Crack the eggs into the skillet, season with a pinch of salt, and cover. Cook the eggs until the whites are set and the yolks are runny, 2 to 3 minutes. If you like very firm whites with set yolks, cook for an additional 30 to 90 seconds.
4. Garnish with green onion slices, if desired.

note

Chili crisp, aka chili crunch, is a spicy, crunchy condiment made from fried chili peppers, garlic, and other aromatics, generally in oil. It is typically found in the Asian food aisle of the grocery store or near other condiments, like sauces, oils, and spices.

CALORIES: **243** | PROTEIN: **12.6g** | FAT: **19.5g** | TOTAL CARBS: **0.7g** | NET CARBS: **0.7g** | FIBER: **0g**

OMELET IN A MUG

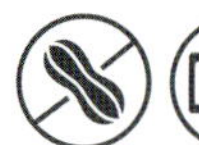
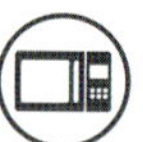

SERVES 1

PREP TIME: 5 minutes (not including time to cook bacon)

COOK TIME: 2 minutes or 30 minutes, depending on method

When I want an omelet but don't feel like breaking out my skillet or channeling my inner French chef, I just whip up an omelet in a mug! Using the microwave, you can enjoy all the savory goodness of your favorite omelet without any flipping or fuss and in less than 10 minutes. Customize your creation with different veggies, proteins, cheeses, and seasonings. If you prefer to use an oven to make this omelet, you'll find instructions below the recipe.

---

3 large eggs

2 slices thick-cut bacon, cooked and crumbled

2 tablespoons shredded cheddar cheese

1 tablespoon thinly sliced green onions

¼ teaspoon ground black pepper

⅛ teaspoon salt

MICROWAVE INSTRUCTIONS:

1. Spray an 8-ounce microwave-safe ramekin or mug with cooking oil.
2. Put all the ingredients in the ramekin and whisk to combine.
3. Microwave for 30 seconds, then stir to keep the bacon and onions from sinking to the bottom. Continue microwaving in 30-second intervals until the egg is set and cooked through. It may take about 2 minutes depending on your microwave and its wattage.

OVEN INSTRUCTIONS:

Use an 8-ounce oven-safe ramekin. After spraying it with cooking oil and filling it with the ingredients, place in a preheated 350°F oven for 30 minutes, or until the omelet is set around the edges but still slightly jiggly in the center. Remove from the oven and let rest for 5 minutes to allow the omelet to set completely in the center.

CALORIES: **399** | PROTEIN: **30.9g** | FAT: **28.8g** | TOTAL CARBS: **3.9g** | NET CARBS: **3.1g** | FIBER: **0.8g**

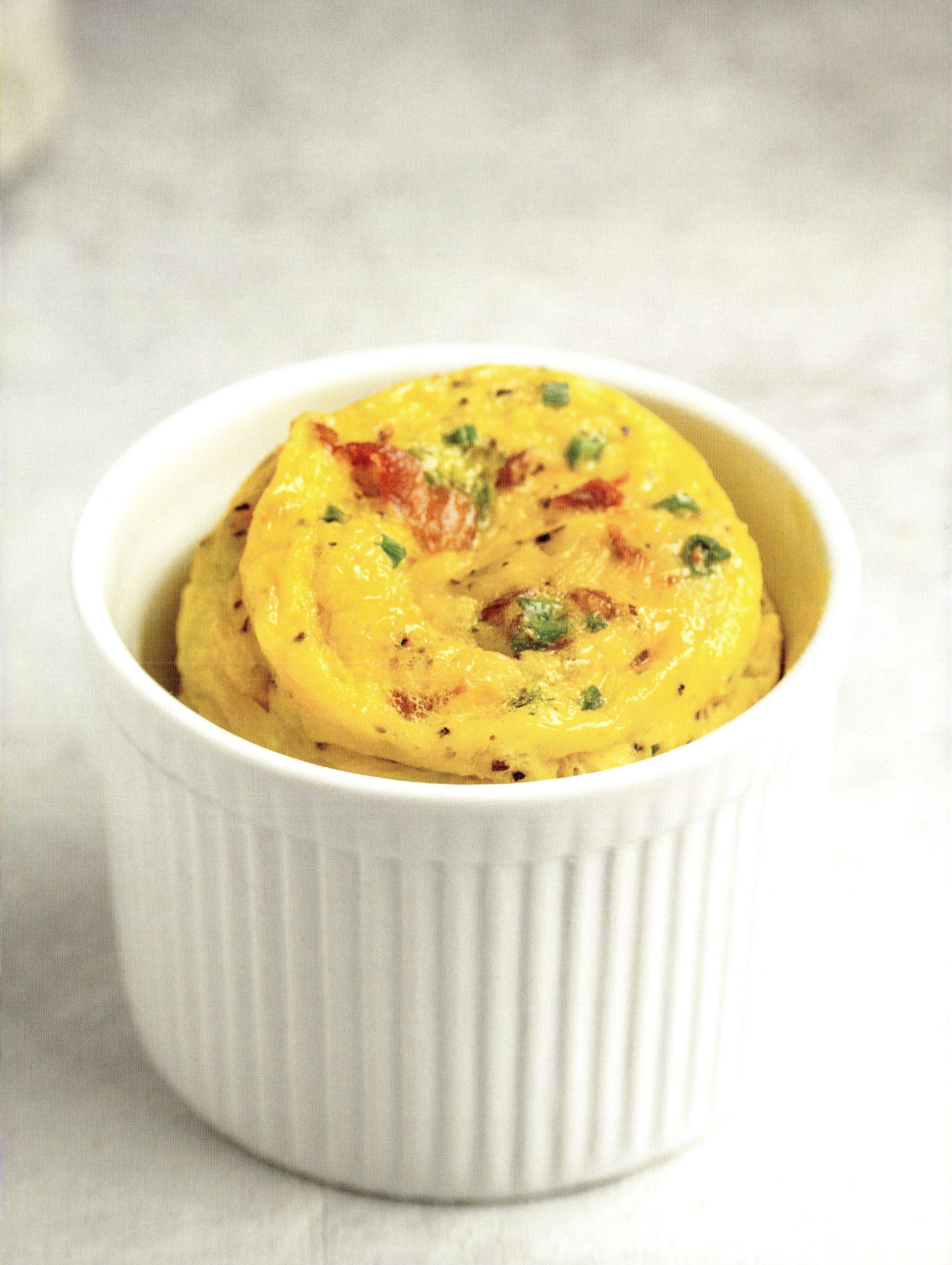

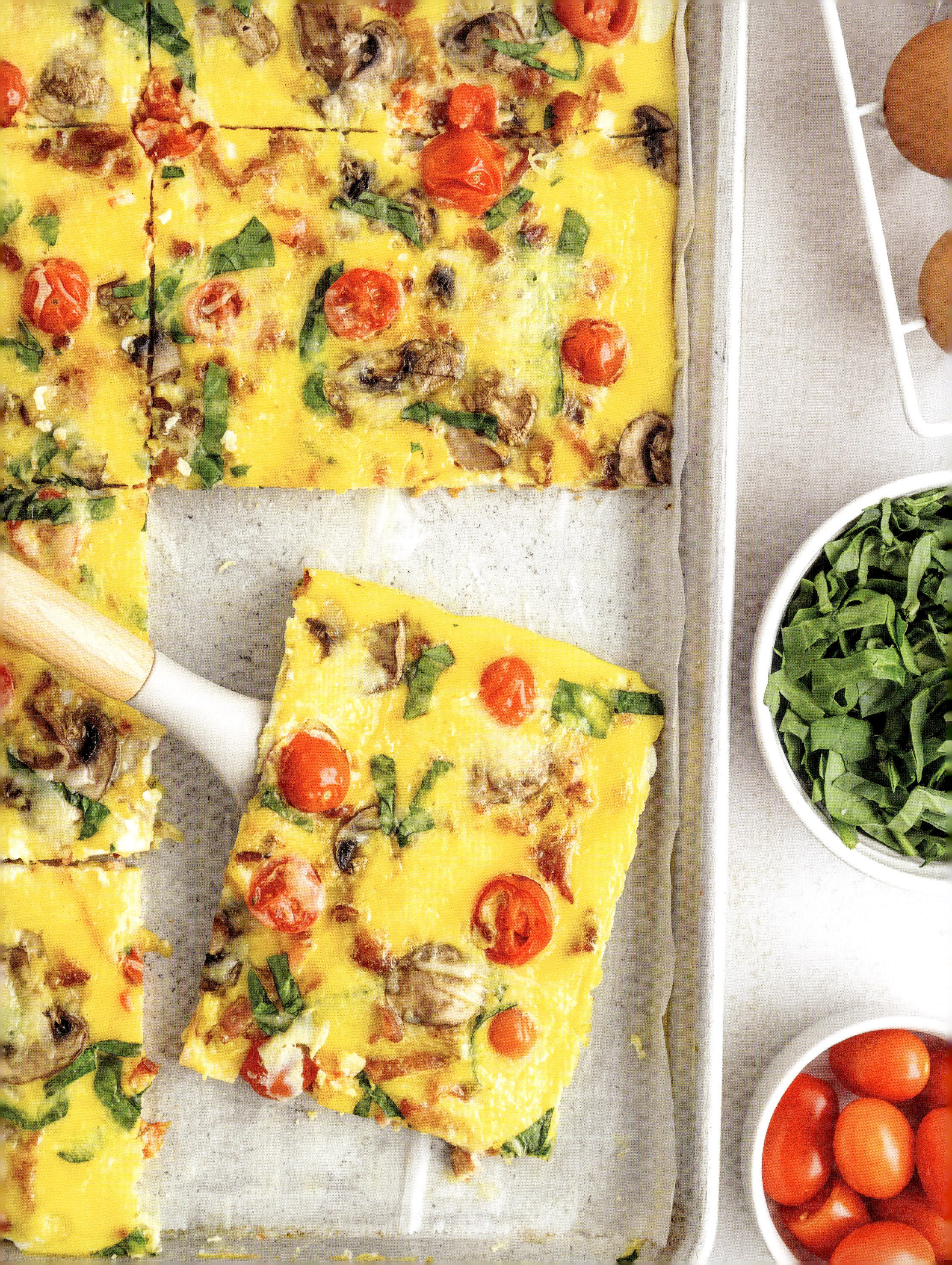

SHEET PAN OMELET

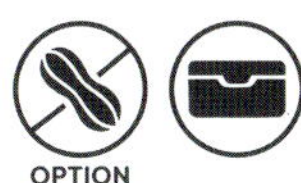

SERVES 4

PREP TIME: 10 minutes (not including time to cook bacon)

COOK TIME: 15 minutes

I love using a sheet pan to cook eggs. Not only do I not have to hover around the stovetop making sure my eggs don't overcook, but I can easily customize my breakfast by using different veggies, cheeses, and proteins. It's perfect for feeding a crowd or for when you want to meal prep your breakfast for the week.

1 dozen large eggs

¼ cup nut or seed milk of choice (unflavored and unsweetened)

1 teaspoon salt

½ teaspoon ground black pepper

½ cup chopped baby spinach

6 slices thick-cut bacon, cooked and chopped

½ cup thinly sliced mushrooms

⅓ cup halved cherry tomatoes

½ cup shredded Swiss cheese

1. Preheat the oven to 350°F. Spray a rimmed baking sheet with cooking oil. Lay a sheet of parchment paper on the oiled pan. Set aside.
2. In a large bowl, whisk together the eggs, milk, salt, and pepper. Pour the egg mixture into the prepared baking tray.
3. Evenly scatter the spinach, bacon, mushrooms, tomatoes, and cheese over the top of the egg mixture.
4. Bake until the eggs are set and no longer jiggly, 14 to 15 minutes.

(per serving)
CALORIES: **370** | PROTEIN: **28.9g** | FAT: **26.6g** | TOTAL CARBS: **3g** | NET CARBS: **2.5g** | FIBER: **0.5g**

BREAKFAST BOWLS

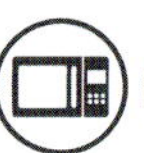

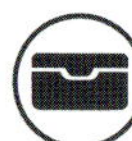

SERVES 10

PREP TIME: 15 minutes

COOK TIME: 15 minutes

These hearty and filling breakfast bowls will save you time in the morning. In just 20 minutes, you can prep ten breakfast bowls to stash in your fridge or freezer. When you roll out of bed in the morning, simply crack in a couple of eggs and microwave! Experiment with different proteins, cheeses, and veggies to add variety each week.

2 pounds bulk breakfast sausage

Salt

1 teaspoon onion powder

½ teaspoon ground black pepper

1 red bell pepper

1 green bell pepper

1 medium onion

3 cloves garlic

1 tablespoon avocado oil

8 ounces sharp cheddar cheese, shredded

20 large eggs

Fresh chives or green onions, thinly sliced, for garnish (optional)

1. Have on hand ten pint-size microwave-safe mason jars or meal prep containers with lids. If planning to freeze the breakfast bowls, make sure the jars or containers you use are freezer-safe as well.
2. Heat a large skillet over medium-high heat. Crumble in the sausage and cook, continuing to break it up, until almost cooked through, 5 to 6 minutes. Stir in 1 teaspoon of salt along with the onion powder and black pepper. Continue cooking until the sausage is browned and cooked through, 2 to 4 minutes more. Scrape the sausage into a large bowl and set aside; do not clean the skillet.
3. While the sausage is cooking, prepare the vegetables and garlic: Remove the stems and seeds from the bell peppers, then dice them. Dice the onion and mince the garlic. Set aside.
4. Pour the oil into the same pan you used to cook the sausage and set over medium-high heat. Put the bell peppers and onion in the pan and season with a pinch or two of salt, stirring to distribute it evenly. Sauté until the vegetables are tender, 3 to 5 minutes.
5. Return the cooked sausage to the pan and add the garlic. Stir to combine and cook for 1 minute more, until the garlic is fragrant. Remove the pan from the heat and set aside to cool.
6. To assemble the bowls, put about 1 cup of the sausage and veggie mixture in each container. Evenly divide the cheese among the containers, adding about 3 tablespoons to each one. Secure the lids and store in the refrigerator for up to 5 days or in the freezer for up to 2 months.
7. When ready to serve, crack two eggs into one of the prepped containers. Stir to combine. Microwave on high for 1 minute. Stir to distribute the contents. Microwave for 45 more seconds, or until the eggs are cooked through. Garnish with chives, if desired.

(per bowl)

CALIORIES: **548** | PROTEIN: **33g** | FAT: **44g** | TOTAL CARBS: **3.8g** | NET CARBS: **3.3g** | FIBER: **0.5g**

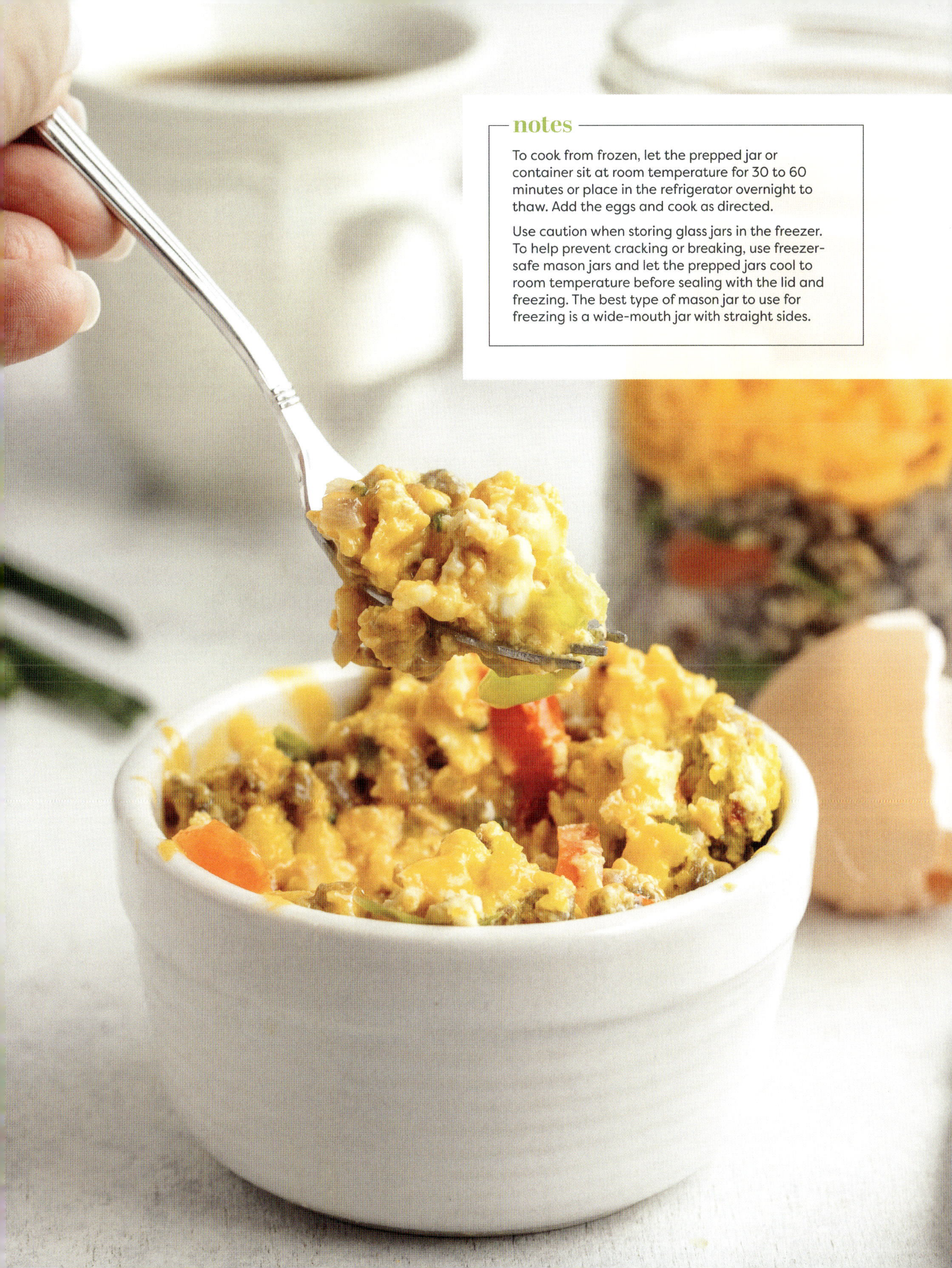

notes

To cook from frozen, let the prepped jar or container sit at room temperature for 30 to 60 minutes or place in the refrigerator overnight to thaw. Add the eggs and cook as directed.

Use caution when storing glass jars in the freezer. To help prevent cracking or breaking, use freezer-safe mason jars and let the prepped jars cool to room temperature before sealing with the lid and freezing. The best type of mason jar to use for freezing is a wide-mouth jar with straight sides.

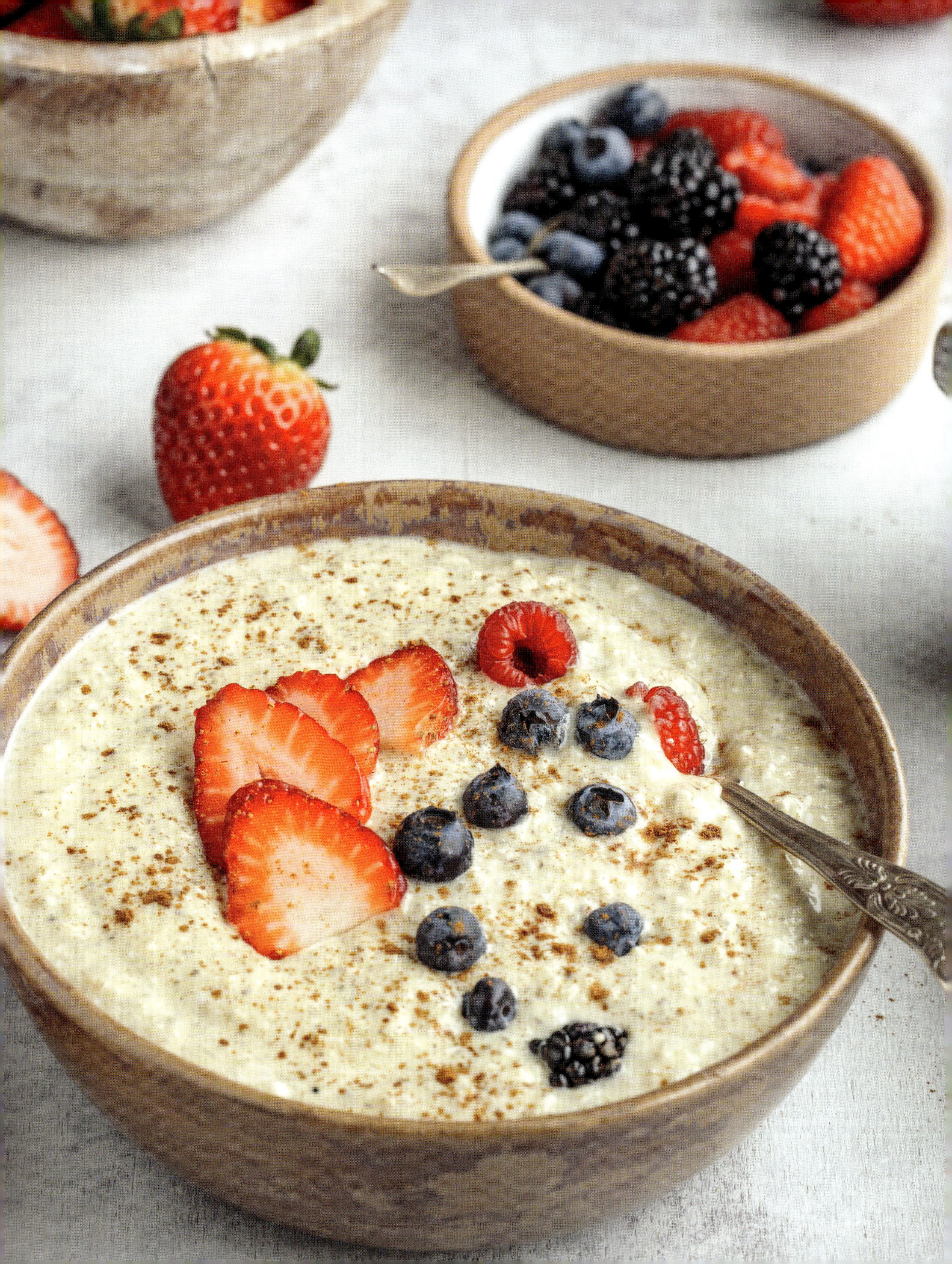

NOATMEAL

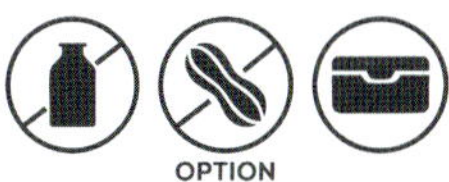

SERVES 1

PREP TIME: 5 minutes

COOK TIME: 15 minutes

Hot "oats" are no longer off-limits in a low-carb lifestyle. This keto oatmeal recipe captures the flavor and texture of your favorite hot cereal without using oats. That's why it's called NOatmeal! Customize this quick and easy meal prep–friendly recipe with your favorite toppings and mix-ins. Two of my favorite flavor variations are listed below.

---

1 teaspoon chia seeds

¾ cup frozen cauliflower rice

½ cup nut or seed milk of choice (unflavored and unsweetened)

1 large egg, beaten

1½ tablespoons coconut oil

½ scoop unflavored or vanilla-flavored protein powder

2 to 3 teaspoons granulated sugar-free sweetener

½ teaspoon ground cinnamon

Pinch of salt

Mixed fresh berries, for topping (optional)

1. Crush the chia seeds by grinding them with a mortar and pestle or in a coffee grinder.
2. Put the frozen cauliflower rice in a small saucepan. Heat over medium heat until most of the moisture has evaporated. Stir in the chia seeds and milk and continue to heat until simmering.
3. Reduce the heat to low. Slowly stir in the beaten egg and cook until thickened, stirring occasionally. This will take 5 to 8 minutes.
4. Remove the pan from the heat. Stir in the coconut oil, protein powder, sweetener, cinnamon, and salt. Top with fresh berries, if desired.

FLAVOR VARIATIONS:

- **Strawberries & Cream:** Add 2 sliced strawberries, a teaspoon of vanilla extract, and a splash of nut or seed milk.
- **Maple Pecan:** Instead of adding sweetener, stir in 2 tablespoons of sugar-free maple syrup. Toss in 2 tablespoons of chopped pecans.

MEAL PREP INSTRUCTIONS: Double or triple the recipe. Then portion into meal prep containers and refrigerate for up to 5 days. To reheat, microwave for 30 to 45 seconds, or until warmed. Or reheat on the stovetop.

notes

Grinding the chia seeds helps release their thickening agent, so your NOatmeal will be thick right away. If you are unable to grind the whole seeds, refrigerate the NOatmeal overnight to thicken.

To keep this dairy free, make sure the protein powder you're using isn't whey based.

CALORIES: **305** | PROTEIN: **19g** | FAT: **23.6g** | TOTAL CARBS: **7g** | NET CARBS: **3.1g** | FIBER: **3.9g**

LOW-CARB PROTEIN FRENCH TOAST

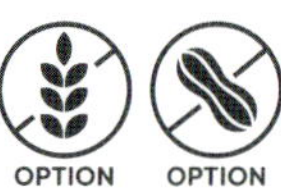

SERVES 2

PREP TIME: 6 minutes

COOK TIME: 12 minutes

When I'm craving something on the sweet side for breakfast, I turn to this easy protein-packed French toast recipe. With almost 30 grams of protein per serving, this delicious breakfast satisfies my need for something sweet and keeps me full all morning long. I top my French toast with butter, sugar-free maple syrup, and fresh berries.

---

1 large egg

1 large egg white

½ cup plain Greek or low-carb yogurt

¼ cup nut or seed milk of choice (unflavored and unsweetened)

½ scoop unflavored or vanilla-flavored protein powder

½ teaspoon vanilla extract

¼ teaspoon ground cinnamon

6 slices keto bread, preferably stale (see note)

FOR SERVING (OPTIONAL)

Butter

Sugar-free maple syrup

Fresh berries of choice

1. Preheat a griddle or large nonstick skillet over medium heat.
2. Using a mini processor or blender, mix the egg, egg white, yogurt, milk, protein powder, vanilla, and cinnamon until smooth.
3. Pour the batter into a shallow bowl. Set one slice of bread in the batter. Let soak for 30 to 60 seconds on each side. Remove from the batter, allowing excess to drip off, and set aside on a plate. If your griddle or skillet is large enough to accommodate two slices at once without crowding, soak a second slice of bread in the batter.
4. Spray the hot griddle or skillet with cooking oil. Place two slices of batter-soaked bread on the griddle (or in the skillet) and cook on each side for 90 seconds to 2 minutes, until golden brown.
5. Repeat with the remaining bread slices and batter, spraying the griddle or skillet with cooking oil before each batch.
6. Evenly divide the French toast between two plates and serve with butter, syrup, and fresh berries, if desired.

Pack It with Protein: Spread on your favorite nut or seed butter.

note

Keto bread can be found in the bread section of the grocery store. If you avoid gluten, make sure the keto bread you're using is gluten free (not all are). Gluten-free keto breads are generally kept in the freezer section. Older bread is ideal for soaking up all the batter.

(per serving)

CALORIES: **214** | PROTEIN: **28.9g** | FAT: **6.5g** | TOTAL CARBS: **37.7g** | NET CARBS: **4.5g** | FIBER: **33.2g**

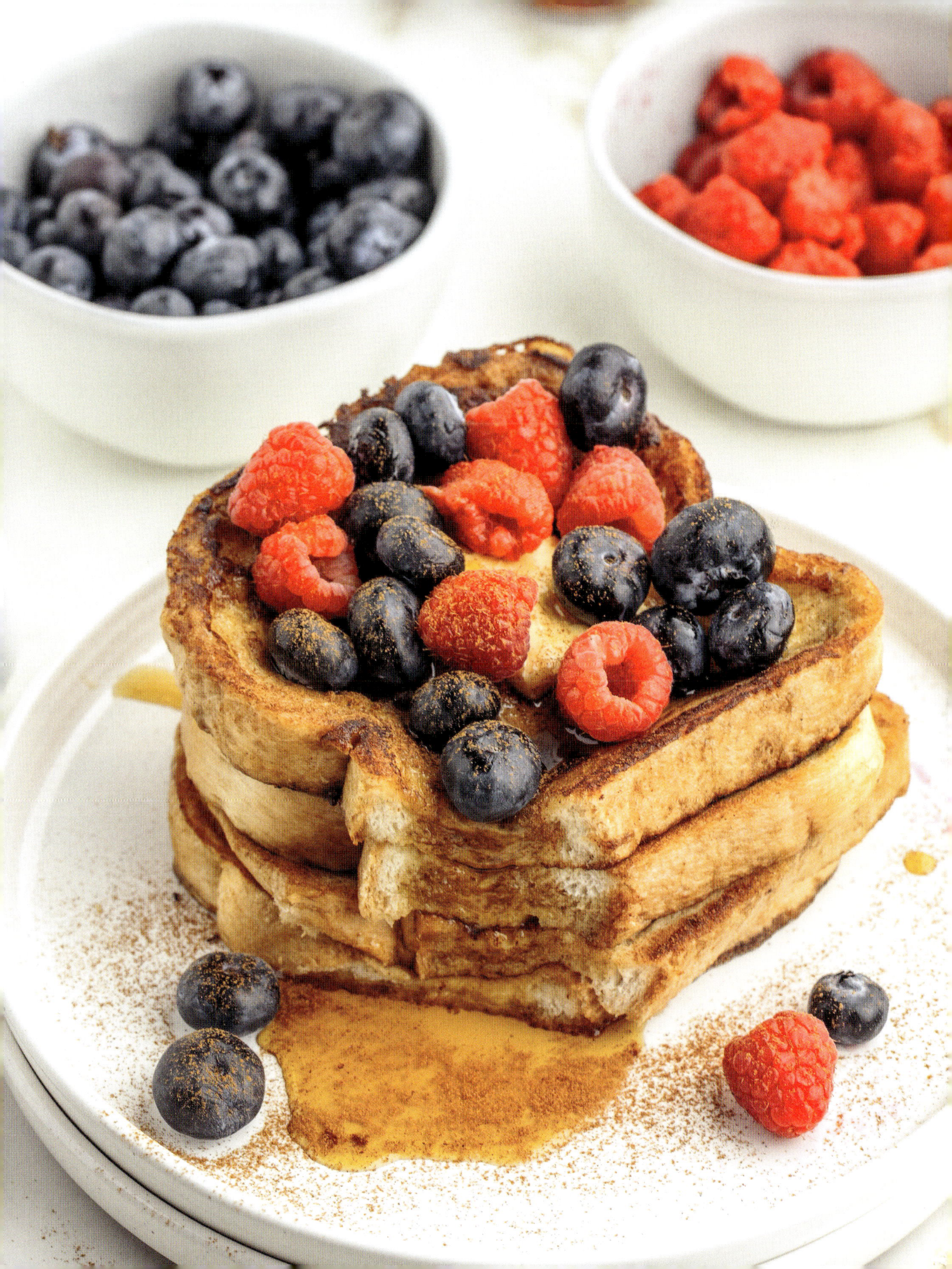

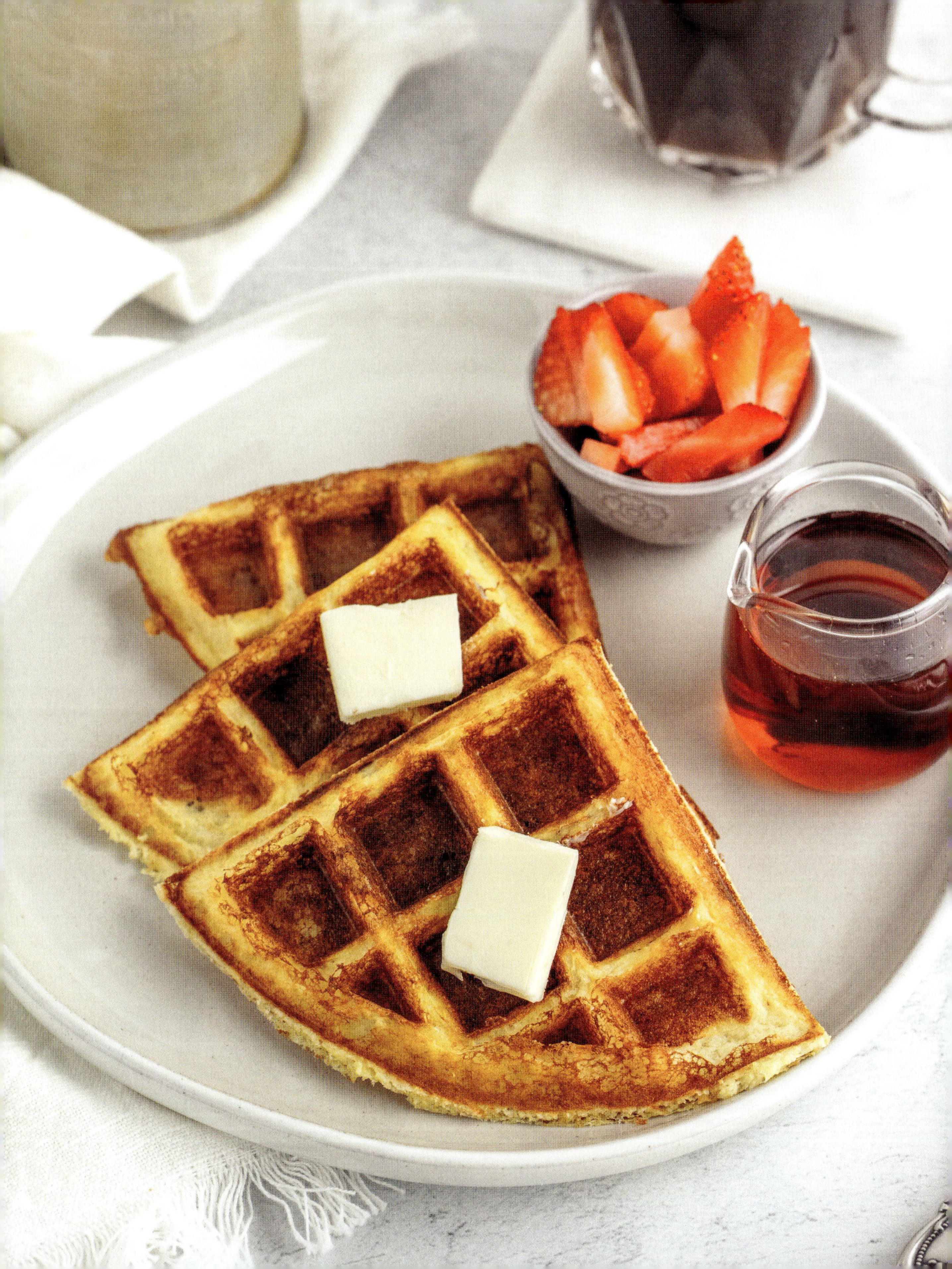

LOW-CARB PROTEIN WAFFLES

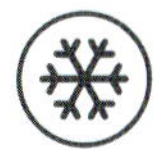
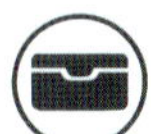

SERVES 1

PREP TIME: 10 minutes

COOK TIME: 9 minutes

I'm in love with these high-protein waffles! With over 40 grams of protein, these crispy yet fluffy waffles are dreamy when topped with butter and sugar-free maple syrup, or even a dollop of sweetened whipped cream and fresh strawberries. Double or triple the recipe to make a bunch now to freeze for later.

¼ cup blanched, super-fine almond flour

1 scoop unflavored protein powder

1 teaspoon baking powder

Pinch of salt

1 large egg

⅓ cup plain Greek or low-carb yogurt

½ teaspoon vanilla extract

FOR SERVING (OPTIONAL)

Butter

Sugar-free maple syrup

Fresh berries of choice

1. Preheat a waffle iron.
2. In a medium bowl, whisk together the almond flour, protein powder, baking powder, and salt.
3. Add the egg, yogurt, and vanilla. Stir until smooth. Let sit for 5 minutes while the waffle maker heats up.
4. Spray the waffle iron with cooking oil. Pour in one-third to one-half of the batter, depending on the size of your waffle maker. (If your waffle iron makes 4-inch waffles, use about one-third of the batter at a time; if it makes larger waffles, use half of the batter.) Close the lid and cook for 2 to 3 minutes, until the waffle is crispy on the outside and releases easily. Repeat with the remaining batter, spraying the waffle iron with cooking oil before making each waffle. Depending on the size of your waffle iron, you'll end up with 2 larger or 3 smaller waffles.
5. Serve with butter, syrup, and fresh berries, if desired.

FREEZING INSTRUCTIONS: Once cool, place the waffles on a plate or baking sheet and into the freezer to flash freeze. Once frozen, remove and stack in a freezer-safe bag or container. Freeze for 1 to 2 months.

REHEATING INSTRUCTIONS: Put frozen waffles directly in the toaster on a medium setting. Toast until warm and crisp, 2 to 3 minutes.

Pack It with Protein: Spread on your favorite nut butter or top with cottage cheese or a fried egg.

note

For a nut-free version, use 2 tablespoons coconut flour in place of the almond flour.

CALORIES: **394** | PROTEIN: **43.5g** | FAT: **20.6g** | TOTAL CARBS: **8g** | NET CARBS: **3g** | FIBER: **5g**

LOW-CARB PROTEIN PANCAKES

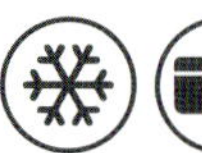 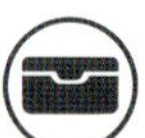

SERVES 2

PREP TIME: 5 minutes

COOK TIME: 20 minutes

I whip up these protein pancakes at least once a week to satisfy my hungry growing teenage boys. Each serving packs over 25 grams of protein and enough healthy fats to keep them full all morning. Top these fluffy, dreamy pancakes with butter, sugar-free syrup, fresh berries, or even a dollop of sweetened whipped cream. If you're meal prepping, you can easily double or triple this recipe. Using a griddle is recommended for cooking multiple pancakes at once. These pancakes freeze and reheat well, so you can store them and reheat for a quick, delicious breakfast later. The cooking time listed is based on using a skillet.

1⅓ cups blanched, super-fine almond flour

1 teaspoon baking powder

¼ teaspoon salt

¼ cup plain Greek or low-carb yogurt

2 large eggs

3 tablespoons nut or seed milk of choice (unflavored and unsweetened), plus more if needed

1 tablespoon unsalted butter, melted

1 tablespoon granulated sugar-free sweetener

1 teaspoon vanilla extract

FOR SERVING (OPTIONAL)

Butter

Sugar-free maple syrup

Fresh berries of choice

1. Preheat a griddle or large nonstick skillet over medium heat. Spray with cooking oil.
2. In a large bowl, mix together the almond flour, baking powder, and salt.
3. Stir in the yogurt, eggs, milk, melted butter, sweetener, and vanilla. The batter will be slightly thicker than regular pancake batter.
4. Once the greased griddle or skillet is heated, pour on enough batter to make a 4-inch pancake. If the size of your griddle or skillet allows you to cook more than one pancake at a time without crowding, repeat to make additional pancakes. Cook until the underside is golden brown and you can easily release the pancake with a spatula, 2 to 3 minutes. Flip and cook for 1 to 2 more minutes, or until golden brown on both sides. Repeat with the remaining batter, respraying the griddle or skillet with cooking oil before each batch.
5. The batter may continue to thicken as it sits. If this happens, add an additional tablespoon of milk to thin it out a bit.
6. Top the pancakes with butter, syrup, and fresh berries, if desired.

FREEZING INSTRUCTIONS: Once cool, place the pancakes on a plate or baking sheet and into the freezer to flash freeze. Once frozen, stack them in a freezer-safe bag or container and freeze for 1 to 2 months.

REHEATING INSTRUCTIONS: Place four frozen pancakes in a single layer on a microwave-safe plate and microwave on high for 30 to 40 seconds.

(per serving)
CALORIES: **626** | PROTEIN: **25.6g** | FAT: **51g** | TOTAL CARBS: **15g** | NET CARBS: **7g** | FIBER: **8g**

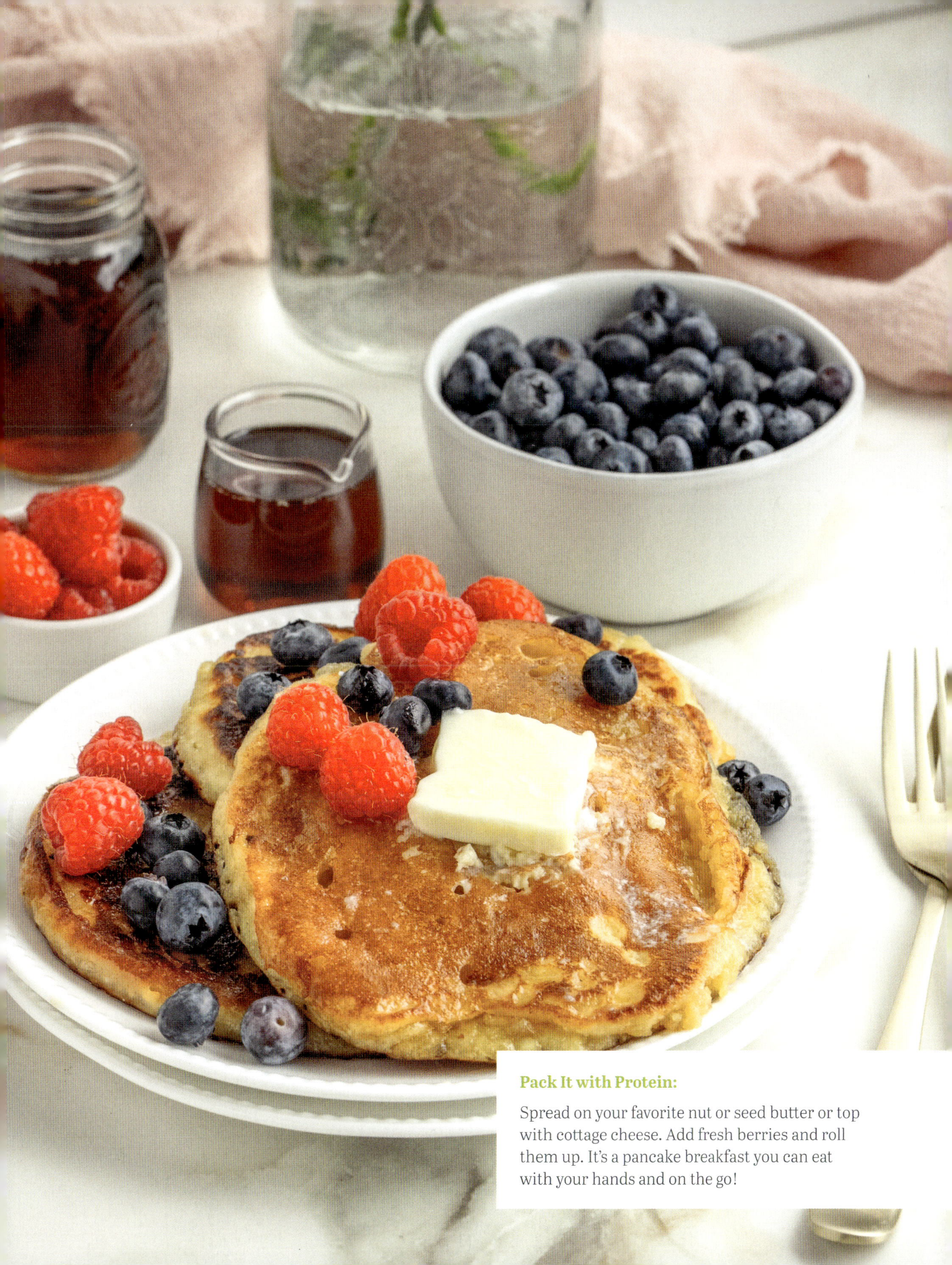

Pack It with Protein:

Spread on your favorite nut or seed butter or top with cottage cheese. Add fresh berries and roll them up. It's a pancake breakfast you can eat with your hands and on the go!

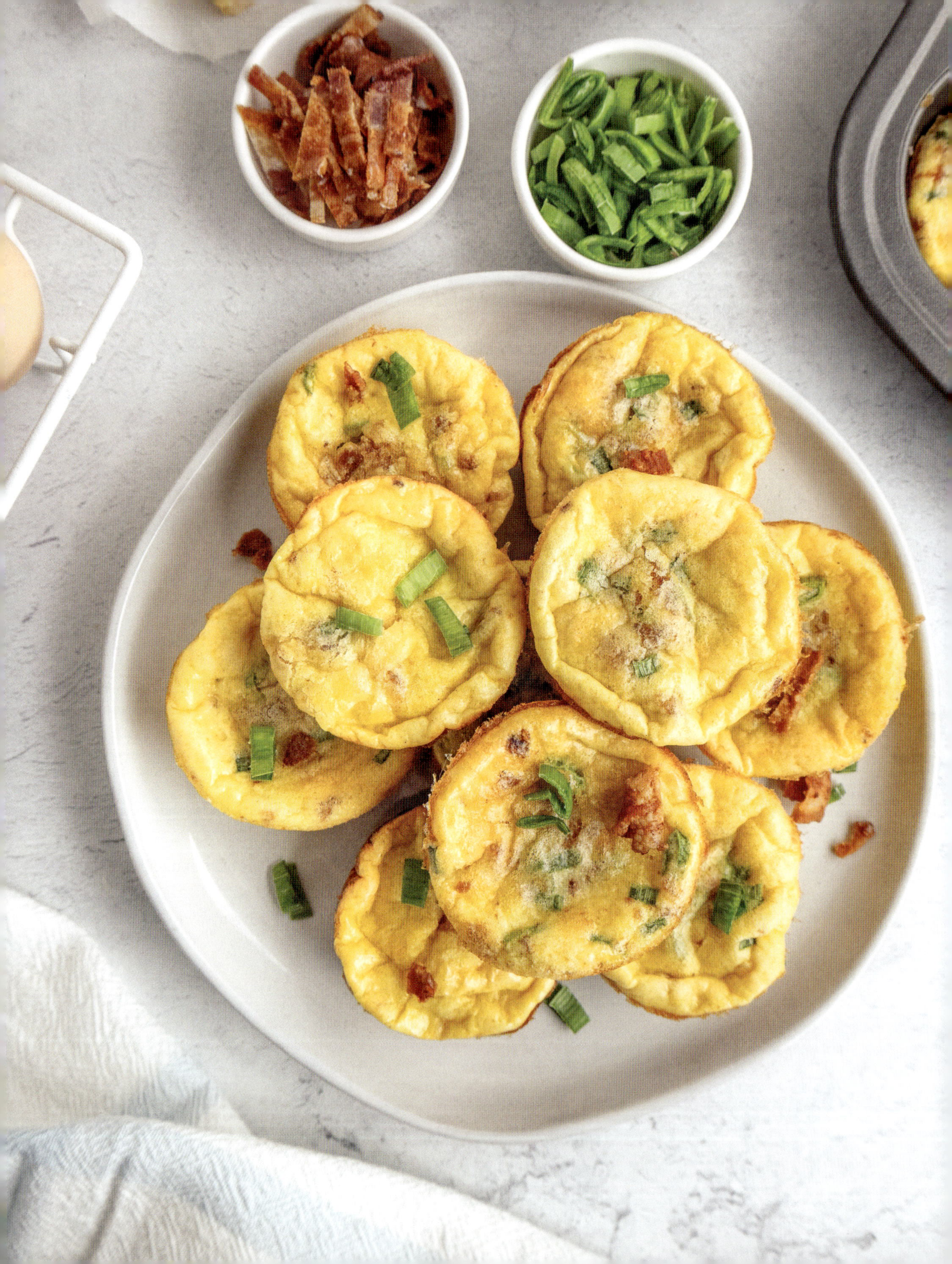

MUFFIN PAN EGG BITES

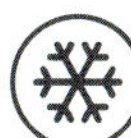
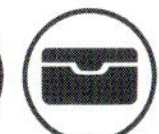

MAKES 12 egg bites (3 per serving)

PREP TIME: 10 minutes (not including time to cook bacon)

COOK TIME: 30 minutes

One of my favorite savory grab-and-go breakfasts is packed with protein, healthy fats, and flavor. They're perfect fresh from the oven, but they also keep well in the fridge for a couple of days or in the freezer for longer, and they reheat nicely. Enjoy two or three or more for a quick breakfast at home or pack them up for a meal or snack later. Mix in a few veggies or change up the meat and cheeses for endless variations.

---

1 cup cottage cheese (4% milkfat)

8 large eggs

1 teaspoon salt

½ teaspoon ground black pepper

6 slices regular-cut bacon, cooked and crumbled

4 ounces Gruyère cheese, shredded

2 tablespoons thinly sliced fresh chives or green onions

1. Preheat the oven to 350°F and spray a standard-size 12-cup muffin pan with cooking oil.
2. In a mini food processor or blender, blend the cottage cheese until smooth. Then scoop into a large bowl.
3. To the bowl, add the eggs, salt, pepper, bacon, cheese, and chives. Using a fork, mix until evenly combined.
4. Divide the egg mixture evenly among the prepared muffin wells, filling them almost to the top.
5. Bake until each egg bite is set in the center, 25 to 30 minutes. Remove from the oven and let cool for a few minutes before removing the bites from the pan. Enjoy while fresh or store for later.

FREEZING INSTRUCTIONS: Allow the egg bites to cool to room temperature, then seal them in an airtight container or freezer bag. Store them in the freezer for up to 2 months.

REHEATING INSTRUCTIONS:

- **From refrigerated:** Place on a microwave-safe plate and microwave on high for 20 to 30 seconds.
- **From frozen:** Place on a microwave-safe plate and microwave on high for 45 to 60 seconds.

(per serving)
CALORIES: **362** | PROTEIN: **32.1g** | FAT: **25.8g** | TOTAL CARBS: **2.5g** | NET CARBS: **2.4g** | FIBER: **0.1g**

PROTEIN GRANOLA

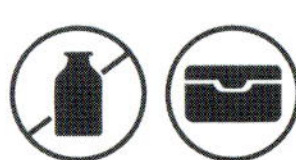

MAKES 3 cups (¾ cup per serving)

PREP TIME: 20 minutes

COOK TIME: 50 minutes

The secret to getting crunchy granola with big clusters is to use egg whites. The protein from the egg whites helps glue together those granola clusters and creates a desirable crunch when baked. This protein granola recipe is customizable. Don't care for some of the nuts or seeds listed below? Replace them with your own favorites. Change up the flavor by adding cocoa powder or pumpkin pie spice (see opposite). Plus, it's easy to make big batches all at once by doubling the recipe and using two sheet pans. Enjoy by the handful, over yogurt, or with a hefty splash of your favorite nut or seed milk.

---

1 cup chopped macadamia nuts

½ cup chopped pecans

½ cup sliced almonds

¼ cup pumpkin seeds

2 tablespoons dry roasted and salted sunflower kernels

2 tablespoons chia seeds

2 tablespoons hemp hearts

2 tablespoons granulated sugar-free sweetener

2 tablespoons brown sugar substitute

½ teaspoon ground cinnamon

¼ teaspoon ground nutmeg

Pinch of salt

2 large egg whites

1. Preheat the oven to 250°F. Line a rimmed baking sheet with parchment paper.
2. Put the macadamia nuts, pecans, almonds, and pumpkin seeds in a large dry skillet. Cook over medium heat until the nuts and seeds are lightly toasted, stirring the nuts and seeds or shaking the pan often. Remove the skillet from the heat.
3. To the skillet, add the sunflower kernels, chia seeds, hemp hearts, both sweeteners, spices, and salt. Stir to combine. Set aside.
4. Put the egg whites in a medium bowl. Using an electric mixer, beat until soft peaks form. You know you have soft peaks when you lift up the beater and the tips of the whites have a peak shape, but they curl a bit and quickly flop down back into the mixture.
5. Gently fold the nut and seed mixture into the egg whites.
6. Spread the granola mixture into an even layer in the prepared pan. Bake until golden, about 45 minutes.
7. Remove from the oven and let cool completely in the pan. The granola will still be soft right out of the oven but will harden as it cools. Once cooled, break into bite-size pieces.

STORAGE INSTRUCTIONS: Store the granola in an airtight container at room temperature for 1 to 2 weeks.

MEAL PREP INSTRUCTIONS: To make a larger batch, double the recipe and bake on two rimmed baking sheets. Swap the positions of the baking sheets halfway through to ensure even cooking.

(per serving)
CALORIES: **535** | PROTEIN: **13.2g** | FAT: **48.5g** | TOTAL CARBS: **14g** | NET CARBS: **3.5g** | FIBER: **10.5g**

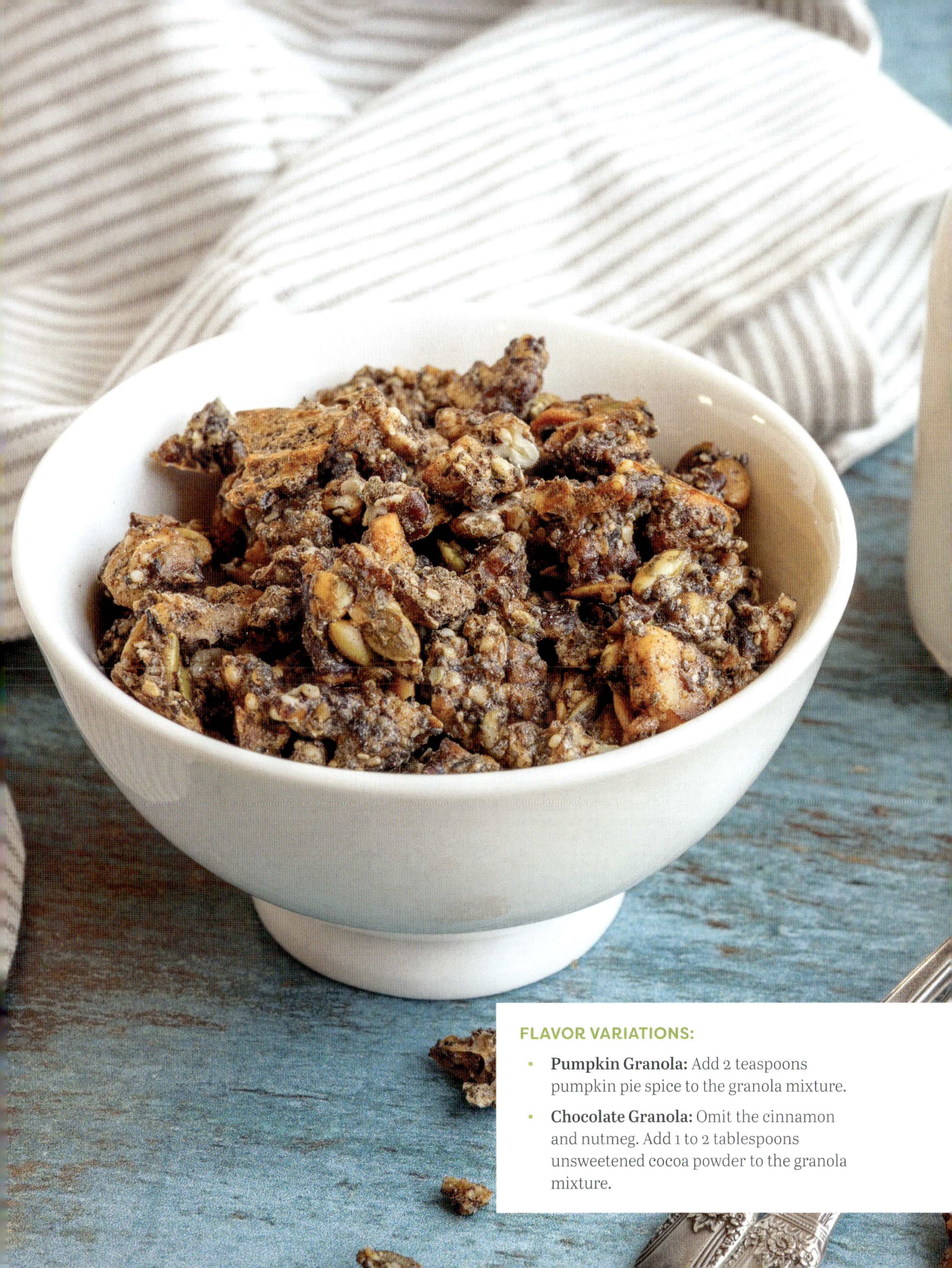

FLAVOR VARIATIONS:

- **Pumpkin Granola:** Add 2 teaspoons pumpkin pie spice to the granola mixture.
- **Chocolate Granola:** Omit the cinnamon and nutmeg. Add 1 to 2 tablespoons unsweetened cocoa powder to the granola mixture.

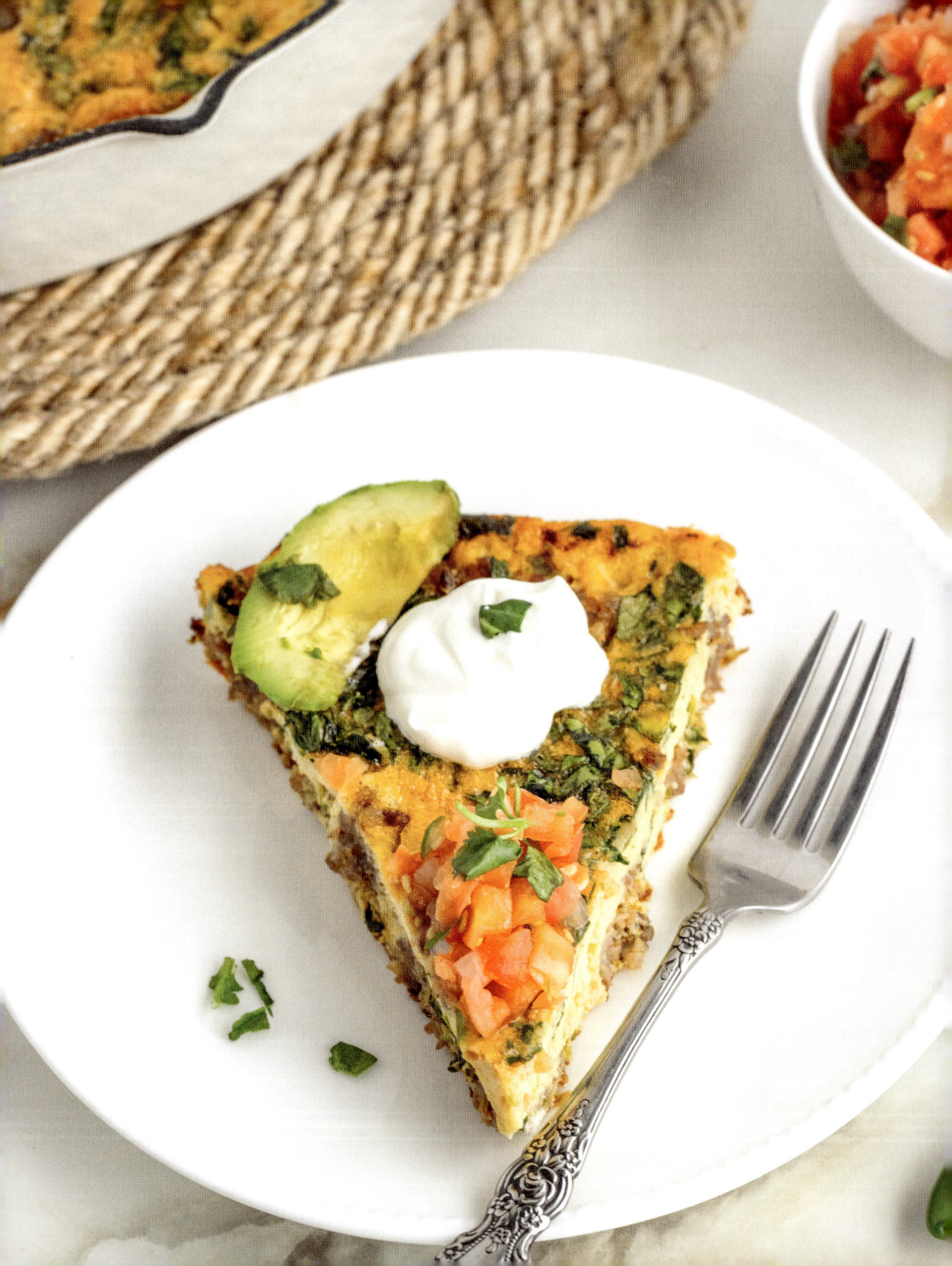

SOUTHWEST SAUSAGE FRITTATA

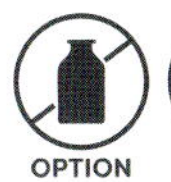

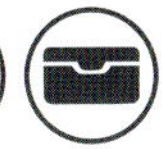

SERVES 6

PREP TIME: 15 minutes

COOK TIME: 45 minutes

For mornings when I need to feed the whole family and don't want to spend too much time, I make frittatas. It's easy to get in a lot of protein with each serving since we use almost a whole carton of eggs and a pound of meat. Loaded with peppers (sweet and hot), onions, and a blend of Southwest spices, the bold flavors of this frittata are a nice change of pace from the classic.

1 tablespoon avocado oil

2 tablespoons chopped onions

1 green bell pepper, chopped

1 jalapeño pepper, seeded and finely diced

1 pound bulk pork sausage of choice

1 tablespoon chili powder

1 teaspoon garlic powder

½ teaspoon ground cumin

½ teaspoon salt, divided

¼ cup salsa verde

10 large eggs

3 tablespoons heavy cream or unflavored, unsweetened seed milk of choice

2 large handfuls baby spinach, chopped

FOR SERVING (OPTIONAL)

Sour cream

Pico de gallo

Avocado slices

1. Preheat the oven to 375°F.
2. Heat a 10- or 11-inch oven-safe nonstick skillet over medium heat and pour in the oil. Add the onions, bell pepper, and jalapeño and cook until softened, 3 to 4 minutes.
3. Add the sausage to the pan, break it into crumbles, and cook until it's no longer pink but not yet browned, 4 to 5 minutes. Season with the chili powder, garlic powder, cumin, and ¼ teaspoon of the salt and continue cooking until the sausage is cooked through and browned, another 2 to 4 minutes. Do not drain the fat.
4. Remove the pan from the heat and stir in the salsa; set aside to cool.
5. In a large bowl, whisk the eggs, cream, spinach, and remaining ¼ teaspoon of salt until well combined.
6. Once the sausage pan is no longer hot (warm is okay), pour in the egg mixture.
7. Place the pan in the oven and bake until the eggs have set in the center, 25 to 30 minutes.
8. Top with sour cream, pico de gallo, and/or avocado slices, if desired.

note

For a dairy-free version, use seed milk instead of heavy cream and skip the sour cream on top.

(per serving)
CALORIES: **468** | PROTEIN: **31.4g** | FAT: **35.4g** | TOTAL CARBS: **5.3g** | NET CARBS: **3.6g** | FIBER: **1.7g**

PROTEIN-PACKED BREAKFAST BURRITOS

MAKES 6 burritos

PREP TIME: 30 minutes

COOK TIME: 20 minutes

A make-ahead breakfast burrito packed with protein from the inside and out! When the traditional flour tortilla is replaced by an egg wrap, as here, you can easily get 20 grams of protein in a single burrito. You can mix up the protein in this burrito by swapping the ground pork, sausage, or bacon for ground turkey or diced ham. Customize it by adding diced onion, bell pepper, or zucchini. Stock your freezer with these and breakfast becomes a breeze! You can easily reheat the burritos from frozen.

FOR THE SAUCE

⅓ cup plain Greek or low-carb yogurt

2 tablespoons mayonnaise

1 tablespoon diced chipotle peppers (see note, opposite)

1 tablespoon distilled white vinegar

½ teaspoon granulated sugar-free sweetener

½ teaspoon onion powder

½ teaspoon garlic powder

FOR THE BURRITOS

½ pound ground pork or bulk breakfast sausage, or 3 slices regular-cut bacon, diced

5 large eggs

¼ teaspoon salt

6 egg wraps, store-bought or homemade (page 245)

¾ cup shredded cheddar cheese

½ avocado, sliced

3 Campari tomatoes, diced

2 tablespoons chopped fresh cilantro

1. In a small bowl, whisk together the ingredients for the sauce and set aside.
2. Heat a large nonstick skillet over medium-high heat. If using ground pork or sausage, put it in the skillet, break it into crumbles, and cook until browned, 4 to 5 minutes. If using bacon, cook the bacon in the skillet until crispy, 5 to 6 minutes. Once cooked, remove the meat with a slotted spoon, leaving behind the grease to cook the eggs.
3. Reduce the heat under the skillet to low.
4. In a medium bowl, whisk together the eggs and salt. Pour the eggs into the preheated skillet and scramble until curds form and the egg is cooked through, 3 to 5 minutes depending on how firm you like your eggs. Transfer the eggs to a plate. Wipe the pan clean and return it to the stovetop over medium heat.
5. Set one egg wrap in the preheated skillet. Take 2 tablespoons of the cheese and sprinkle it from the center to one edge of the wrap. The cheese at the edge will serve as the glue to hold the burrito together once folded.
6. Cover the pan with a lid and let sit until the cheese is melted. Remove the wrap from the pan and set on a clean work surface, positioned so that the edge with the melted cheese is at the top.
7. To assemble the burrito, spread about 2 tablespoons of sauce on top of the melted cheese. Then add one-sixth of the cooked meat and scrambled eggs, about one-sixth of the avocado and tomato, and a sprinkling of cilantro. Roll up like a burrito, rolling toward the melted cheese edge, folding the sides of the wrap over the filling and rolling and tucking in the edges as you go. Press the melted cheese edge into the wrap to seal the burrito shut.
8. Repeat Steps 5 through 7 using the remaining wraps, sauce, and fillings to make a total of six burritos. Use any leftover sauce as a dip for the burritos.

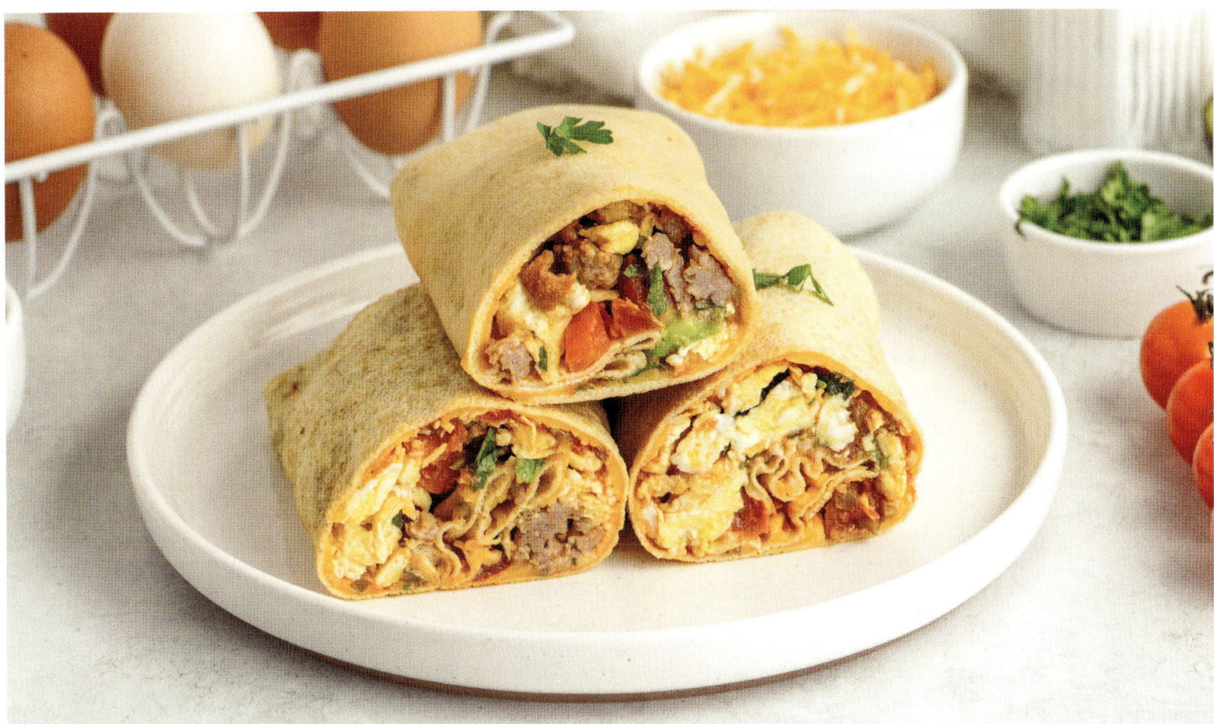

note

If you can't find diced chipotle peppers, you can buy a can or jar of whole chipotle peppers in adobo sauce and finely dice them yourself, mixing some of the sauce in with them.

STORAGE INSTRUCTIONS:

Wrap the burritos with aluminum foil. Store in the refrigerator for up to 5 days. If freezing, put the foil-wrapped burritos in a freezer-safe bag or container and freeze for up to 3 months.

REHEATING INSTRUCTIONS:

- **Microwave:** Remove the foil wrapping from the frozen or refrigerated burrito and place on a microwave-safe plate. Microwave a frozen burrito at 70 percent power for about 4 minutes; microwave a refrigerated burrito on high for about 45 seconds. Allow to rest for 2 minutes before eating.
- **Oven:** Preheat the oven to 300°F. Leave the frozen or refrigerated burrito wrapped in foil. Place on a rimmed baking sheet. Bake until heated through, about 30 minutes for a frozen burrito or 10 to 12 minutes for a refrigerated burrito. Allow to rest for 2 minutes before eating.
- **Air fryer:** Preheat the air fryer to 400°F. Peel back the foil from the frozen or refrigerated burrito, but leave the burrito sitting on the foil. Lightly spray the top of the burrito with cooking oil. Air-fry a frozen burrito for 7 to 8 minutes, then flip and air-fry for 5 to 6 more minutes; air-fry a refrigerated burrito for 2 to 3 minutes. Allow to rest for 2 minutes before eating.

(per pork/sausage burrito)
CALORIES: **302** | PROTEIN: **21.7g** | FAT: **21.7g** | TOTAL CARBS: **3.2g** | NET CARBS: **2.1g** | FIBER: **1.1g**

(per bacon burrito)
CALORIES: **238** | PROTEIN: **17.3g** | FAT: **16.2g** | TOTAL CARBS: **3.7g** | NET CARBS: **2.6g** | FIBER: **1.1g**

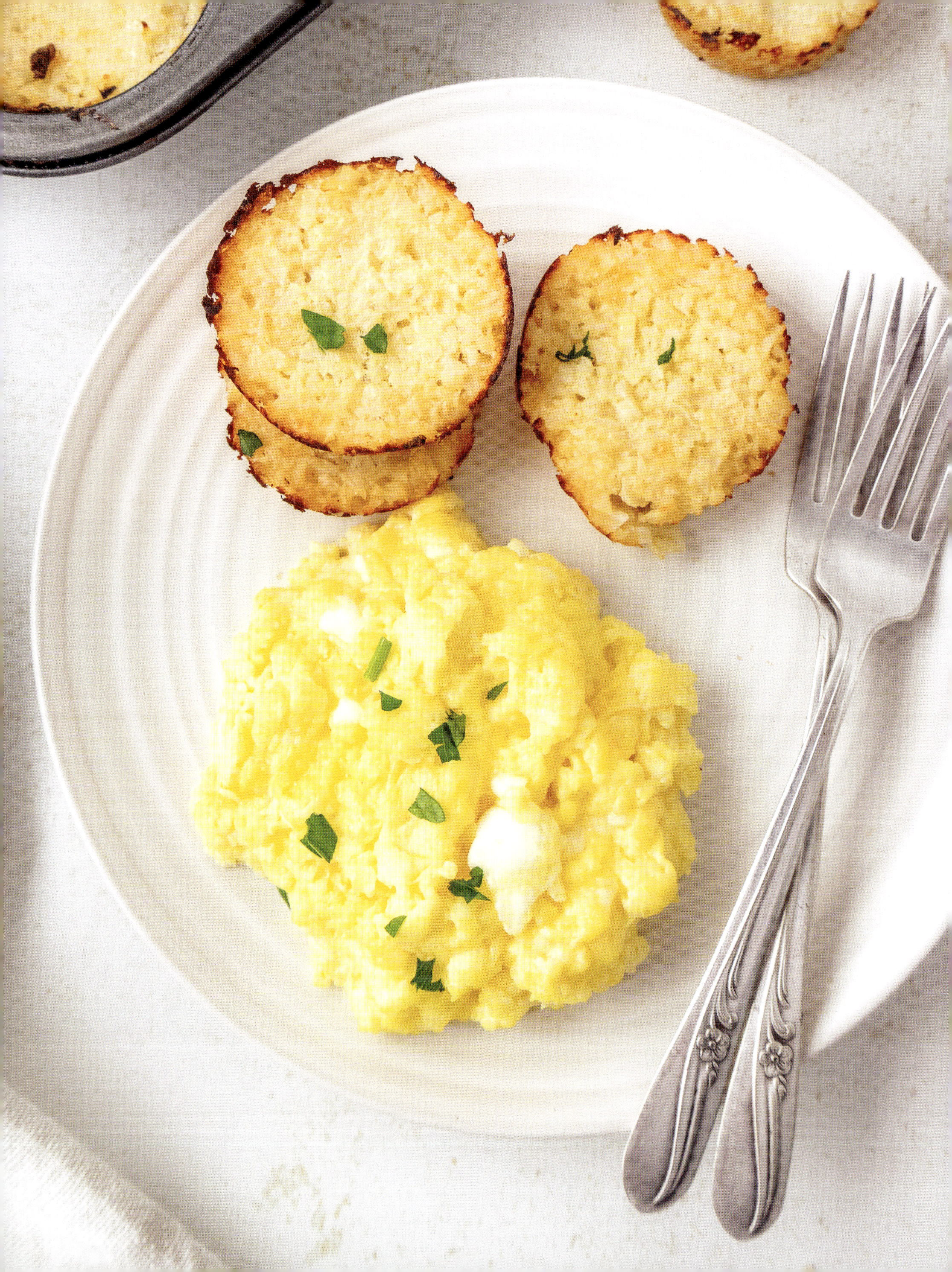

COTTAGE CHEESE SCRAMBLED EGGS

SERVES 1

PREP TIME: 2 minutes

COOK TIME: 3 minutes

The perfect way to add more protein to your eggs is to add cottage cheese. Not only does adding ¼ cup of cottage cheese to one serving of eggs give an additional 7 grams of protein, but it also makes the scrambled eggs extra fluffy and creamy. Pair with a few Protein Cauli Hash Brown Patties (page 84) for a complete meal.

---

2 large eggs

¼ cup cottage cheese (4% milkfat)

Pinch of salt

Sliced green onions, for garnish (optional)

1. Preheat a small nonstick skillet over medium-low heat. Spray the skillet with cooking oil.
2. In a small bowl, whisk together the eggs, cottage cheese, and salt.
3. Pour the egg mixture into the skillet and scramble until set and fluffy, about 3 minutes.
4. Top with sliced green onions, if desired.

CALORIES: **198** | PROTEIN: **19.4g** | FAT: **12.3g** | TOTAL CARBS: **2.5g** | NET CARBS: **2.5g** | FIBER: **0g**

PROTEIN CAULI HASH BROWN PATTIES

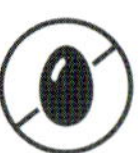  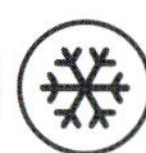 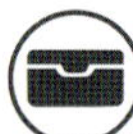

MAKES 12 patties (3 per serving)

PREP TIME: 5 minutes

COOK TIME: 35 minutes

These high-protein hash brown patties use cottage cheese for added protein and structure while keeping them low carb. Made with cauliflower rice instead of potatoes, they cook up crispy in the oven. Pair with Cottage Cheese Scrambled Eggs (page 83) for a complete meal.

1 (10-ounce) bag frozen cauliflower rice

1 cup cottage cheese (4% milkfat)

¼ cup shredded whole milk mozzarella cheese

1 tablespoon grated Parmesan cheese

½ teaspoon garlic powder

¼ teaspoon salt

1. Preheat the oven to 400°F and spray a standard-size 12-cup muffin pan with cooking oil.
2. Heat a large nonstick skillet over medium heat. Pour the frozen cauliflower rice into the dry skillet. Stirring occasionally, cook until the majority of the moisture has evaporated and the cauliflower rice is fluffy, 5 to 7 minutes. When done, remove the skillet from the heat.
3. While the rice is cooking, put the cottage cheese in a blender or food processor and blend until smooth and creamy.
4. In a large bowl, use a wooden spoon to combine the cooked cauliflower rice, blended cottage cheese, mozzarella, Parmesan, garlic powder, and salt.
5. Scoop 2 tablespoons of the cauliflower mixture into each cavity in the prepared muffin pan.
6. Bake for 25 to 30 minutes, until golden brown on top. Remove from the oven and let cool in the pan for a few minutes before serving.

STORAGE INSTRUCTIONS: Store hash brown patties in the refrigerator for up to 5 days. If freezing, place in a freezer-safe bag or container and freeze for up to 3 months.

REHEATING INSTRUCTIONS:

- **From refrigerated:** Place on a microwave-safe plate and microwave on high for 30 to 45 seconds.
- **From frozen:** Place on a microwave-safe plate and microwave on high for 1½ to 2 minutes.

(per serving)
CALORIES: **101** | PROTEIN: **11.3g** | FAT: **4.3g** | TOTAL CARBS: **5g** | NET CARBS: **3.5g** | FIBER: **1.5g**

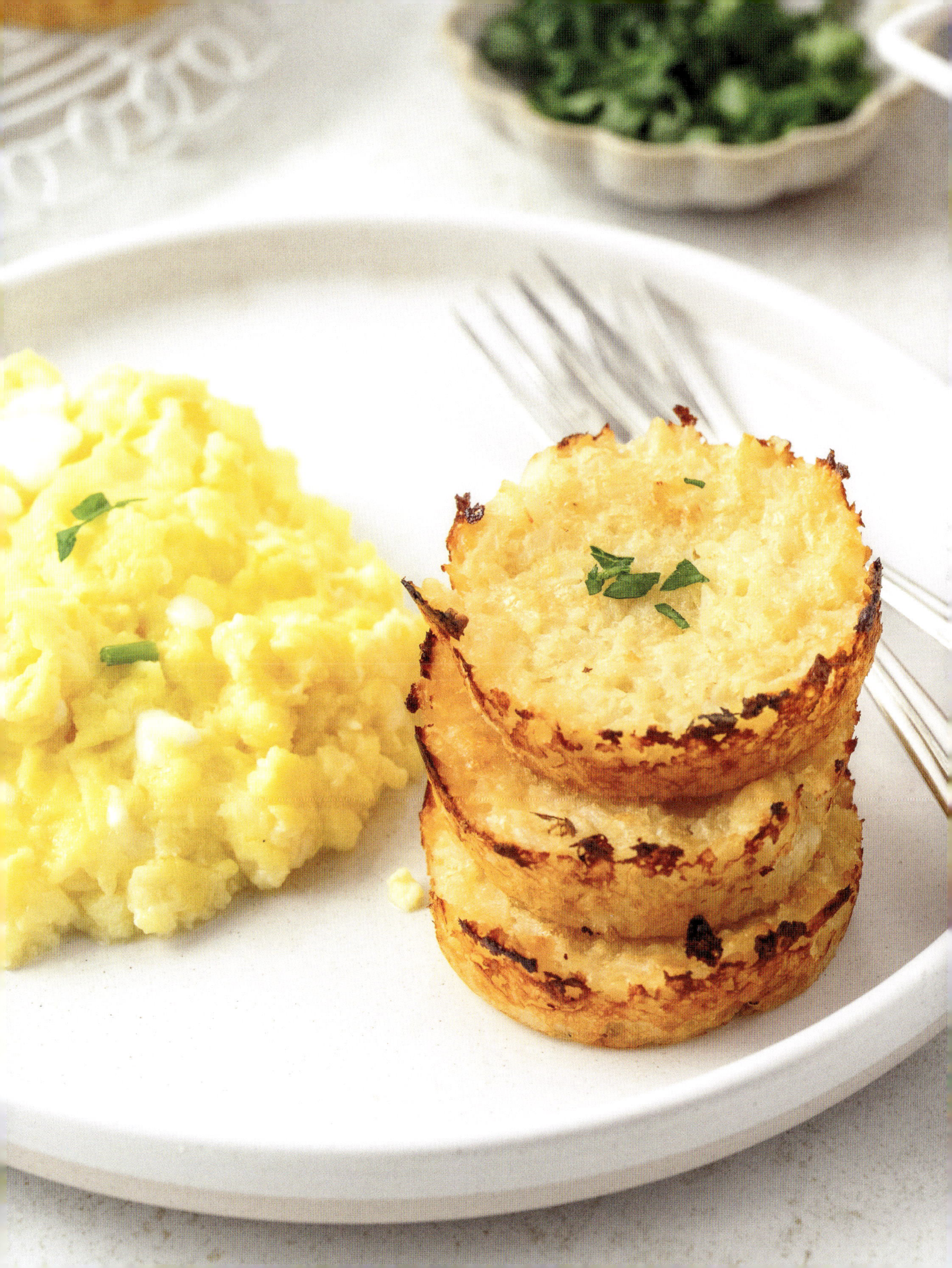

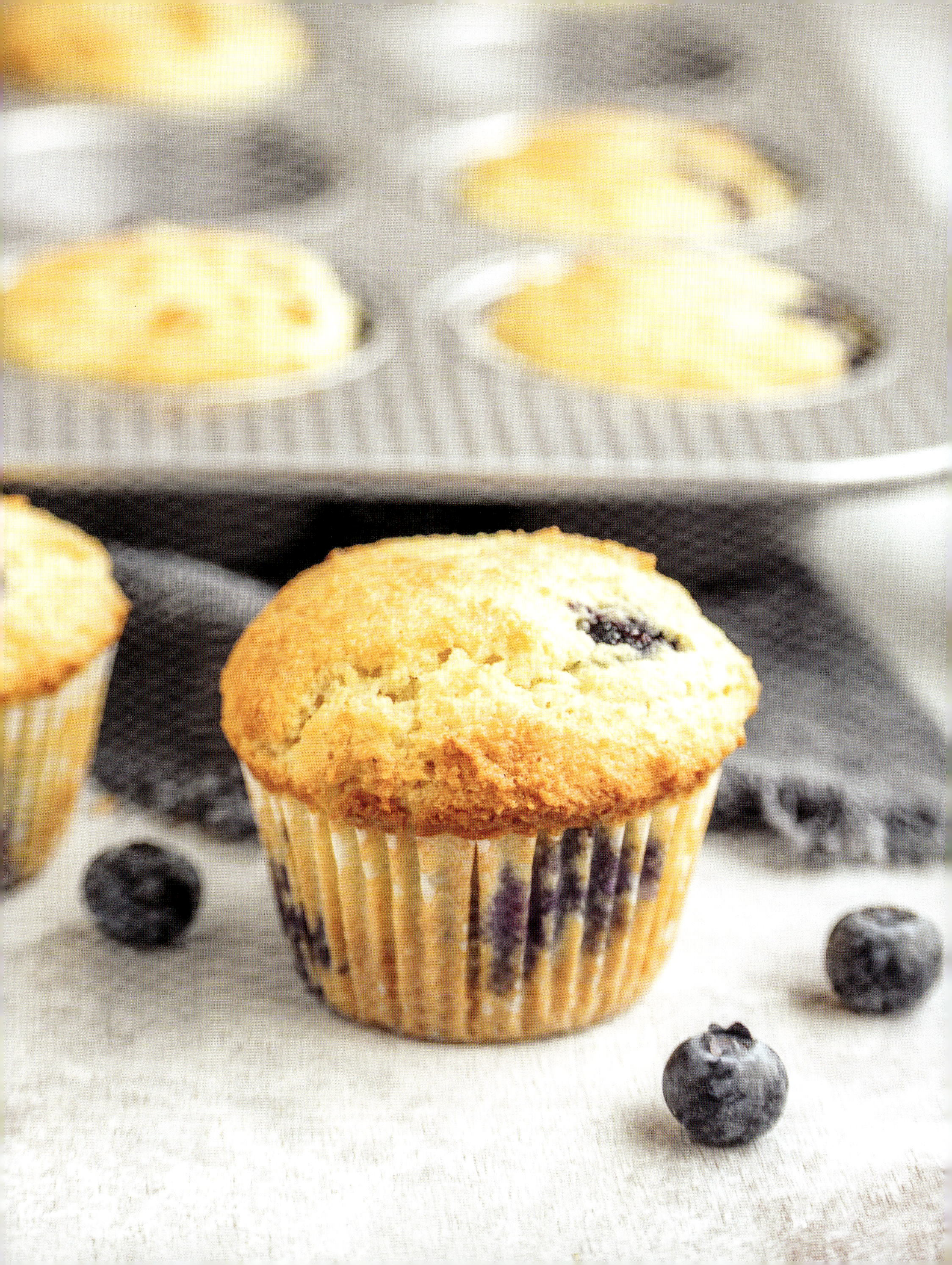

BLUEBERRY PROTEIN MUFFINS

MAKES 12 muffins
PREP TIME: 10 minutes
COOK TIME: 25 minutes

Made with eggs, Greek yogurt, and protein powder, these muffins combine that classic blueberry flavor with a healthy, high-protein twist. (Each muffin is packed with 10 grams of protein, with less than 3 grams of net carbs.) This recipe is quick and easy and yields fluffy, bakery-style muffins that are perfect for breakfast, a snack, or meal prep.

2½ cups blanched, super-fine almond flour

½ cup unflavored protein powder

2 teaspoons baking powder

¼ teaspoon salt

3 tablespoons unsalted butter, melted

½ cup granulated sugar-free sweetener

¼ cup plain Greek or low-carb yogurt

3 large eggs

1 teaspoon vanilla extract

1 cup fresh blueberries

1. Preheat the oven to 350°F. Line a standard-size 12-cup muffin pan with liners.
2. In a large bowl, thoroughly combine the almond flour, protein powder, baking powder, and salt.
3. Add the melted butter, sweetener, yogurt, eggs, and vanilla. Mix with a wooden spoon or electric mixer to combine. Stir in the blueberries.
4. Evenly divide the batter among the prepared muffin cups, filling each one nearly to the top. Bake for 23 to 25 minutes, until a toothpick inserted into the center comes out clean. Let cool in the pan for a few minutes. Then remove and allow to sit and cool for a few more minutes before enjoying.

(per muffin)
CALORIES: **211** | PROTEIN: **9.9g** | FAT: **16.6g** | TOTAL CARBS: **13.5g** | NET CARBS: **2.9g** | FIBER: **2.6g**
SUGAR ALCOHOLS: **8g**

DOUBLE CHOCOLATE ZUCCHINI PROTEIN MUFFINS

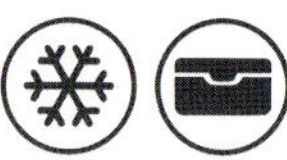

MAKES 12 muffins

PREP TIME: 10 minutes

COOK TIME: 25 minutes

These chocolate zucchini muffins are a high-protein, low-carb sweet treat with about 10 grams of protein per muffin. Made with zucchini for moisture and packed with cocoa powder and chocolate chips, these fluffy, bakery-style muffins let you enjoy that chocolaty flavor you crave while getting your fill of protein.

---

1 medium zucchini (about 3½ ounces)

2½ cups blanched, super-fine almond flour

½ cup unflavored protein powder

½ cup granulated sugar-free sweetener

⅓ cup unsweetened cocoa powder

2 teaspoons baking powder

½ teaspoon salt

3 large eggs

⅓ cup plain Greek or low-carb yogurt

3 tablespoons unsalted butter, melted

½ cup sugar-free chocolate chips

1. Preheat the oven to 350°F and line a standard-size 12-cup muffin pan with liners.
2. Using a box grater, shred the zucchini. You will need about 1½ cups of shredded zucchini for this recipe. (If you have extra, save it for another use.) Set aside.
3. In a large bowl, thoroughly combine the almond flour, protein powder, sweetener, cocoa powder, baking powder, and salt.
4. To the dry ingredients, add the eggs, yogurt, melted butter, and zucchini. Beat with an electric mixer on medium speed to combine. Stir in the chocolate chips.
5. Evenly divide the batter among the prepared muffin cups, filling each one nearly to the top. Bake for 25 minutes, or until a toothpick inserted into the center comes out clean. Remove from the oven and let cool in the pan for a few minutes before removing.

(per muffin)
CALORIES: **204** | PROTEIN: **10.2g** | FAT: **15.7g** | TOTAL CARBS: **19.3g** | NET CARBS: **3.7g** | FIBER: **7.1g**
SUGAR ALCOHOLS: **8.5g**

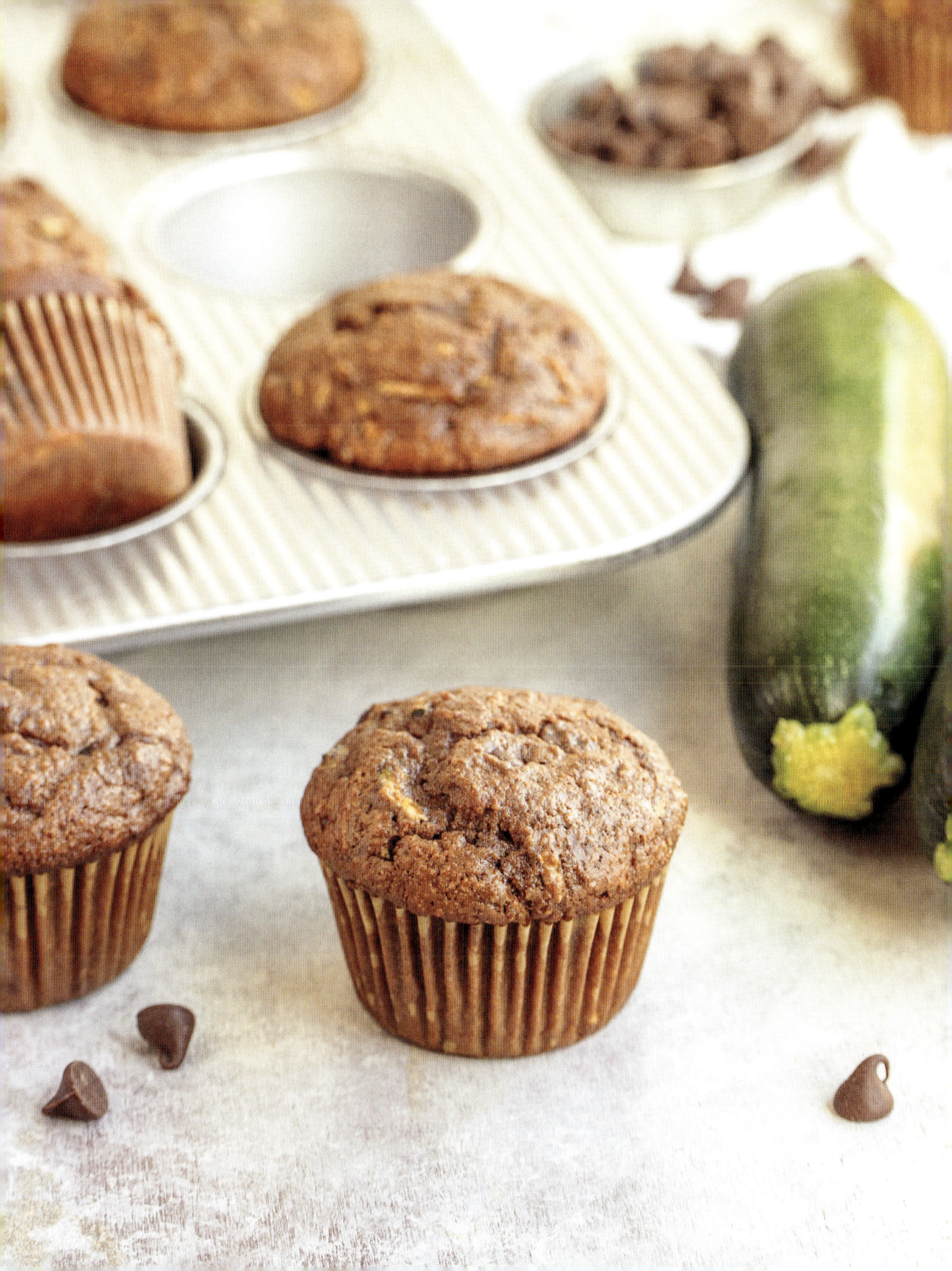

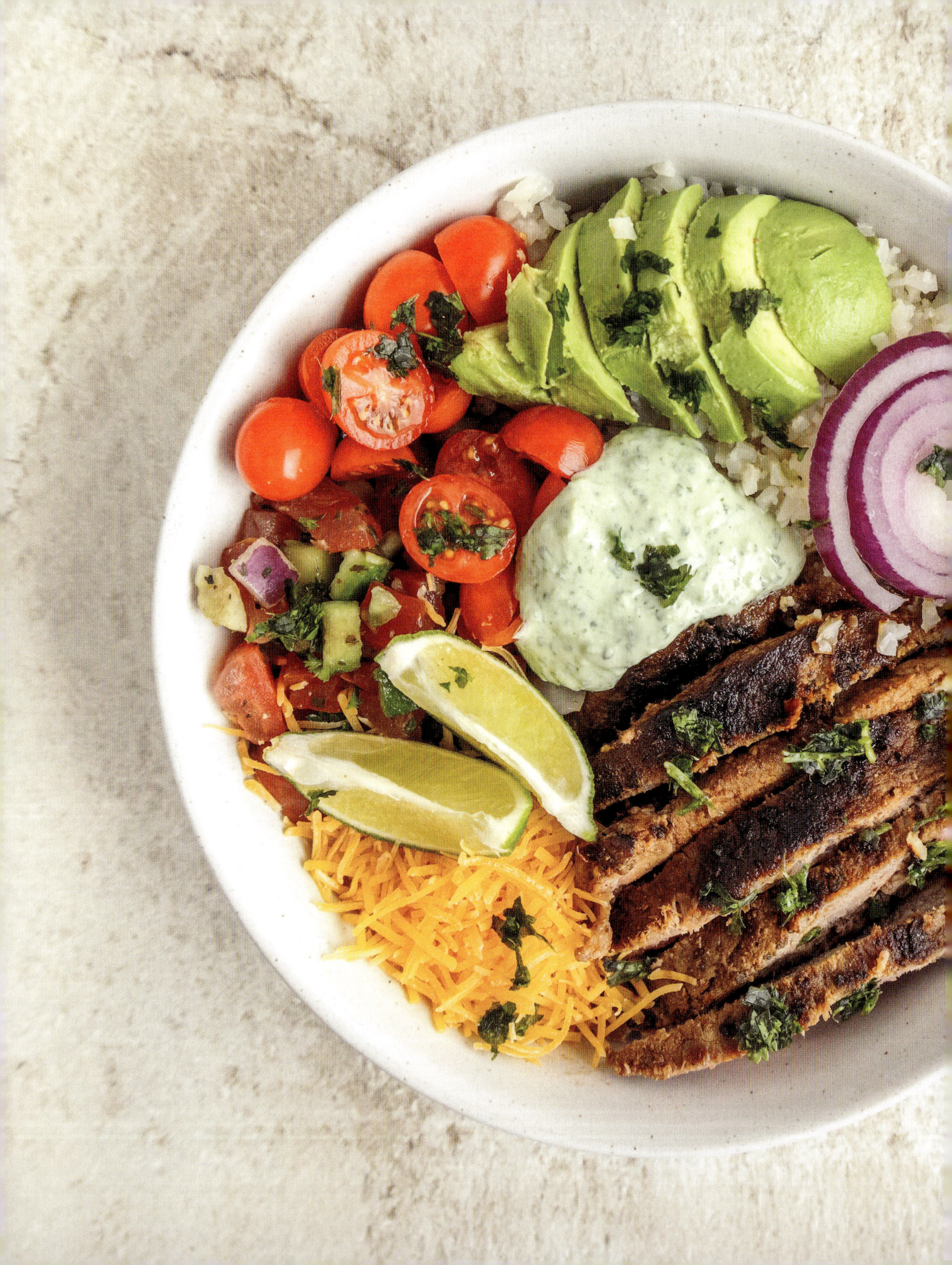

BEEF & LAMB

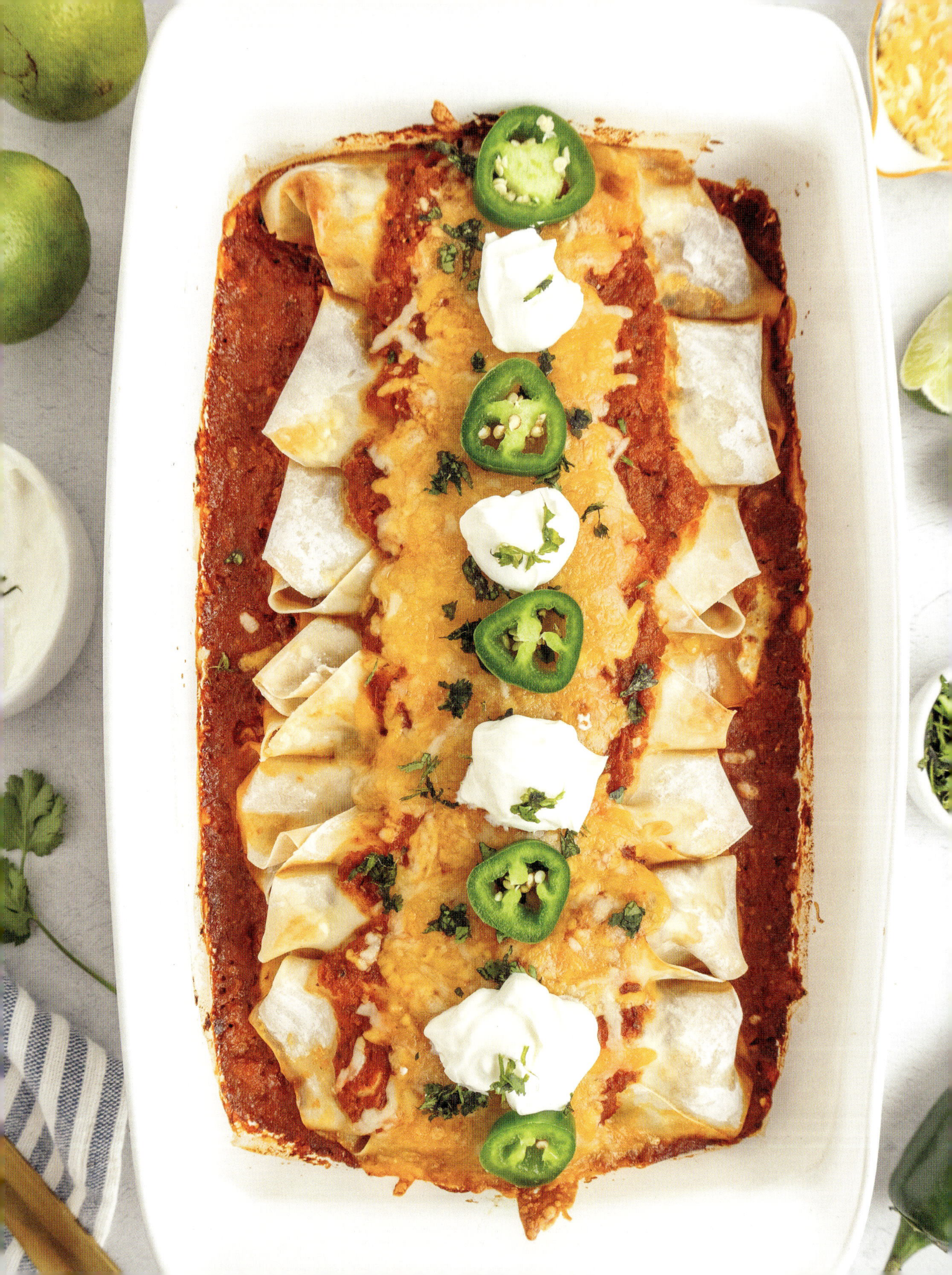

BEEF EGGCHILADAS

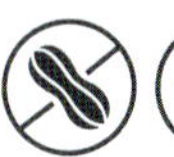
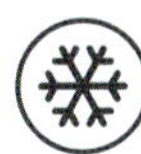
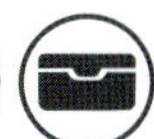

SERVES 4
PREP TIME: 20 minutes
COOK TIME: 50 minutes

This recipe is appropriately named Beef Eggchiladas since I've swapped out the traditional tortillas for egg wraps to keep it low in carbs and high in protein, but don't worry, it won't taste eggy. This dish maintains its classic enchilada flavor from a simple recipe of ground beef, onion, garlic, diced tomatoes, broth, chipotle chiles, and cumin, which, once rolled in the wraps, is covered in a blanket of melted Colby Jack cheese.

1 (14.5-ounce) can diced tomatoes

1 cup beef broth

3 chipotle chiles in adobo sauce

1½ teaspoons ground cumin, divided

1 pound ground beef (85/15)

½ cup diced onions

½ teaspoon salt

6 cloves garlic, minced

3 tablespoons chopped fresh cilantro

8 ounces Colby Jack cheese, shredded, divided

8 egg wraps, store-bought or homemade (page 245)

SUGGESTED TOPPINGS

Sour cream

Pico de gallo

Jalapeño slices

Chopped fresh cilantro

1. Preheat the oven to 400°F.
2. To make the enchilada sauce, combine the diced tomatoes (plus their juices), broth, chipotle chiles, and 1 teaspoon of the cumin in a large skillet. Cook over medium-high heat until bubbly and slightly reduced, about 15 minutes.
3. Remove from the heat and carefully pour the sauce into a blender or food processor. Puree until smooth.
4. In the same skillet, cook the ground beef, stirring occasionally to break it into crumbles, over medium-high heat until only slightly pink, 6 to 8 minutes. Add the onions, salt, and remaining ½ teaspoon of cumin and cook until the onions have softened and the beef is no longer pink, 1 to 2 minutes. Stir in the garlic and continue to cook until fragrant, 30 to 60 seconds. Remove the pan from the heat.
5. Stir the cilantro, about three-quarters of the cheese, and ¼ cup of the enchilada sauce into the beef mixture.
6. To assemble, pour in enough of the enchilada sauce to cover the bottom of a 13 by 9-inch casserole dish (about ½ cup). Spoon some of the beef mixture (½ to 2/3 cup) into the center of an egg wrap and roll it up like a tortilla. Place in the dish, seam side down, and repeat with the remaining egg wraps and filling. Pour the remaining sauce on top. Sprinkle with the remaining cheese.
7. Bake for 15 to 20 minutes, until the cheese is bubbly. Let cool for 3 to 5 minutes before serving. Top with sour cream, pico de gallo, sliced jalapeño, and fresh cilantro, if desired.

note

To freeze for meal prep, assemble the casserole and cover tightly with plastic wrap and foil. Freeze for up to 3 months. When ready to bake, thaw overnight in the refrigerator, remove the plastic wrap and re-cover with the foil, and bake in a preheated 400°F oven for 25 to 35 minutes, removing the foil for the last 10 minutes.

(per serving)
CALORIES: **565** | PROTEIN: **45.6g** | FAT: **35g** | TOTAL CARBS: **13g** | NET CARBS: **9.7g** | FIBER: **3.3g**

BAKED BEEFY ZITI

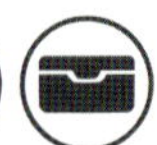

SERVES 8
PREP TIME: 10 minutes
COOK TIME: 65 minutes

The whole family will enjoy this baked ziti. Here, I've swapped regular noodles for low-carb pasta and used a low-sugar marinara sauce to keep the carbs down. Adding cottage cheese and eggs to the beef and pork mixture packs this meal with extra protein. The pasta I recommend isn't just low carb; it gives 20 grams of extra protein per serving. To make this dish truly delicious, I've added a blend of aromatics from my mom's secret recipe, adding that special depth of flavor we all love—it's comfort food with a healthy twist.

---

1 tablespoon extra-virgin olive oil

¼ medium onion, diced

3 cloves garlic, minced

1 pound ground beef (85/15)

1 pound ground pork

1 (14.5-ounce) can diced tomatoes

1 (25-ounce) jar low-carb marinara sauce (see notes)

2 teaspoons Italian seasoning

¾ teaspoon salt

½ teaspoon ground black pepper

¼ teaspoon anise seeds

2 cups shredded mozzarella cheese, divided

1 cup cottage cheese (4% milkfat)

⅓ cup grated Parmesan cheese

2 large eggs

16 ounces high-protein, low-carb ziti pasta (see notes)

Chopped fresh parsley, for garnish (optional)

1. Preheat a large skillet over medium heat. Pour in the olive oil. Add the diced onion and garlic. Sauté for 2 to 3 minutes, until softened.
2. Stir in the ground beef and pork, breaking it up with a spatula. Cook until browned, 7 to 8 minutes. Drain off some of the fat, leaving 2 to 3 tablespoons behind for moisture.
3. Stir in the diced tomatoes (plus their juices), marinara sauce, Italian seasoning, salt, pepper, and anise seeds. Bring to a simmer, then reduce the heat to low and continue to simmer, stirring occasionally, for 20 to 25 minutes to deepen the flavors. When done, transfer 2½ cups of the sauce to a heatproof bowl and set aside for faster cooling; leave the rest in the pan, but slide the pan off the heat.
4. While the sauce is simmering, in a large bowl, mix together 1½ cups of the mozzarella, the cottage cheese, Parmesan, and eggs.
5. Preheat the oven to 375°F.
6. Cook the pasta according to the instructions on the box, not longer. Otherwise, the pasta may break and get mushy when mixed with the sauce. Drain the pasta and run cold water over it to cool it down and keep it from sticking.
7. Pour the drained pasta into the bowl with the cheese mixture or vice versa (whichever pot/bowl is larger) and stir to coat.
8. Stir the 2½ cups of cooled meat sauce into the pasta mixture.
9. To assemble, spoon half of the sauced pasta into a 13 by 9-inch baking pan, spreading it into an even layer. Spoon half of the remaining meat sauce over the top, then top with ¼ cup of the remaining mozzarella. Repeat the layers with the remaining pasta, sauce, and cheese.
10. Bake for 20 to 30 minutes, until the cheese is bubbly and melted. Remove from the oven and let sit for 5 minutes before serving. Garnish with parsley, if desired.

(per serving)
CALORIES: **622** | PROTEIN: **54g** | FAT: **39.4g** | TOTAL CARBS: **29.8g** | NET CARBS: **13.4g** | FIBER: **16.4g**

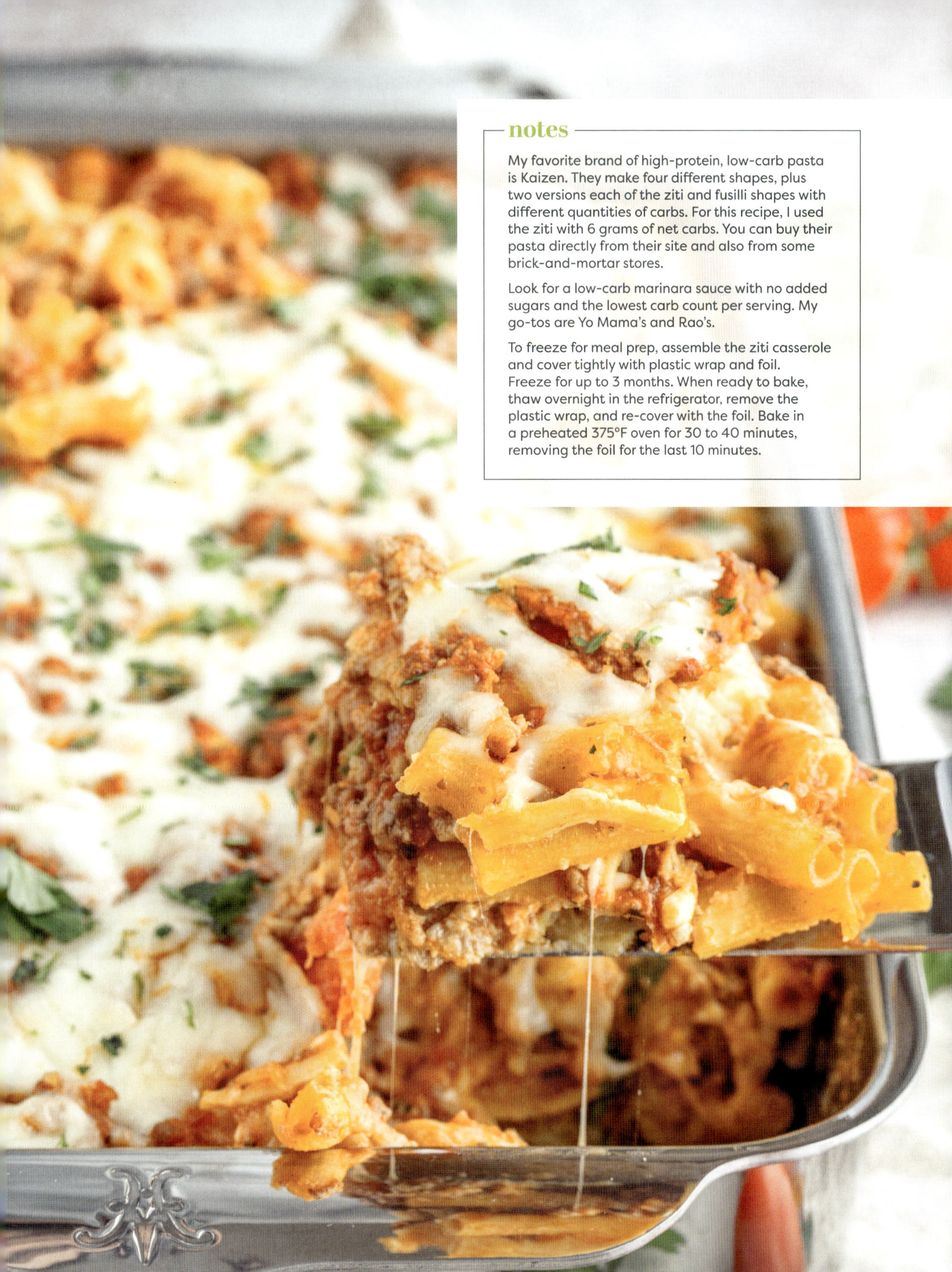

notes

My favorite brand of high-protein, low-carb pasta is Kaizen. They make four different shapes, plus two versions each of the ziti and fusilli shapes with different quantities of carbs. For this recipe, I used the ziti with 6 grams of net carbs. You can buy their pasta directly from their site and also from some brick-and-mortar stores.

Look for a low-carb marinara sauce with no added sugars and the lowest carb count per serving. My go-tos are Yo Mama's and Rao's.

To freeze for meal prep, assemble the ziti casserole and cover tightly with plastic wrap and foil. Freeze for up to 3 months. When ready to bake, thaw overnight in the refrigerator, remove the plastic wrap, and re-cover with the foil. Bake in a preheated 375°F oven for 30 to 40 minutes, removing the foil for the last 10 minutes.

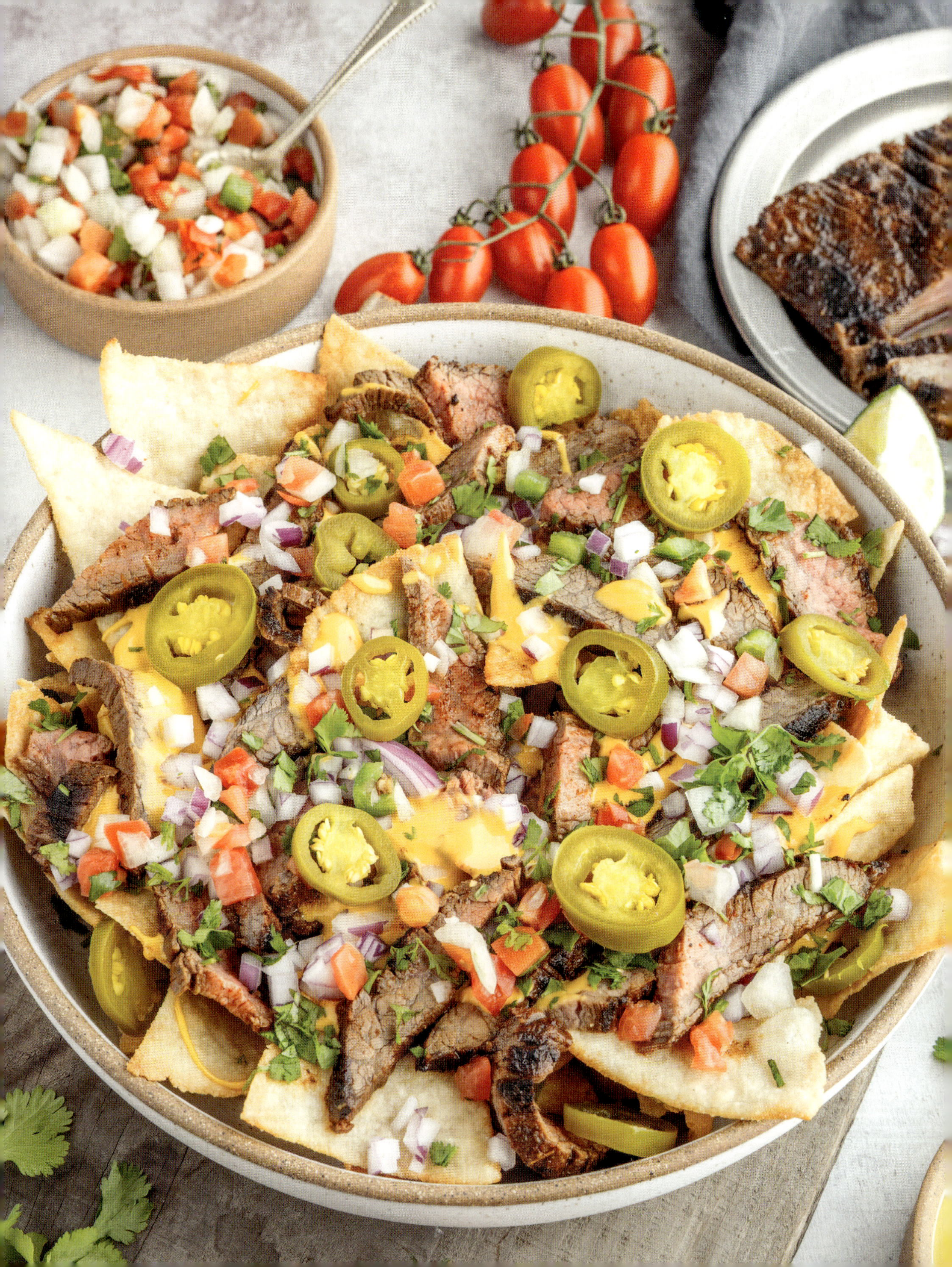

CARNE ASADA NACHOS

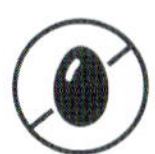

SERVES 4

PREP TIME: 15 minutes, plus 30 minutes to marinate steak

COOK TIME: 7 minutes

These nachos are loaded with grilled marinated steak, creamy queso, and toppings like pico de gallo and pickled jalapeños. This simple base recipe allows for plenty of flexibility—add extras like olives, shredded cheese, tomatoes, guacamole, or sour cream. I like to prepare the chips and nacho cheese sauce ahead of time, but I do use store-bought versions on occasion for an easy weeknight dinner.

---

3 tablespoons lime juice

2 tablespoons avocado oil

2 tablespoons chili powder

1 teaspoon ground cumin

1 teaspoon dried oregano leaves

1 teaspoon garlic powder

1 teaspoon salt

½ teaspoon ground black pepper

2 pounds skirt or flank steak

1 batch Low-Carb Tortilla Chips (page 312) (see notes)

½ cup low-carb nacho cheese sauce, store-bought or homemade (page 317), heated (see notes)

¾ cup pico de gallo

¼ cup chopped fresh cilantro

¼ cup sliced pickled jalapeños

3 tablespoons finely diced red onions

1. In a small bowl, whisk together the lime juice, avocado oil, chili powder, cumin, oregano, garlic powder, salt, and pepper.
2. Put the steak in a baking dish or gallon-size zip-top bag and pour the marinade over it. Rub the marinade all over the steak. Cover or seal the bag and refrigerate for at least 30 minutes or up to overnight. The longer the steak marinates, the more flavorful it will be.
3. To cook the steak, preheat a grill to high heat (425°F to 450°F). Remove the steak from the marinade and discard the marinade. Place the meat on the grill over direct heat, close the lid, and cook for 3 to 5 minutes. Flip the steak and cook for 2 to 4 more minutes, until the internal temperature reaches 125°F to 130°F. Remove from the grill and let rest for 5 minutes before slicing into thin strips, cutting across the grain.
4. To assemble the nachos, spread the tortilla chips on a serving dish and top with the sliced steak. Drizzle the warmed nacho cheese sauce over the chips and steak. Top with the pico de gallo, cilantro, pickled jalapeños, and red onions. Serve right away.

notes

Instead of making your own nacho cheese sauce and/or tortilla chips, you can buy them from the grocery store. Nacho cheese sauce is generally low in carbs (around 5 grams per serving) and can be found next to the salsa and tortillas or in the chip aisle. Some brands of low-carb tortilla chips that I enjoy are Mr. Tortilla Keto Chips (not gluten free) and Beyond Chipz (gluten free). For this recipe, you will need 4 cups of chips.

(per serving, using homemade chips and cheese sauce)
CALORIES: **658** | PROTEIN: **60g** | FAT: **40.8g** | TOTAL CARBS: **11g** | NET CARBS: **5.5g** | FIBER: **5.5g**

CHEESEBURGER MEATLOAF

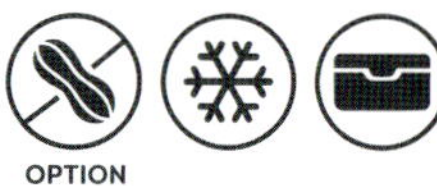

SERVES 8

PREP TIME: 10 minutes

COOK TIME: 1 hour 5 minutes

This meatloaf was one of the first low-carb recipes my family fell in love with. Ground beef, savory low-carb BBQ sauce, and melty cheese create that signature burger flavor. To keep it low in carbs and high in protein, pork panko (ground pork rinds) replaces traditional breadcrumbs. The result is a juicy, flavorful meatloaf with all the best parts of a cheeseburger. It's still a meal that my kids request regularly.

---

1 tablespoon avocado oil

½ cup diced onions

6 cloves garlic, minced

2 pounds ground beef (85/15)

2 large eggs

2 cups pork panko

2 cups shredded Colby Jack cheese

½ cup heavy cream or nut or seed milk of choice (unflavored and unsweetened)

¼ cup low-carb BBQ sauce

2 tablespoons chopped fresh parsley, plus more for garnish if desired

2 teaspoons dried oregano leaves

2 teaspoons salt

1 teaspoon ground black pepper

1 teaspoon smoked paprika

FOR TOPPING (OPTIONAL)

2 to 3 tablespoons low-carb BBQ sauce

¼ cup shredded Colby Jack cheese

1. Preheat the oven to 350°F. Spray an 8½ by 4½-inch loaf pan with cooking oil. If you don't have a loaf pan, line a rimmed baking sheet with foil. Set aside.
2. Pour the avocado oil into a large skillet and set over medium-high heat. When the oil is hot, add the onions and cook until softened. Stir in the garlic and continue cooking until fragrant. Remove from the heat and transfer to a large bowl.
3. To the bowl, add the remaining ingredients and mix with a wooden spoon or clean hands until fully combined.
4. Press the meatloaf mixture into the prepared loaf pan or mold into a meatloaf shape on the foil-lined pan. Bake for 45 to 60 minutes, until the internal temperature of the meatloaf reaches 160°F.
5. If using the optional toppings, brush the meatloaf with the BBQ sauce and top with the cheese. Set the oven to broil on high. Broil the meatloaf on the top rack for 2 to 3 minutes, until the cheese is melted.
6. Allow the meatloaf to cool slightly before serving. If desired, garnish with parsley.

note

To freeze for meal prep, assemble the meatloaf as instructed. Cover tightly with plastic wrap and foil. Freeze for up to 3 months. To bake from frozen, remove the plastic wrap and foil and bake in a preheated 350°F oven for 90 to 120 minutes, until the internal temperature of the meatloaf reaches 160°F.

(per serving)

CALORIES: **591** | PROTEIN: **47.7g** | FAT: **41.8g** | TOTAL CARBS: **4.1g** | NET CARBS: **3.4g** | FIBER: **0.7g**

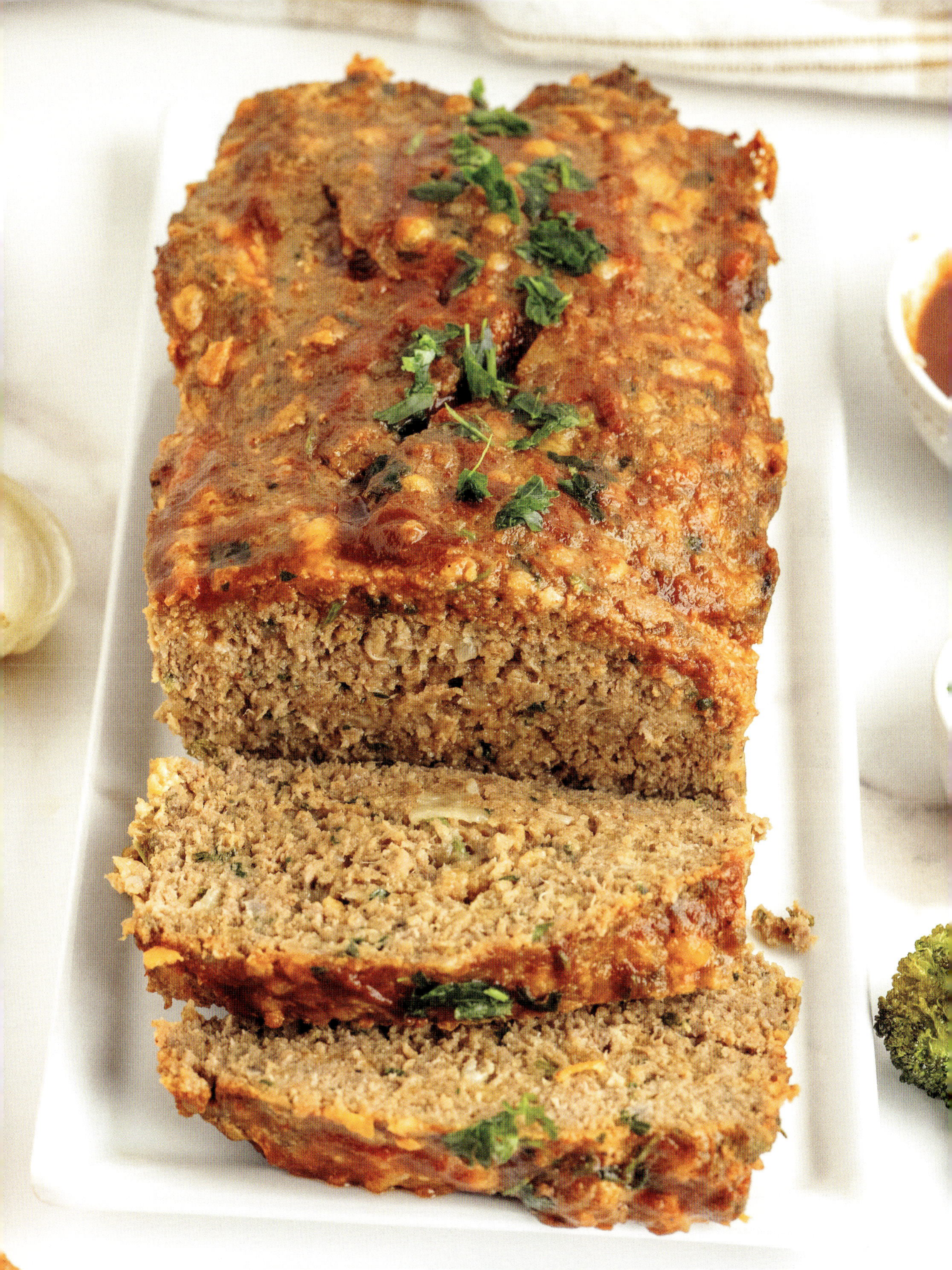

CITRUS BEEF & SPINACH STEW

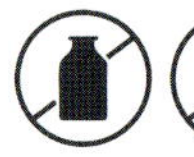
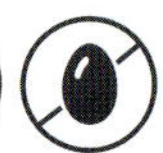
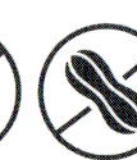
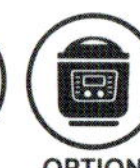

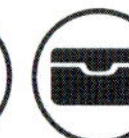
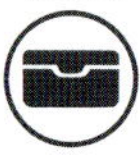

SERVES 4

PREP TIME: 15 minutes, plus 30 minutes to rest beef

COOK TIME: 45 minutes to 3 hours 15 minutes, depending on method

This is not your usual beef stew. It has bright notes of lemon and a fresh, herbaceous flavor that sets it apart. Packed with tender chunks of beef, celery, onion, fennel bulb, carrot, turnip, and spinach, it brings a vibrant medley of flavor. Whether you cook it on the stovetop, in a slow cooker, or in an Instant Pot, this dish is easy to prepare for a comforting dinner any night of the week.

---

2 pounds beef stew meat, cut into ½-inch cubes

2 teaspoons salt

1 teaspoon ground black pepper

3 tablespoons extra-virgin olive oil, plus more if needed

4 cloves garlic, minced

3 celery stalks, sliced

½ medium onion, diced

1 fennel bulb, diced

½ teaspoon paprika

4 cups beef broth

1 cup water

½ teaspoon dried rosemary needles

½ teaspoon rubbed dried sage, or 1½ teaspoons finely chopped fresh sage

2 bay leaves

2 medium carrots, sliced

2 medium turnips, peeled and cut into ½-inch dice

5 ounces baby spinach

Grated zest of 1 lemon, plus more for garnish if desired

2 tablespoons lemon juice

Chopped fresh parsley, for garnish (optional)

STOVETOP INSTRUCTIONS:

1. Season the beef with the salt and pepper. Let stand for 30 minutes.
2. Heat the olive oil in a stockpot or Dutch oven over medium-high heat. Working in batches, add enough beef to sear the meat without overcrowding the pot, which would cause it to steam instead of sear. Cook, turning occasionally, until well browned on all sides. Add more oil if the pan gets too dry. Transfer the seared meat to a paper towel–lined plate. Lower the heat under the pot to medium.
3. Put the garlic, celery, onion, and fennel in the now-empty pot. Cook until softened, stirring occasionally. Stir in the paprika.
4. Return the beef to the pot. Pour in the broth and water. Add the rosemary, sage, and bay leaves. Bring the liquid to a boil, reduce the heat to medium, and simmer, partly covered, for 1 hour.
5. Add the carrots and turnips. Continue to simmer until the meat is tender and the vegetables have softened, 15 to 20 minutes. Discard the bay leaves.
6. Remove the pot from the heat. Stir in the spinach leaves, lemon zest, and lemon juice. Stir until the spinach is wilted. Taste and add more salt and pepper if needed. Garnish servings with lemon zest and chopped parsley, if desired.

(recipe continues)

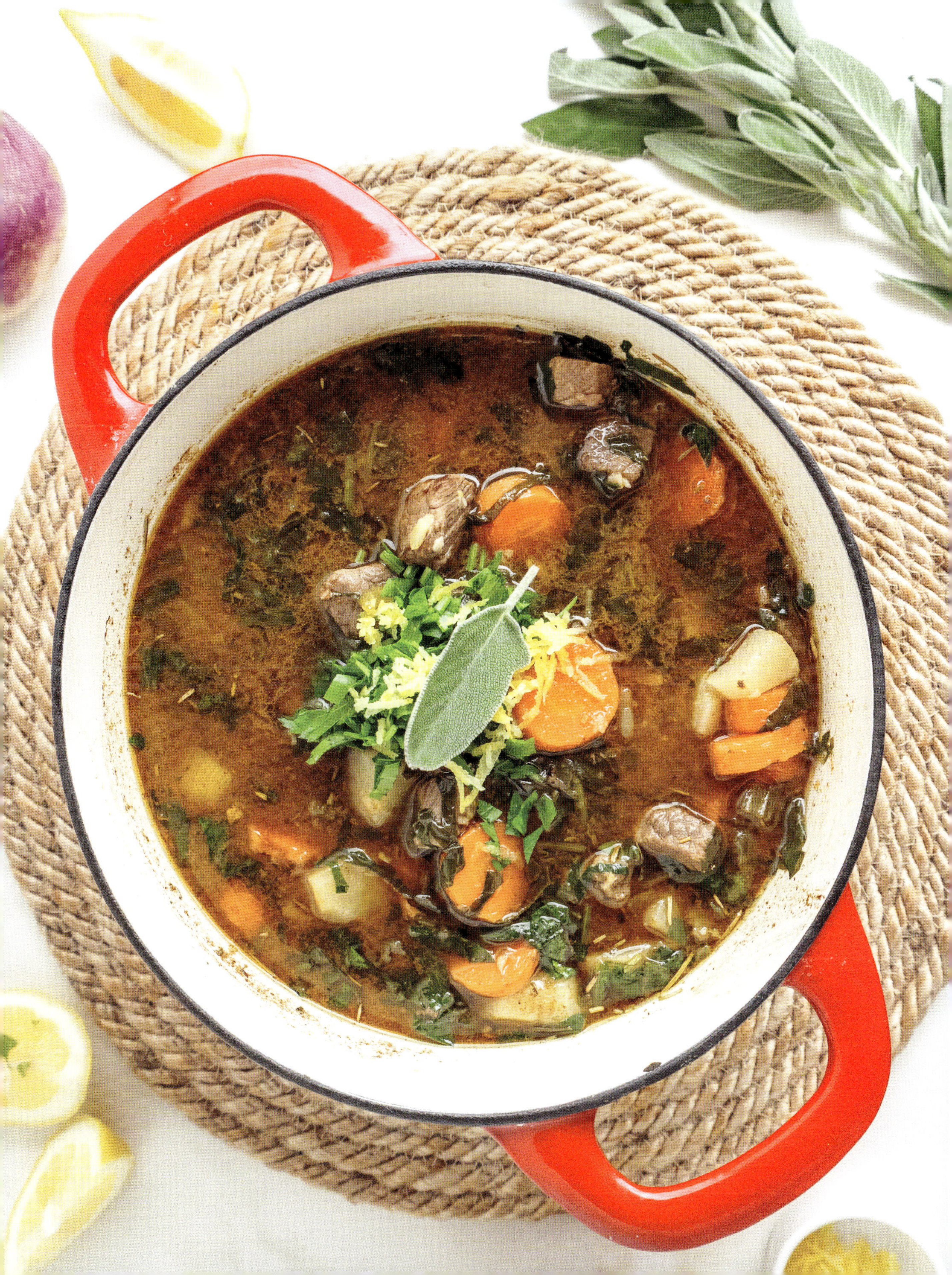

SLOW COOKER INSTRUCTIONS:

1. Follow Steps 1 and 2 of the stovetop instructions, using a large skillet for Step 2. Transfer the seared beef to the slow cooker.
2. Deglaze the skillet with the water, stirring well to get all the flavorful brown bits from the bottom of the pan. Pour the liquid into the slow cooker.
3. Add all the remaining ingredients to the slow cooker except the spinach and lemon zest and juice. Stir, cover, and cook on low for 6 hours or high for 3 hours, until the meat is tender and the vegetables have softened.
4. Remove the lid and discard the bay leaves. Stir in the spinach, lemon zest, and lemon juice. Gently stir until the spinach is wilted. Garnish servings with lemon zest and chopped parsley, if desired.

INSTANT POT INSTRUCTIONS:

1. Follow Step 1 of the stovetop instructions.
2. Turn the Instant Pot to the Sauté function. Pour the olive oil into the liner of the Instant Pot. Working in batches, add enough beef to evenly sear the meat without overcrowding (which would cause it to steam instead of sear). Turn occasionally and cook until well browned on all sides. Add more oil if the liner gets too dry. Transfer the meat to a paper towel–lined plate once evenly seared.
3. Add the garlic, celery, onion, and fennel to the Instant Pot. Continue cooking in Sauté mode until softened. Stir in the paprika.
4. Return the beef to the pot. Pour in the broth and water. Add the rosemary, sage, bay leaves, carrots, and turnips.
5. Secure the lid and pressure-cook on high for 25 minutes. Allow the Instant Pot to vent naturally for 20 minutes before turning or pressing the vent to release the remaining pressure.
6. Remove the lid and stir in the spinach, lemon zest, and lemon juice until the spinach is wilted. Garnish servings with lemon zest and chopped parsley, if desired.

(per serving)
CALORIES: **460** | PROTEIN: **32.6g** | FAT: **31g** | TOTAL CARBS: **12.7g** | NET CARBS: **7.4g** | FIBER: **5.3g**

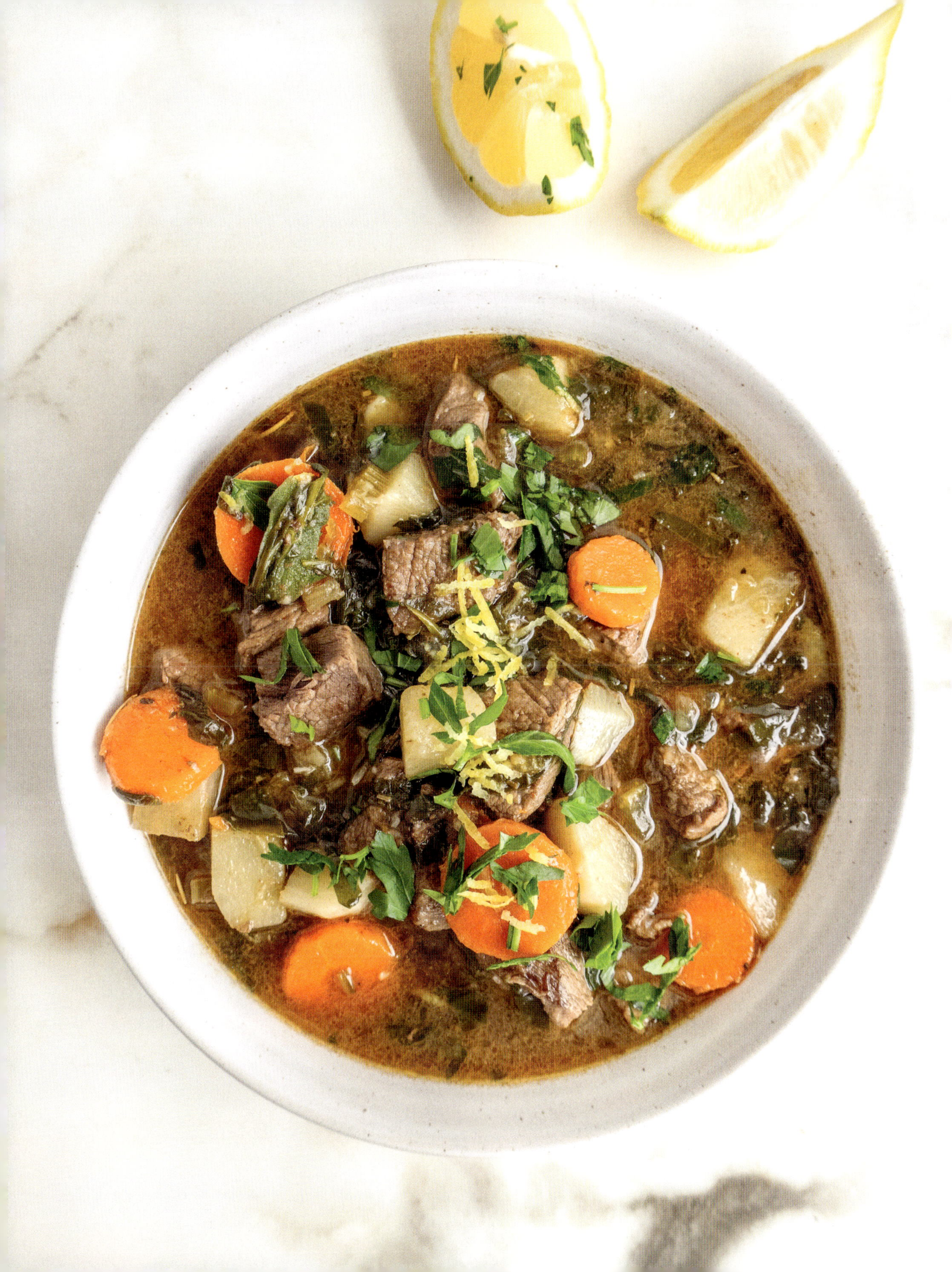

CREAMY BEEF & CHEESE BURRITOS

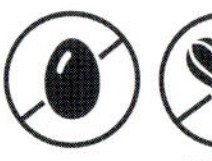
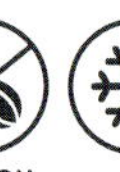
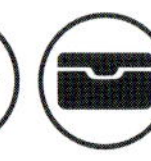

OPTION

MAKES 8 burritos
PREP TIME: 15 minutes
COOK TIME: 25 minutes

Each of these creamy burritos delivers over 30 grams of protein, wrapped in a low-carb tortilla and loaded with a velvety, cheesy beef filling that satisfies your taste buds and your hunger. Perfect for meal prep, they can be made ahead of time, frozen, and reheated for a quick high-protein meal.

---

1 tablespoon avocado oil

¼ cup diced onions

1½ pounds ground beef (90/10)

3 cloves garlic, minced

1 teaspoon chili powder

1 teaspoon salt

1 teaspoon ground black pepper

1 teaspoon dried oregano leaves

1 teaspoon garlic powder

1 teaspoon ground cumin

½ teaspoon onion powder

2 tablespoons tomato paste

4 ounces (½ cup) cream cheese, cubed

2 cups shredded cheddar cheese, divided

8 (8-inch) low-carb tortillas, store-bought or homemade (page 249)

1 cup low-carb nacho cheese sauce, store-bought or homemade (page 317)

FOR SERVING/GARNISH (OPTIONAL)

Chopped fresh cilantro

Diced tomato

Lime wedges

1. Heat the avocado oil in a large skillet over medium-high heat. Add the onions and cook until softened. Add the ground beef, breaking it up until crumbled, and cook for about 5 minutes, until only slightly pink. Then add the garlic, chili powder, salt, pepper, oregano, garlic powder, cumin, and onion powder. Continue to cook until the beef is no longer pink, 3 to 5 minutes.
2. Stir in the tomato paste, cubed cream cheese, and 1 cup of the cheddar. Continue to cook, stirring often, until the cheese is melted. Remove the pan from the heat.
3. To assemble, evenly divide the beef mixture among the tortillas, placing about ⅓ cup on the bottom half of each tortilla, leaving space around the edge. Add 2 tablespoons of nacho cheese and 2 tablespoons of the remaining shredded cheddar to each burrito.
4. To roll up a burrito, fold the sides of the tortilla inward over the filling. Next, lift the bottom edge of the tortilla over the filling and begin to roll it tightly away from you, tucking the filling as you go. Continue rolling until the burrito is fully wrapped, ensuring it's snug and secure.
5. Heat a medium nonstick skillet over medium heat. Place one or two burritos seam-side down in the pan and cook for 30 to 60 seconds, until the bottom is browned and toasted. Flip and repeat on the other side.
6. Garnish with cilantro and diced tomato and serve with lime wedges, if desired.

STORAGE INSTRUCTIONS: Wrap the burritos in aluminum foil. Store in the refrigerator for up to 5 days. If freezing, place in a freezer-safe bag or container and freeze for up to 3 months.

note

To make this nut free, opt for store-bought nut-free tortillas; my tortilla recipe uses almond flour.

(per burrito, using Mission Carb Balance flour tortillas and homemade cheese sauce)

CALORIES: **491** | PROTEIN: **34.5g** | FAT: **33.7g** | TOTAL CARBS: **23.9g** | NET CARBS: **8.3g** | FIBER: **15.6g**

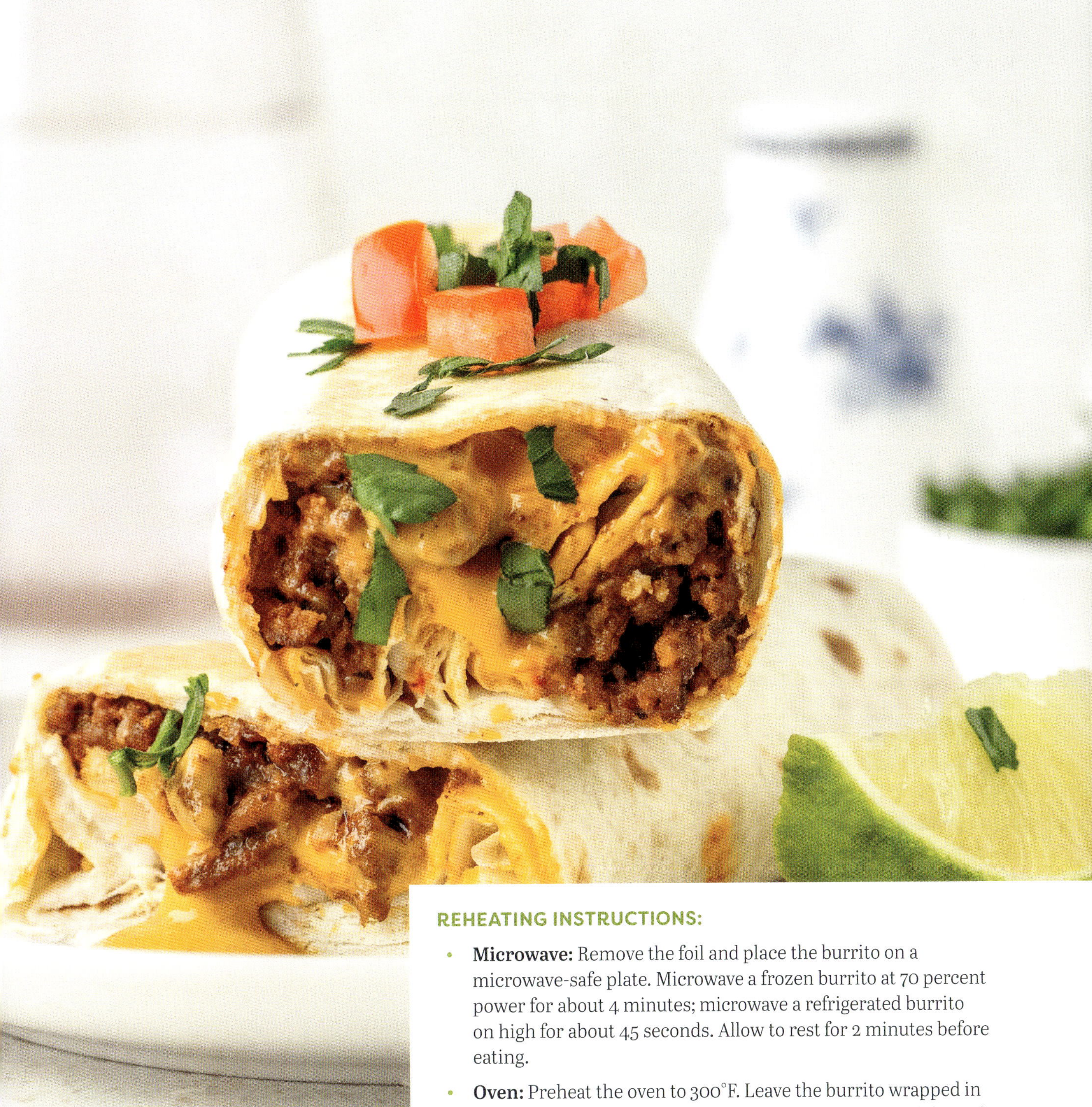

REHEATING INSTRUCTIONS:

- **Microwave:** Remove the foil and place the burrito on a microwave-safe plate. Microwave a frozen burrito at 70 percent power for about 4 minutes; microwave a refrigerated burrito on high for about 45 seconds. Allow to rest for 2 minutes before eating.
- **Oven:** Preheat the oven to 300°F. Leave the burrito wrapped in foil. Place on a rimmed baking sheet. Bake until heated through, about 30 minutes for a frozen burrito or 10 to 12 minutes for a refrigerated burrito. Allow to rest for 2 minutes before eating.
- **Air fryer:** Preheat the air fryer to 400°F. Peel back the foil, but leave the burrito sitting on the foil. Lightly spray the top of the burrito with cooking oil. Air-fry a frozen burrito for 7 to 8 minutes, then flip and air-fry for 5 to 6 more minutes; air-fry a refrigerated burrito for 2 to 3 minutes. Allow to rest for 2 minutes before eating.

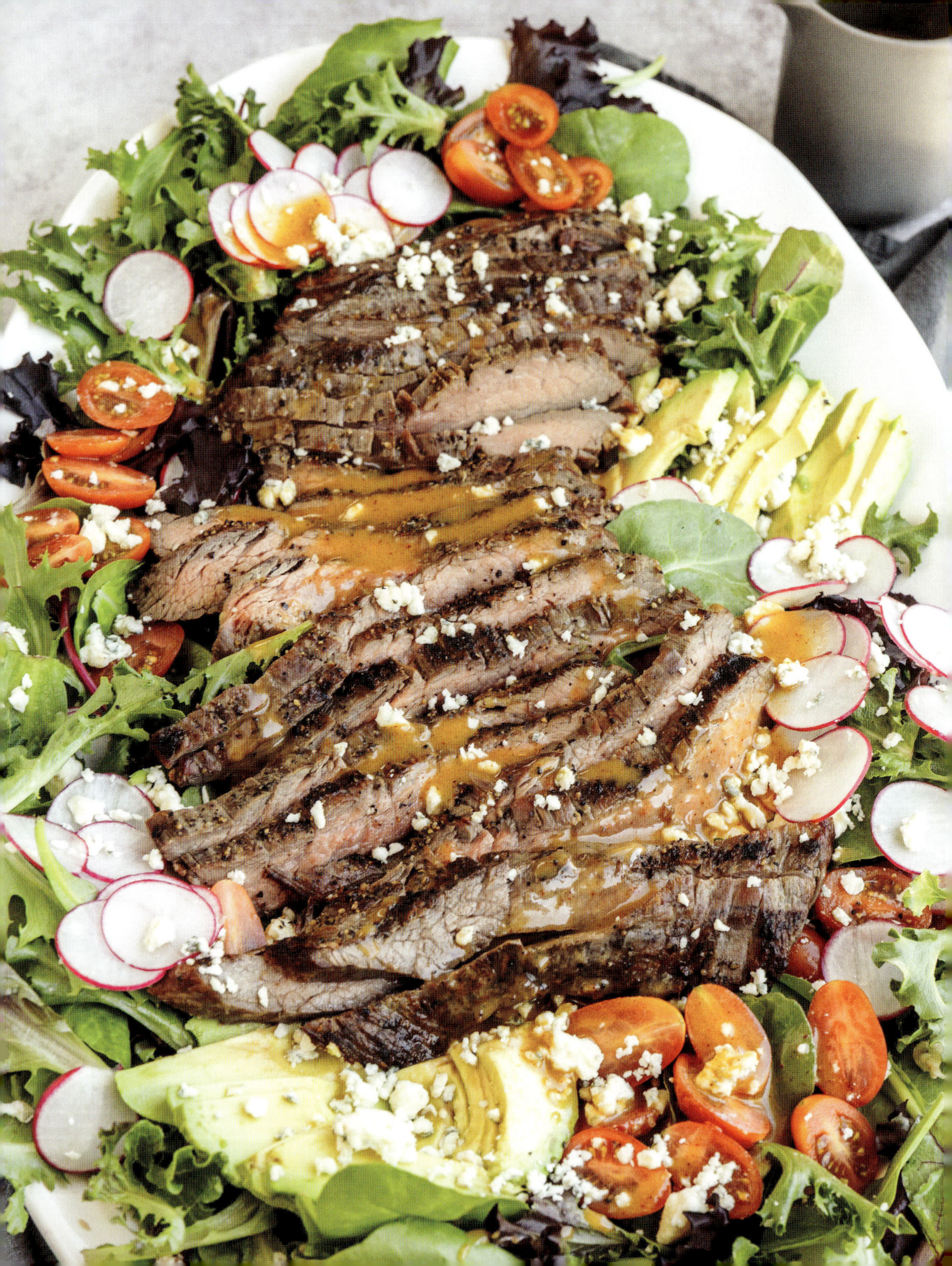

GRILLED STEAK SALAD WITH HOT HONEY MUSTARD DRESSING

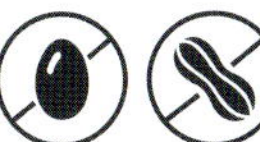

SERVES 4

PREP TIME: 20 minutes

COOK TIME: 9 minutes

Packed with flavor and freshness, this quick and easy salad comes together in less than 30 minutes. Juicy grilled flank steak is sliced and served over a bed of mixed greens, crisp radishes, grape tomatoes, creamy avocado, and gorgonzola cheese. The salad is topped with spicy, tangy hot honey mustard dressing made with sugar-free imitation honey for a low-carb option. You can use regular honey if you prefer; just remember that it will increase the net carbs.

- 1½ pounds flank or skirt steak
- 2 teaspoons salt
- ½ teaspoon ground black pepper
- ⅓ cup extra-virgin olive oil
- 3 tablespoons Dijon mustard
- 3 tablespoons sugar-free honey
- 2 tablespoons lemon juice
- 1 tablespoon apple cider vinegar
- ½ teaspoon chili powder
- ¼ teaspoon cayenne pepper
- 8 cups mixed greens
- 2 radishes, thinly sliced
- ½ cup halved grape tomatoes
- 1 medium avocado, sliced
- ¾ cup crumbled gorgonzola cheese

1. Preheat a grill to high heat (400°F to 450°F).
2. Pat the steak dry with a paper towel and season both sides with the salt and black pepper.
3. Place the seasoned steak on the grill over direct heat, close the lid, and cook for 5 minutes. Flip over and grill for another 3 to 4 minutes, until the internal temperature reaches 125°F (medium-rare). Remove from the grill and let rest for 15 minutes before slicing into thin strips against the grain.
4. Meanwhile, prepare the dressing. In a small bowl, whisk together the olive oil, mustard, honey, lemon juice, vinegar, chili powder, and cayenne. Set aside.
5. To assemble the salad, place the mixed greens in a large bowl. Toss the greens with the radishes, tomatoes, avocado, and gorgonzola cheese. Top with the sliced steak and drizzle the dressing on top. For a more formal presentation, place the mixed greens on a platter, arrange the other vegetables around the perimeter of the platter, set the steak strips in the center, and then drizzle with the dressing.

(per serving)
CALORIES: **615** | PROTEIN: **44.1g** | FAT: **45g** | TOTAL CARBS: **19.1g** | NET CARBS: **3.1g** | FIBER: **8.5g**
SUGAR ALCOHOLS: **7.5g**

KOREAN BEEF "RICE" BOWL

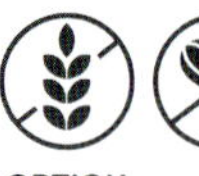

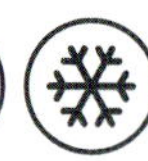
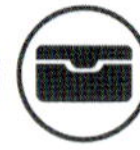

OPTION

SERVES 4
PREP TIME: 10 minutes
COOK TIME: 30 minutes

This Korean beef "rice" bowl is an easy lunch or dinner meal you can prep for the week. It features tender, seared sirloin steak coated in a savory-sweet sauce made with garlic, toasted sesame oil, brown sugar substitute, garlic chili sauce, and soy sauce. Instead of white rice, I use fluffy cauliflower rice cooked in a special way to reduce the typical cauliflower smell and flavor. A creamy sriracha mayo with a protein boost tops the bowl.

FOR THE "RICE" AND KOREAN BEEF

2 (10-ounce) bags frozen cauliflower rice

2 tablespoons avocado oil

1½ pounds boneless sirloin steak, thinly sliced

⅓ cup soy sauce or tamari

4 cloves garlic, minced

2 tablespoons brown sugar substitute

1½ tablespoons garlic chili sauce (like Huy Fung or sambal oelek)

1 tablespoon toasted sesame oil

FOR THE SRIRACHA MAYO

⅓ cup mayonnaise

2½ tablespoons plain Greek or low-carb yogurt

2½ tablespoons sriracha

2 tablespoons water

1 tablespoon lemon juice

½ teaspoon garlic powder

½ teaspoon salt

FOR GARNISH

2 green onions, thinly sliced

1 teaspoon sesame seeds

1. To prepare the cauliflower rice, preheat a medium nonstick skillet over medium heat. Pour the frozen cauliflower rice into the dry skillet. Stirring occasionally, cook until the majority of the moisture has evaporated and the rice is fluffy, 7 to 10 minutes. Remove the pan from the heat, but leave the rice in the pan for a few minutes to allow the residual heat to evaporate the remaining moisture.
2. Meanwhile, prepare the sriracha mayo by combining all the ingredients in a small bowl.
3. Preheat a large skillet over medium-high heat. Pour in 1 tablespoon of the avocado oil. Working in batches, add the sliced steak to the skillet and sear on all sides until a dark, caramelized crust forms on both sides. Don't overcrowd the skillet or the steak will steam instead of sear. Transfer the seared steak to a plate and continue cooking the remaining steak with the remaining tablespoon of oil.
4. While the steak is cooking, whisk together the soy sauce, minced garlic, brown sugar substitute, garlic chili sauce, and sesame oil in a small bowl.
5. Return all the seared steak to the skillet. Lower the heat to medium. Pour in the soy sauce mixture and stir to coat the steak. Cook for about 5 minutes, until the sauce has thickened slightly.
6. To assemble, place about ¾ cup of the prepared cauliflower rice in an individual serving bowl. Top with one-quarter of the Korean beef. Drizzle on about 3 tablespoons of the sriracha mayo. Repeat with the remaining ingredients to make a total of four bowls. Garnish the bowls with the sliced green onions and sesame seeds.

(per bowl)
CALORIES: **558** | PROTEIN: **43.3g** | FAT: **36.4g** | TOTAL CARBS: **18g** | NET CARBS: **8.4g** | FIBER: **3.6g**
SUGAR ALCOHOLS: **6g**

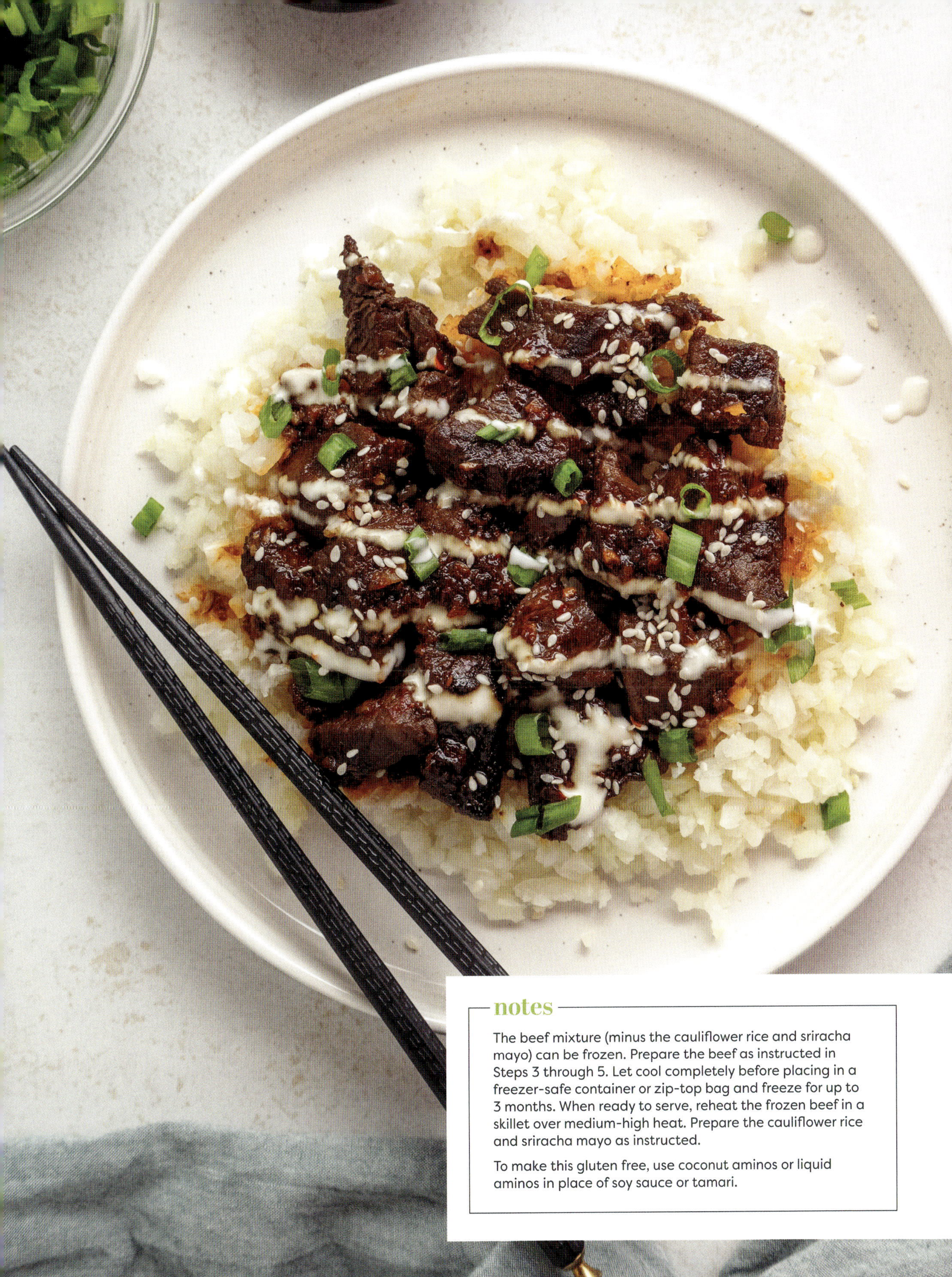

notes

The beef mixture (minus the cauliflower rice and sriracha mayo) can be frozen. Prepare the beef as instructed in Steps 3 through 5. Let cool completely before placing in a freezer-safe container or zip-top bag and freeze for up to 3 months. When ready to serve, reheat the frozen beef in a skillet over medium-high heat. Prepare the cauliflower rice and sriracha mayo as instructed.

To make this gluten free, use coconut aminos or liquid aminos in place of soy sauce or tamari.

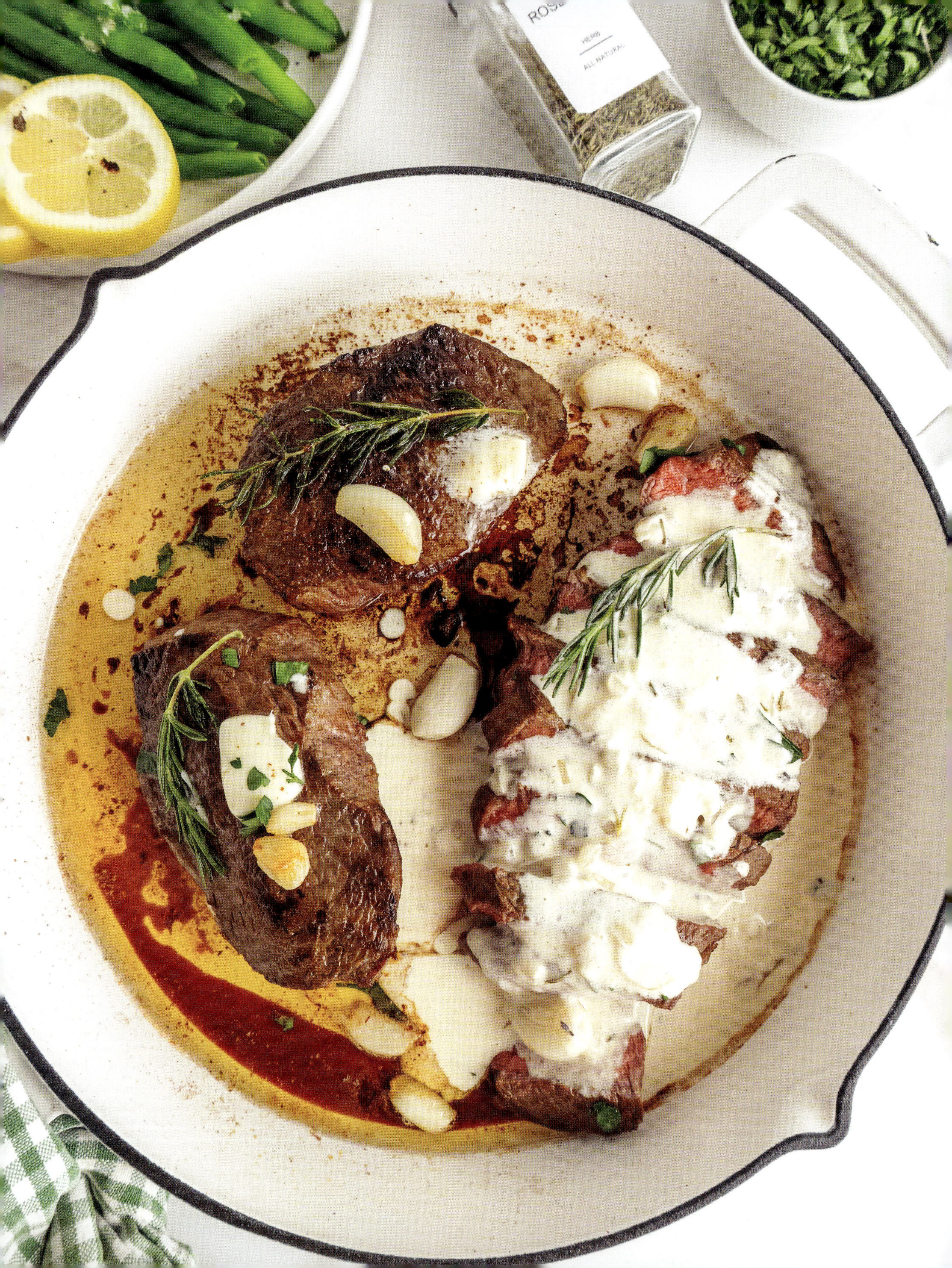
HERB
ALL NATURAL

PAN-SEARED SIRLOIN STEAK WITH ROSEMARY CREAM SAUCE

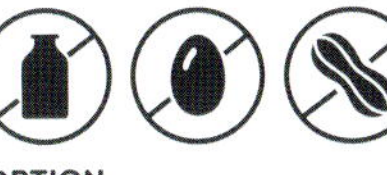

SERVES 4
PREP TIME: 10 minutes
COOK TIME: 35 minutes

Whether you are cooking for a special evening in or looking to make restaurant-quality steak at home, try this recipe for juicy steak with a nice seared-on crust. Then drizzle on a rich, creamy sauce with flavors of rosemary, shallot, and white wine. Don't drink alcohol? Replace the wine with chicken or beef broth. Serve alongside your favorite vegetable side dish. My favorite is steamed and lightly salted green beans with a squeeze of lemon.

---

4 (8-ounce) boneless sirloin steaks (about 1 inch thick)

1½ teaspoons salt

1 tablespoon avocado oil

5 cloves garlic, divided

2 tablespoons unsalted butter

1 shallot, minced

1 tablespoon dried rosemary needles

1 teaspoon ground black pepper

¼ cup dry white wine, such as Sauvignon Blanc or Pinot Grigio

¾ cup heavy cream

2 teaspoons Dijon mustard

Fresh rosemary or parsley sprigs, for garnish

1. Pat the steaks dry with a paper towel and season both sides with the salt.
2. Heat the oil in a large skillet over medium-high heat. Smash three cloves of garlic. Once the oil is almost smoking, add the smashed garlic and the steaks and cook until the internal temperature of each steak is 125°F (for medium-rare). Flip the steaks every 2 to 3 minutes to ensure even cooking. You may have to work in batches so as to not overcrowd the pan. Transfer the steaks to a wire rack, tent with aluminum foil, and let rest for 10 minutes while you work on the cream sauce. (Do not clean the skillet; you will use it for the sauce.)
3. For the sauce, melt the butter in the now-empty skillet over medium heat. While the butter is melting, peel and mince the remaining two cloves of garlic. Stir the shallot, minced garlic, rosemary, and pepper into the melted butter and cook until the shallot is softened, about 3 minutes.
4. Pour in the wine. Stir for about a minute and scrape the bottom of the skillet to dislodge any flavorful brown bits.
5. Stir in the cream and bring to a simmer. Continue to cook until the sauce is slightly thickened, 3 to 6 minutes. Remove the pan from the heat and stir in the mustard. Season to taste with salt and more pepper if needed.
6. Slice the steak and pour the cream sauce over the top. Garnish with rosemary or parsley sprigs.

Make it dairy free! Use more avocado oil or tallow in place of the butter. Replace the heavy cream with ¾ cup seed milk and 1 large egg yolk. Whisk the milk and yolk in a separate bowl and pour in. Continue the recipe as written.

(per serving)
CALORIES: **772** | PROTEIN: **47.6g** | FAT: **59.3g** | TOTAL CARBS: **5g** | NET CARBS: **4g** | FIBER: **1g**

SHEET PAN LASAGNA 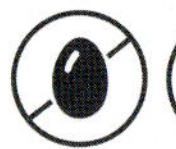  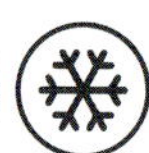 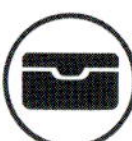

SERVES 8

PREP TIME: 10 minutes

COOK TIME: 45 minutes

I love to make this sheet pan lasagna when I'm craving the flavors of a classic Italian dish but want a quick, hassle-free option. Using a sheet pan and not layering the noodles cuts the cooking time to just 15 minutes while still giving all the hearty layers of ground beef, spinach, and cheese. Plus, using hearts of palm lasagna noodles instead of traditional noodles keeps it low carb.

---

2 pounds ground beef (93/7)

1 tablespoon Italian seasoning

1 teaspoon salt

1 teaspoon ground black pepper

1 teaspoon garlic powder

1 (14.5-ounce) can crushed tomatoes

½ cup tomato sauce

3 cups baby spinach

2 (9-ounce) packages hearts of palm lasagna noodles (see note)

1 cup cottage cheese (4% milkfat)

8 ounces whole milk mozzarella cheese, shredded

¼ cup grated Parmesan cheese, plus more for garnish if desired

Chopped fresh parsley, for garnish (optional)

1. Preheat the oven to 375°F. Spray a rimmed baking sheet with cooking oil. Set aside.
2. In a large skillet, brown the ground beef over medium-high heat, 5 to 7 minutes. Stir the beef occasionally during cooking to crumble it. Drain off the fat. Add the Italian seasoning, salt, pepper, and garlic powder. Mix until combined. Adjust the seasoning to taste if needed.
3. Stir in the crushed tomatoes and tomato sauce. Bring to a simmer and cook for 3 minutes.
4. Stir in the spinach and simmer until wilted.
5. Add the lasagna noodles and stir to combine.
6. Pour the beef and noodle mixture into the prepared pan and spread evenly. Dollop the cottage cheese evenly across the top of the mixture. Top with the mozzarella and Parmesan cheeses.
7. Bake for 14 to 15 minutes, until the cheese is melted and bubbly.
8. Top with chopped parsley and/or more grated Parmesan, if desired.

FREEZER MEAL-PREP INSTRUCTIONS:

To freeze this lasagna, you have two options:

Method 1: Freezing the ground beef, spinach, and noodle mixture

1. Complete Steps 1 through 5 above. Pour the beef, spinach, and noodle mixture into a freezer-safe bag or container. Freeze for up to 3 months.
2. When ready to bake, thaw the mixture in the refrigerator overnight. Pour off any excess liquid. Preheat the oven to 375°F. Spread the thawed mixture on a greased rimmed baking sheet. Add dollops of cottage cheese, then top with the mozzarella and Parmesan cheeses. Bake for 20 to 25 minutes, until the cheese is golden and bubbly.

Method 2: Assembling and freezing the entire dish

1. Complete Steps 1 through 8 above. Once completely cool, wrap tightly with plastic wrap, followed by aluminum foil. Freeze for up to 3 months.
2. To bake from frozen, remove the foil and plastic wrap, then re-cover the pan just with the foil. Bake in a preheated 375°F oven for 30 to 40 minutes. Remove the foil and bake for an additional 10 to 15 minutes, until the cheese is melted and bubbly.

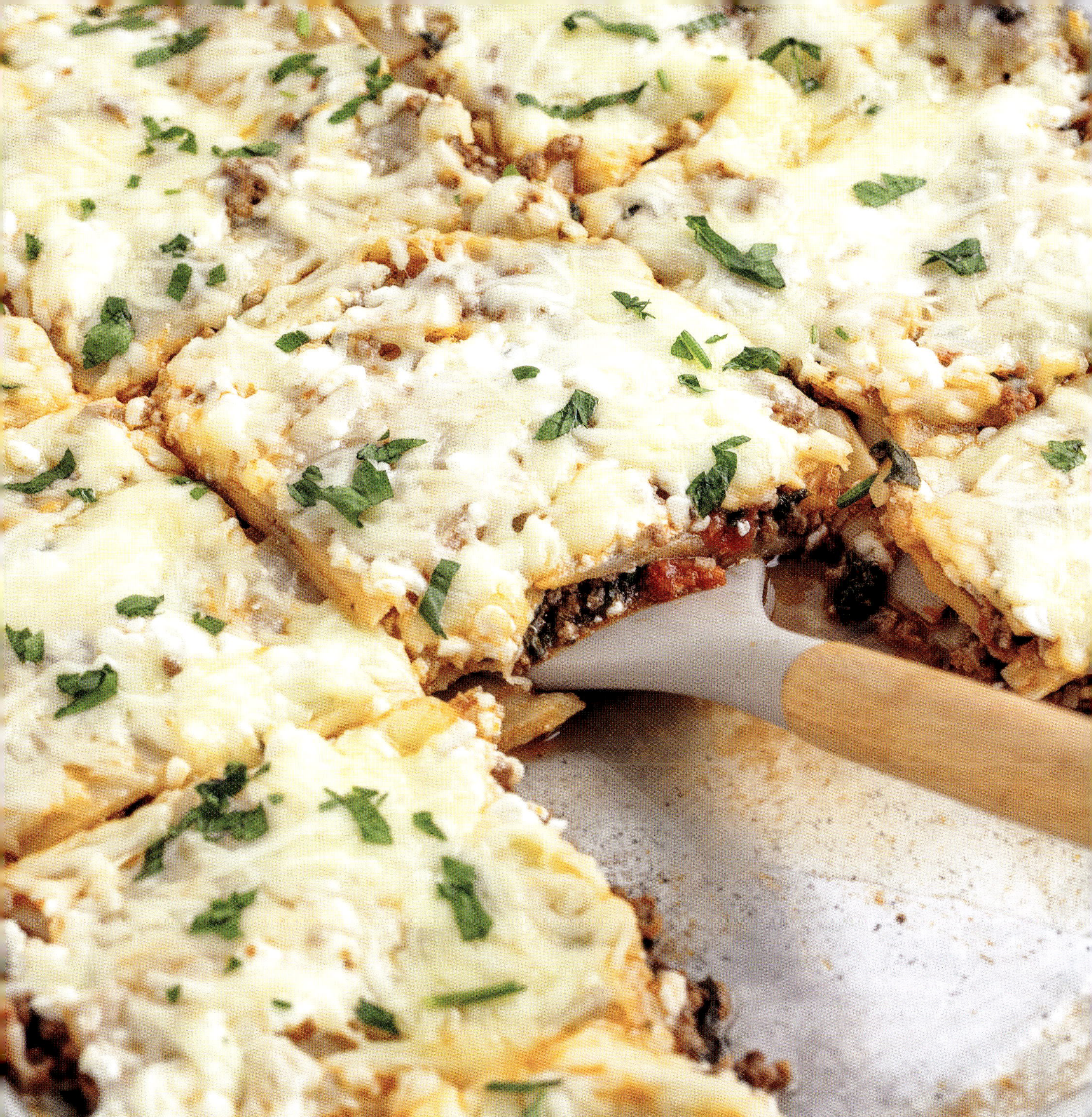

note

The brand of hearts of palm noodles I use is Natural Heaven. They have a tender texture that is more similar to traditional noodles compared to other hearts of palm noodle brands, which can be fibrous and stiff.

(per serving)
CALORIES: **292** | PROTEIN: **33.8g** | FAT: **13.4g** | TOTAL CARBS: **9.8g** | NET CARBS: **6.8g** | FIBER: **3g**

STEAK BURRITO BOWL

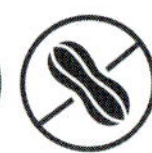
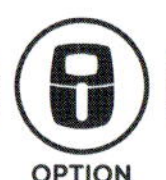
OPTION
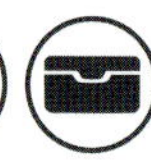

SERVES 4

PREP TIME: 10 minutes, plus 30 minutes to marinate steak

COOK TIME: 30 minutes

This bowl packs all the flavors you love in a burrito but remains low carb by ditching the tortilla and using cauliflower rice instead of traditional rice. Within the bowl, you'll find tender sirloin steak marinated in a smoky Southwest sauce, fresh pico de gallo, cheddar cheese, red onion, avocado, and tomato. It's topped with a zesty protein-packed avocado lime crema.

1½ pounds boneless sirloin steak

3 tablespoons avocado oil

1 tablespoon diced chipotle peppers (see note, page 81)

1 tablespoon chili powder

1 teaspoon garlic powder

1 teaspoon ground cumin

1 teaspoon dried oregano leaves

1 teaspoon salt

½ teaspoon ground black pepper

2 (10-ounce) bags frozen cauliflower rice

1 cup pico de gallo

1 cup shredded cheddar cheese

1 avocado, sliced

¼ medium red onion, thinly sliced

8 to 12 grape tomatoes, halved

FOR THE AVOCADO LIME CREMA

½ avocado

1 cup plain Greek or low-carb yogurt

¼ cup chopped fresh cilantro

1 tablespoon lime juice

½ teaspoon garlic powder

½ teaspoon salt

FOR GARNISH/SERVING

Chopped fresh cilantro

Lime wedges

1. Pat the steak dry with a paper towel. Place the steak in a shallow dish or zip-top bag.
2. To make the marinade, combine the avocado oil, diced chipotle peppers, chili powder, garlic powder, cumin, oregano, salt, and pepper in a small bowl.
3. Brush or rub the marinade all over the steak, until it's well coated. Let marinate for 30 minutes at room temperature.
4. Meanwhile, prepare the avocado lime crema. Put all the ingredients in a mini food processor or blender. Blend until smooth. Place in the refrigerator until ready to use.
5. To prepare the cauliflower rice, preheat a medium nonstick skillet over medium heat. Pour the frozen cauliflower rice into the dry skillet. Stirring occasionally, cook until the majority of the moisture has evaporated and the cauliflower is fluffy, 7 to 10 minutes. Remove the pan from the heat, but leave the rice in the pan for a few minutes to allow the residual heat from the pan to evaporate the remaining moisture.
6. Cook the steak using one of the following three methods:
   - To grill, preheat a grill to high heat (about 400°F). Grill the marinated steak for 2 minutes on each side. Then reduce the heat to medium or move to indirect heat and continue grilling for 9 to 12 minutes, until the internal temperature reaches 125°F to 130°F. Remove and let rest for 5 minutes before slicing into thin strips.
   - To cook on the stovetop, preheat a large cast-iron or other heavy skillet over medium-high heat. Place the steak in the hot skillet, being careful not to overcrowd the pan. Cook the steak for 3 minutes, then flip and cook for 2 minutes on the other side, or until

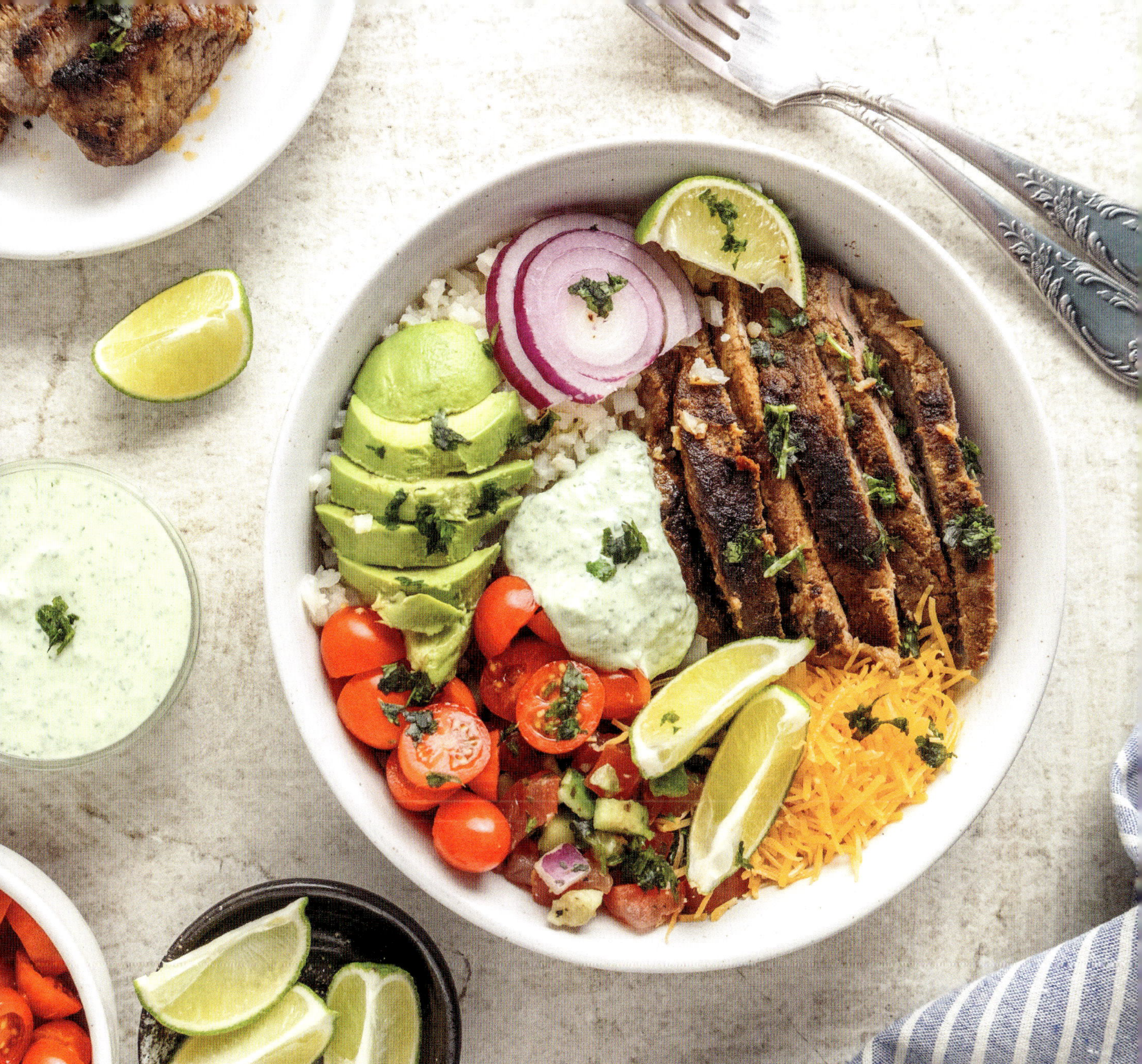

the internal temperature reaches 125°F to 130°F. Remove from the skillet and let rest for 5 minutes before slicing into thin strips.

- To air-fry, preheat the air fryer to 400°F. Put the steak in the air fryer tray or basket, air-fry for 5 minutes, then flip and air-fry for 5 minutes more. Remove and let rest for 5 minutes before slicing into thin strips.

7. To assemble the bowls, layer one-quarter of the cauliflower rice in each bowl. Top each with one-quarter of the sliced steak, pico de gallo, cheese, avocado slices, red onion, tomatoes, cilantro, lime wedges, and avocado lime crema.

(per bowl)
CALORIES: **664** | PROTEIN: **52.1g** | FAT: **41.6g** | TOTAL CARBS: **19.3g** | NET CARBS: **10.3g** | FIBER: **9g**

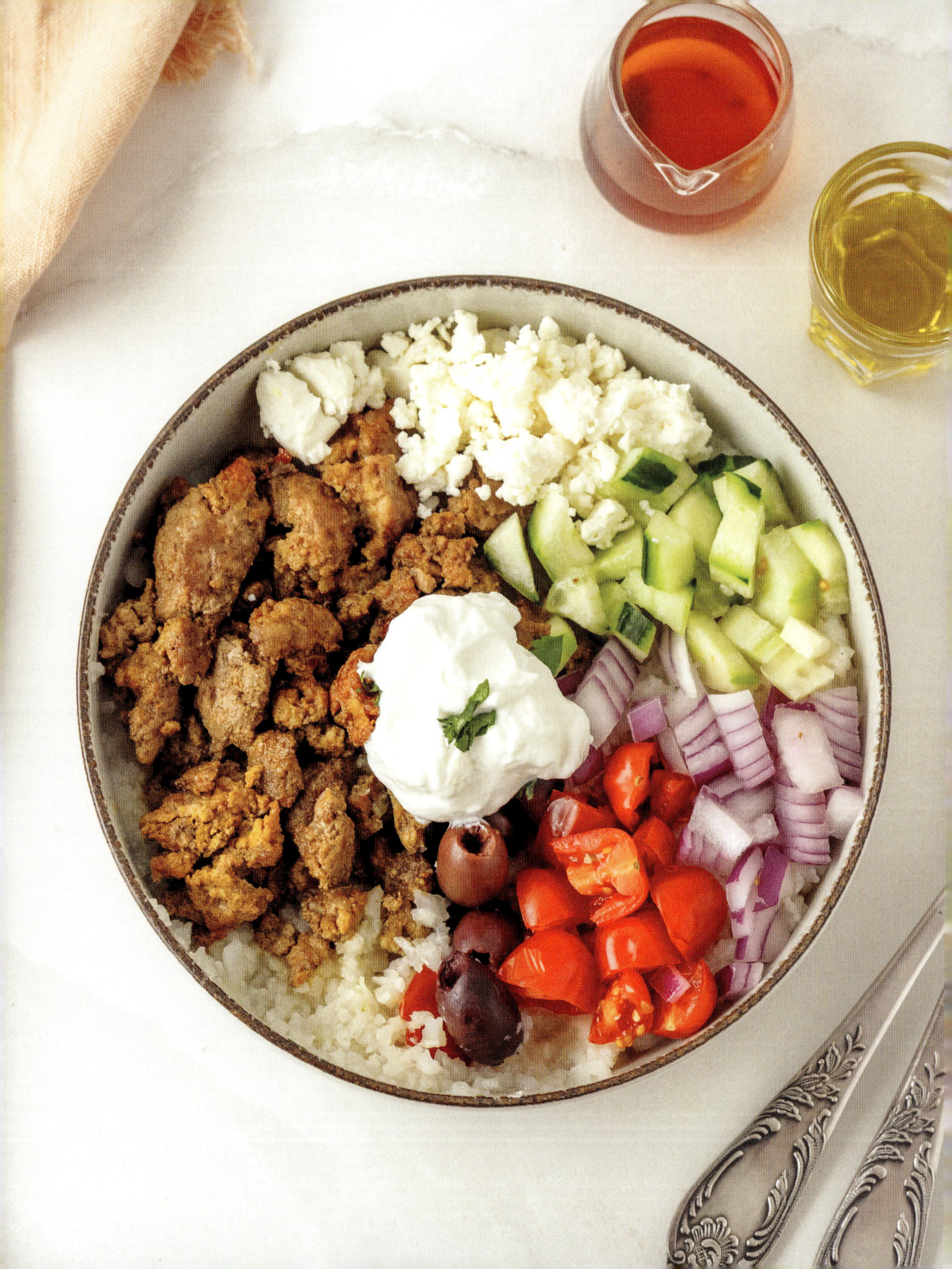

MEDITERRANEAN LAMB & "RICE" BOWLS

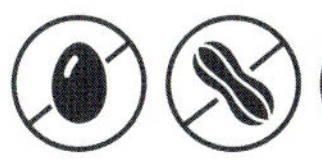
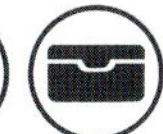

SERVES 3

PREP TIME: 10 minutes

COOK TIME: 20 minutes

These bowls use cauliflower rice in place of white rice and vibrant spices like cumin, turmeric, and allspice to season the lamb. Topped with Kalamata olives, cucumber, feta cheese, tomato, and red onion, each bowl has a distinct mix of Mediterranean flavors. A splash of olive oil and red wine vinegar and a dollop of Greek yogurt add a creamy, tangy finish.

---

1 (10-ounce) bag frozen cauliflower rice

1 tablespoon avocado oil

1 pound ground lamb

1 teaspoon salt

1 teaspoon ground coriander

1 teaspoon paprika

½ teaspoon ground cumin

½ teaspoon turmeric powder

¼ teaspoon ground allspice

¼ teaspoon red pepper flakes

12 pitted Kalamata olives

9 cherry tomatoes, quartered

½ medium cucumber, sliced and quartered

3 tablespoons diced red onions

¾ cup crumbled feta cheese

1½ tablespoons extra-virgin olive oil

1½ tablespoons red wine vinegar

6 tablespoons plain Greek or low-carb yogurt

Chopped fresh cilantro, for garnish (optional)

1. To prepare the cauliflower rice, preheat a medium nonstick skillet over medium heat. Pour the frozen cauliflower rice into the dry skillet and cook, stirring occasionally, until most of the moisture is cooked out, the bottom of the skillet is dry, and the rice is fluffy, 5 to 7 minutes. Transfer the cooked rice to a large bowl and set aside.
2. Wipe the skillet clean with a wet paper towel. Pour in the avocado oil and set over medium heat.
3. When the oil is hot, add the lamb and break it up into crumbles. Add the salt, coriander, paprika, cumin, turmeric, allspice, and red pepper flakes. Stir to combine, then continue cooking for 8 to 9 minutes, until the lamb is browned and cooked through. When done, slide the pan off the heat.
4. To assemble the bowls, divide the prepared cauliflower rice, olives, tomatoes, cucumber, red onions, and feta cheese evenly among three bowls. Drizzle ½ tablespoon of olive oil and ½ tablespoon of red wine vinegar over each bowl. Add one-third of the lamb to each bowl and top each with 2 tablespoons of yogurt. Garnish with cilantro, if desired.

(per bowl)
CALORIES: **657** | PROTEIN: **34.6g** | FAT: **53.2g** | TOTAL CARBS: **12.2g** | NET CARBS: **7.7g** | FIBER: **4.5g**

COCONUT CURRY LAMB MEATBALLS

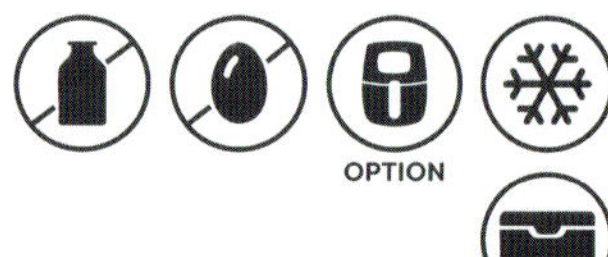

SERVES 5

PREP TIME: 8 to 16 minutes, depending on method

COOK TIME: 40 minutes

These bold-flavored meatballs are easy to cook using an oven, stovetop, or air fryer. After which, they are simmered in a rich, aromatic curry sauce made with Roma tomatoes, onion, coconut milk, and a blend of vibrant spices. Perfect for meal prep, they're easy to portion out with a side of cauliflower rice.

FOR THE MEATBALLS

1 pound ground lamb (80/20)

½ medium onion, grated

¼ cup blanched, super-fine almond flour

1 tablespoon chopped fresh cilantro

1 tablespoon garam masala

1 tablespoon turmeric powder

1 teaspoon salt

½ teaspoon ground black pepper

FOR THE CURRY SAUCE

5 Roma tomatoes

1 tablespoon coconut oil

½ medium onion, diced

3 cloves garlic, minced

1 teaspoon ground coriander

1 teaspoon ground cumin

1 teaspoon garam masala

¾ teaspoon ginger powder

½ teaspoon turmeric powder

¼ teaspoon ground cinnamon

1 (14-ounce) can unsweetened full-fat coconut milk

FOR SERVING (OPTIONAL)

Chopped fresh cilantro

Cooked cauliflower rice

1. Put all the ingredients for the meatballs in a large bowl and mix with clean hands until well combined. Form into twenty 1-inch meatballs.
2. Cook the meatballs using one of the following methods until the internal temperature is 135°F to 145°F:
   - Oven: Preheat the oven to 350°F. Line a rimmed baking sheet with parchment paper. Place the meatballs on the prepared pan and bake for 12 to 15 minutes.
   - Stovetop: Preheat a large skillet over medium-high heat, then place the meatballs in the pan, keeping them from touching each other. Cook for 8 minutes, then flip them and cook for another 8 minutes.
   - Air fryer: Preheat the air fryer to 400°F. Lightly spray the basket with cooking oil, then carefully place the meatballs in the basket. Air-fry for 8 minutes, shaking the meatballs at the 4-minute mark.
3. While the meatballs are cooking, make the sauce. Trim and discard the tomato tops, then put the tomatoes in a food processor or blender and blend until smooth.
4. Pour the coconut oil into a large nonstick skillet over medium heat. Add the onion and sauté for about 2 minutes, until softened.
5. Add the garlic and spices and fry for about 2 minutes, stirring often so the spices don't burn.
6. Add the pureed tomatoes and cook for about 8 minutes to combine the flavors and reduce some water from the tomatoes.
7. Stir in the coconut milk, then simmer for 10 minutes.
8. Add the meatballs and stir, simmering for 3 to 4 minutes.
9. If desired, garnish with cilantro and serve with cauliflower rice.

(per serving)
CALORIES: **561** | PROTEIN: **22.7g** | FAT: **45.8g** | TOTAL CARBS: **13.8g** | NET CARBS: **10.5g** | FIBER: **3.3g**

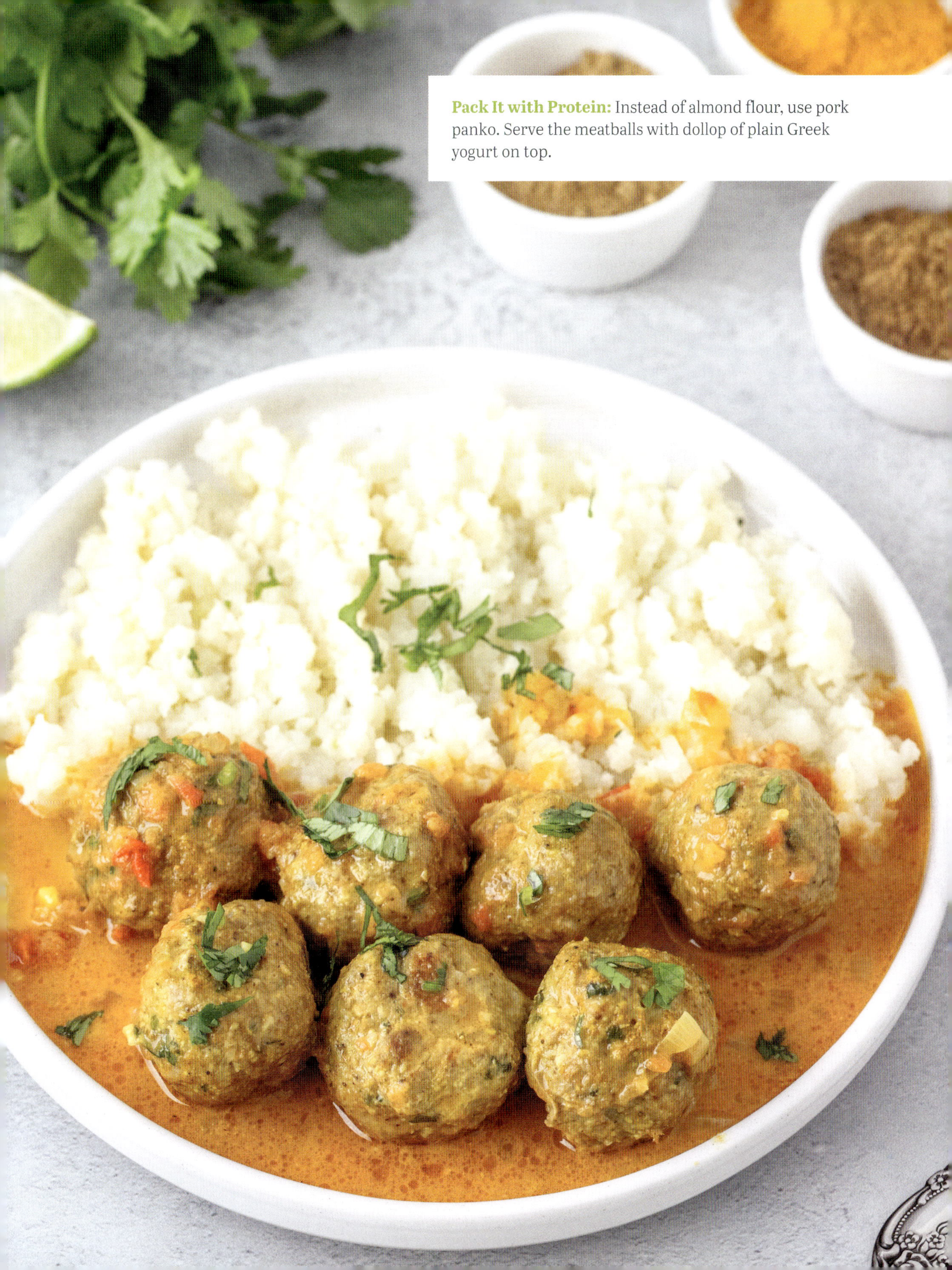

Pack It with Protein: Instead of almond flour, use pork panko. Serve the meatballs with dollop of plain Greek yogurt on top.

MIGHTY GREEK LAMB CHOPS

SERVES 4

PREP TIME: 20 minutes, plus 1 hour to marinate

COOK TIME: 8 or 15 minutes, depending on method

These Greek-inspired lamb chops are marinated in a fragrant mix of herbs and spices and then grilled or seared to create a golden crust with a juicy, medium-rare interior. While the chops are marinating, you'll whip up a high-protein tzatziki sauce from Greek yogurt, cucumber, and a few aromatics, along with a simple salad of tomatoes, cucumbers, mint, onions, garlic, and feta. This is a meal you can save for a special night in or when you are wanting something different.

---

4 bone-in lamb chops (1 inch thick)

FOR THE MARINADE

2 cloves garlic, grated

1 tablespoon dried oregano leaves

1 tablespoon chopped (aka cracked or crushed) dried rosemary needles

1½ teaspoons smoked paprika

½ teaspoon dried thyme leaves

½ teaspoon ground cumin

Grated zest and juice of ½ lemon

2 tablespoons extra-virgin olive oil

1 tablespoon sugar-free honey

1 teaspoon salt

FOR THE TZATZIKI SAUCE

¾ cup plain Greek or low-carb yogurt

½ English cucumber, seeded and finely chopped

3 cloves garlic, minced

1½ tablespoons extra-virgin olive oil

1½ teaspoons lemon juice

1 tablespoon chopped fresh dill, or 1 teaspoon dried dill weed

½ teaspoon salt

½ teaspoon ground black pepper

FOR THE GREEK SALAD

1 cup sliced cherry tomatoes

1 cup diced cucumbers

2 tablespoons minced fresh mint

1 tablespoon diced red onions

1 clove garlic, minced

¼ cup crumbled feta cheese

1 tablespoon extra-virgin olive oil

1 tablespoon Dijon mustard

1 tablespoon lemon juice

Salt and pepper

1. Pat the lamb chops dry with a paper towel and trim the excess fat, if needed. Place in a zip-top bag or shallow baking dish.
2. In a small bowl, combine the grated garlic, oregano, rosemary, smoked paprika, thyme, cumin, lemon zest and juice, olive oil, honey, and salt. Pour the marinade over the chops and turn to evenly coat. Let marinate for 1 hour at room temperature, flipping every 15 minutes to ensure the meat is evenly marinated.
3. While the chops are marinating, prepare the tzatziki sauce and salad. For the sauce, put all the ingredients in a medium bowl and mix well. Cover and chill in the refrigerator for at least 30 minutes, or until ready to eat.
4. For the salad, toss together the tomatoes, cucumbers, mint, onions, garlic, feta, olive oil, mustard, and lemon juice in a large bowl. Season with salt and pepper to taste. Set aside.
5. Remove the lamb chops from the marinade, discarding the marinade. Cook the chops using either of the following methods:
    - Grill: Preheat a grill to medium-high heat (about 400°F). Place the chops on the grill and cook with the lid closed for 2 to 4 minutes per side, until the internal temperature registers 135°F to 140°F. Let rest for 5 minutes before serving.

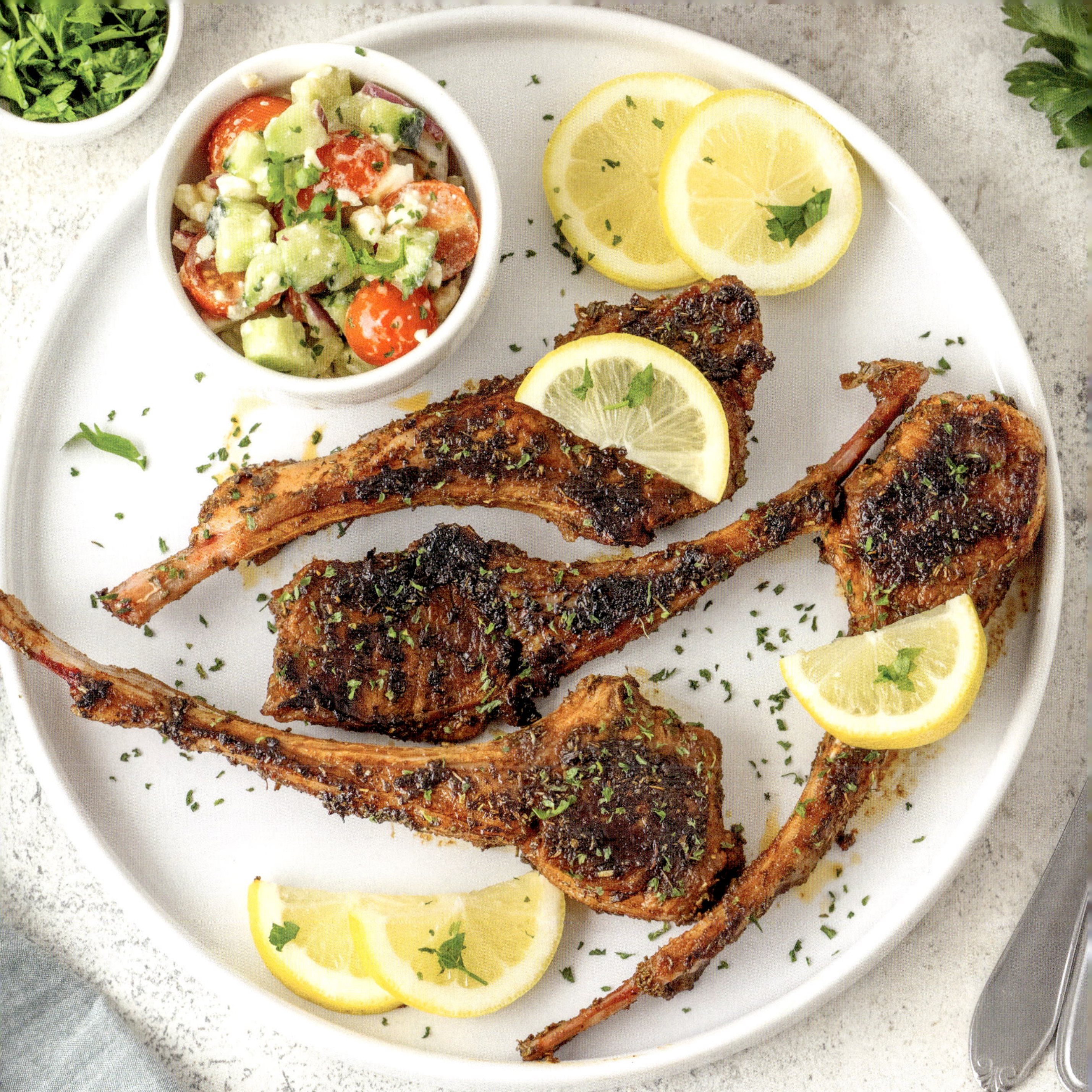

- Stovetop: Preheat a large skillet over medium-high heat. Place the chops in the hot pan and cook for 2 to 4 minutes, flip, and cook for 2 to 4 more minutes. Repeat these steps until the internal temperature reaches 135°F to 140°F. Remove from the pan and let rest for 5 minutes before serving.

6. Serve the chops with the salad and a generous helping of tzatziki.

(per serving)
CALORIES: **661** | PROTEIN: **34.3g** | FAT: **55.7g** | TOTAL CARBS: **11.7g** | NET CARBS: **5.7g** | FIBER: **3.5g**
SUGAR ALCOHOLS: **2.5g**

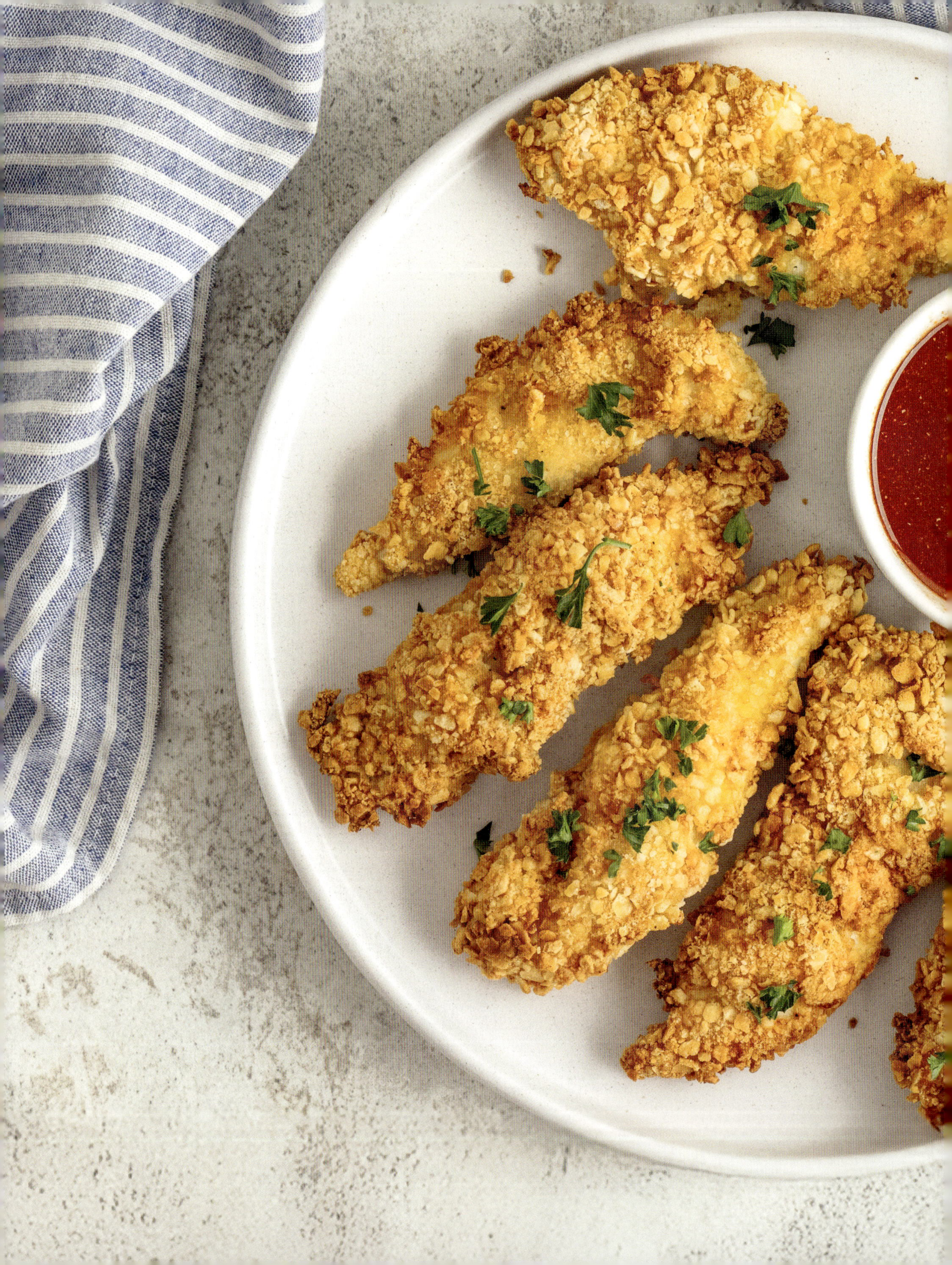

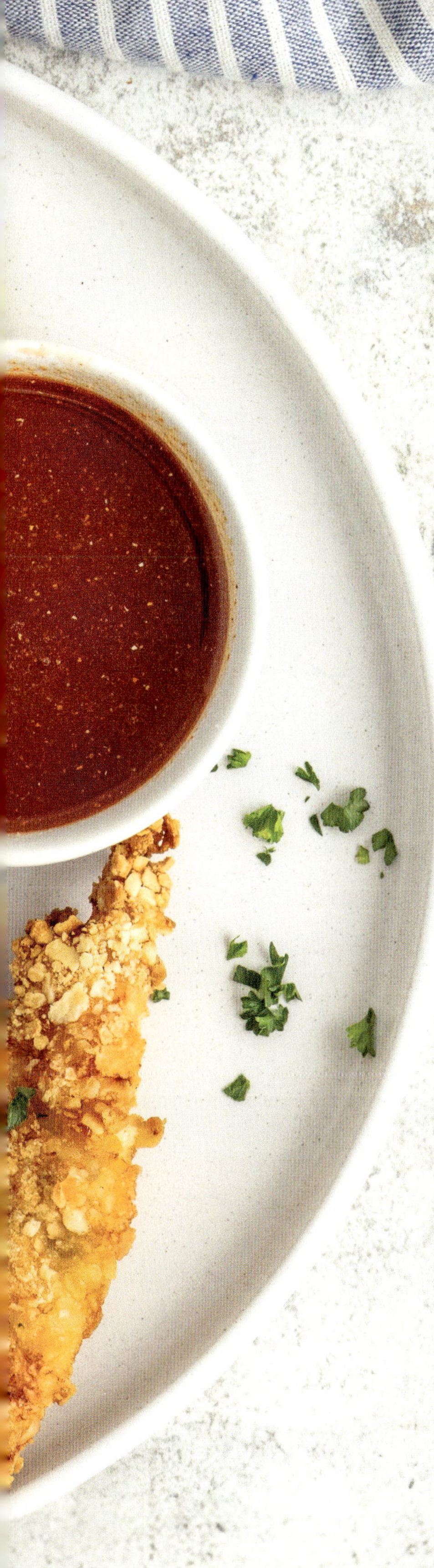

POULTRY

CASHEW CHICKEN & COCONUT RICE

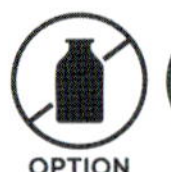

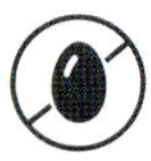
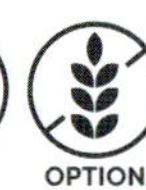

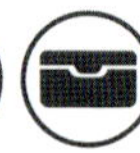

SERVES 6
PREP TIME: 15 minutes
COOK TIME: 25 minutes

When I first made this recipe, I knew I had a winner since my kids ate most of it before I could dish up a portion for myself. I've since adjusted the ingredients to use more protein since that was their favorite part. This dish is a delicious combination of chicken, broccoli, and roasted cashews tossed in a buttery ginger chili sauce. Served over coconut cauliflower rice, it's a perfect balance of savory, nutty, and sweet flavors.

---

4 tablespoons avocado oil, divided

2 pounds boneless, skinless chicken thighs, cubed

1 tablespoon arrowroot powder

1 teaspoon ground black pepper

2 cups broccoli florets, cut into bite-size pieces

1 medium onion, diced, divided

3 tablespoons salted butter

7 cloves garlic, minced, divided

1 teaspoon ginger powder

1 cup whole roasted and salted cashews

⅓ cup soy sauce or tamari

⅓ cup sweet chili sauce

2 tablespoons unseasoned rice vinegar

2 (10-ounce) bags frozen cauliflower rice

½ teaspoon salt

1 cup canned unsweetened full-fat coconut milk

FOR GARNISH (OPTIONAL)

Sesame seeds

Sliced green onions

Grated lime zest

Chopped fresh cilantro

Finely diced jalapeño peppers

1. Preheat a large skillet over medium-high heat. Pour in 2 tablespoons of the avocado oil. Once the oil is rippling, add the cubed chicken, arrowroot powder, and pepper. Stir to evenly coat the chicken in the arrowroot powder and pepper. Sauté until browned and cooked through, 5 to 7 minutes. Remove the chicken from the skillet and set aside.
2. Lower the heat to medium, then put the broccoli florets and half of the diced onion in the skillet. Give it a stir, then mix in the butter, a little more than half of the minced garlic, the ginger powder, and cashews. Cook for 2 minutes, stirring occasionally. Stir in the soy sauce, chili sauce, and vinegar. Cook until the sauce thickens slightly. Stir in the cooked chicken until coated in the sauce. Remove the pan from the heat.
3. Heat the remaining 2 tablespoons of oil in a separate large skillet over medium heat for 1 minute. Add the remaining diced onion and cook for about 2 minutes, stirring constantly. Add the remaining minced garlic and sauté for an additional minute, stirring often so it doesn't burn.
4. Add the cauliflower rice and salt to the skillet and cook, stirring occasionally, for 5 to 7 minutes, until most of the liquid has evaporated and the rice is no longer steaming.
5. Pour in the coconut milk and cook, stirring occasionally, until the liquid has evaporated and the cauliflower rice is cooked through, about 5 minutes.
6. Season with salt and pepper to your liking.
7. Pour the cashew chicken mixture over the coconut rice. Top with your choice of garnishes.

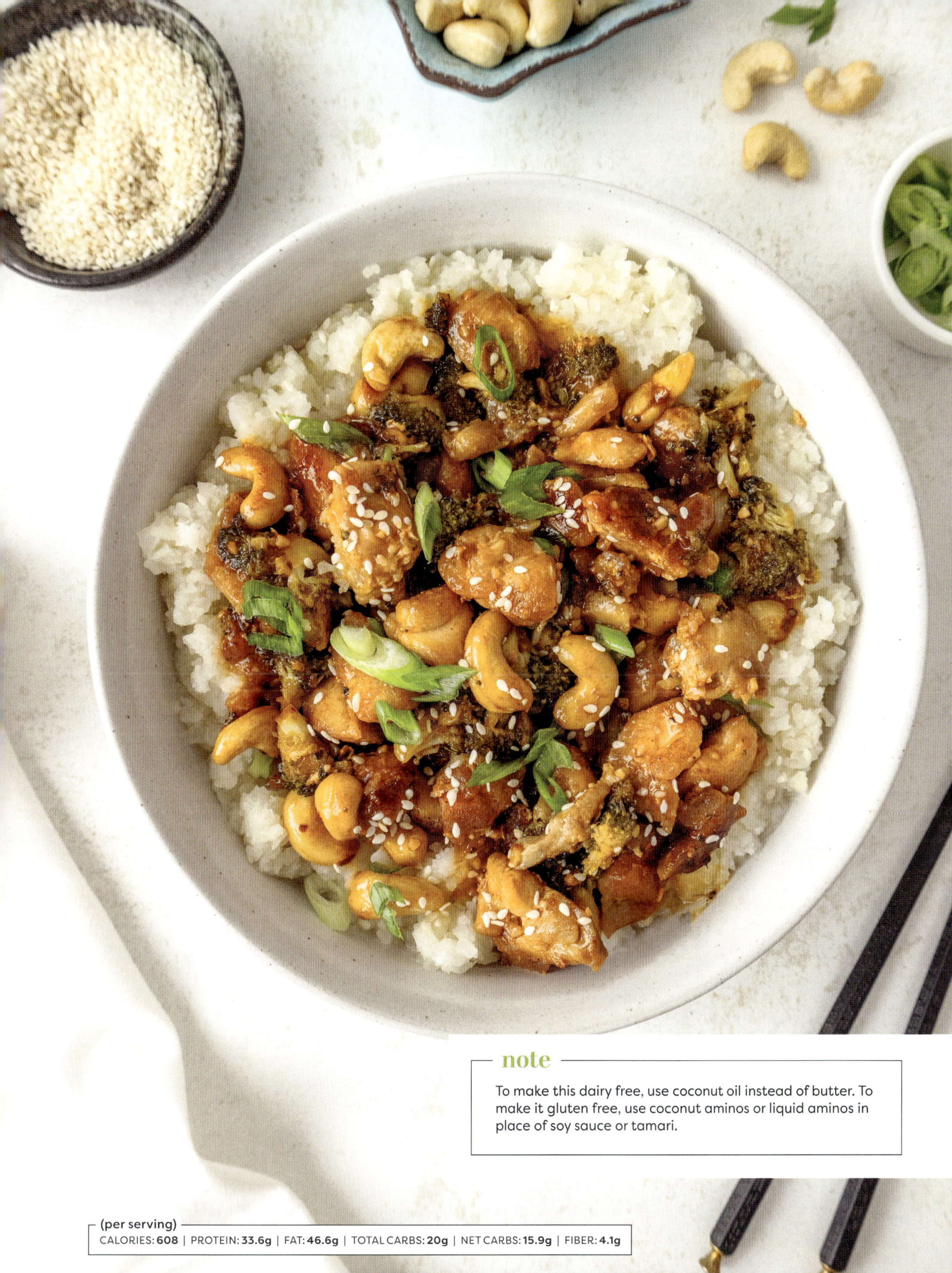

note

To make this dairy free, use coconut oil instead of butter. To make it gluten free, use coconut aminos or liquid aminos in place of soy sauce or tamari.

(per serving)
CALORIES: **608** | PROTEIN: **33.6g** | FAT: **46.6g** | TOTAL CARBS: **20g** | NET CARBS: **15.9g** | FIBER: **4.1g**

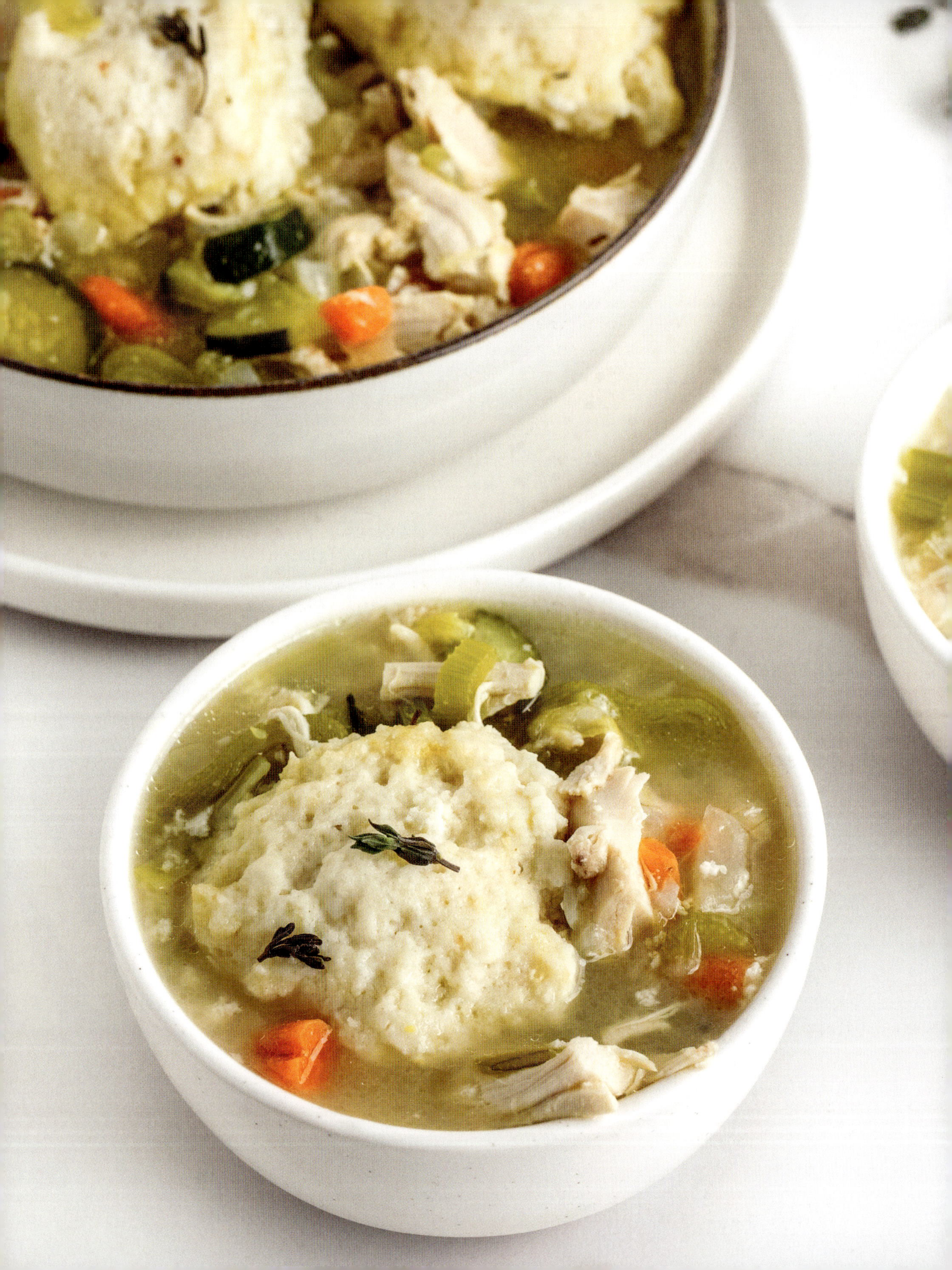

CHICKEN & DUMPLING SOUP

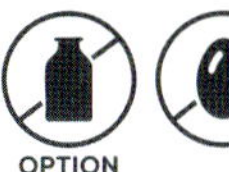

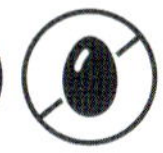

SERVES 6

PREP TIME: 15 minutes (not including time to cook chicken)

COOK TIME: 25 minutes

This soup is the ultimate comfort food for a chilly day when you don't feel like putting in a lot of effort. The low-carb dumplings are made with almond flour and protein powder, which not only helps make them spongy to soak up all that delicious broth but adds extra protein as well. Using precooked rotisserie chicken makes this recipe come together in no time. I used white meat here, but you could also use dark meat or a mix of both.

FOR THE SOUP

¼ cup (½ stick) salted butter

½ leek, cleaned well and sliced (see notes)

4 celery stalks, chopped

½ medium onion, diced

¼ cup chopped carrots

3 cups shredded cooked chicken

1 medium zucchini, cut into half-moons

4 cups chicken broth

½ to 1 teaspoon salt, to taste

½ teaspoon ground black pepper

FOR THE DUMPLINGS

1 cup blanched, super-fine almond flour

½ cup unflavored protein powder

1¼ teaspoons baking powder

1 teaspoon xanthan gum

½ teaspoon salt

¼ teaspoon onion powder

½ cup boiling water

Fresh or dried thyme, for garnish (optional)

1. In an 8-quart stockpot or Dutch oven, melt the butter over medium heat. Add the leek, celery, onion, and carrots and cook until softened, 3 to 5 minutes.
2. Add the chicken, zucchini, broth, ½ teaspoon of the salt, and the pepper. Bring to a boil. Once boiling, turn the heat to low and let simmer while you prepare the dumplings.
3. In a small bowl, mix together the almond flour, protein powder, baking powder, xanthan gum, salt, and onion powder.
4. Pour in the boiling water and stir with a rubber spatula until just combined.
5. To form the dumplings, it's best to use wet hands to keep the dough from sticking. Grab a chunk of dough and roll it into a ball. Repeat with the rest of the dough to make a total of 6 to 8 dumpling balls.
6. Evenly lay the dumpling balls on top of the lightly simmering chicken soup. (*Note:* If your soup is too hot when adding the dumplings, they will not hold up and will dissolve into the soup. You may want to slide the pot off the heat to slightly cool before adding the dumplings, then return the pot to the lowest setting.)
7. Cover the pot and steam the dumplings for 10 minutes, or until set on the outside and spongy inside. Remove the pot from the heat and serve. Garnish with thyme, if desired.

notes

To clean a leek, slice it in half lengthwise. Peel back the first few layers of the white portion and rinse thoroughly under running water to remove any dirt or grit between the layers. Then lay it flat and slice crosswise into thin half-moons.

This soup doesn't freeze well because of the dumplings, but you can refrigerate it and enjoy the leftovers over the next few days.

To make this dairy free, use avocado oil instead of butter.

(per serving)
CALORIES: **401** | PROTEIN: **42.7g** | FAT: **19.8g** | TOTAL CARBS: **12.6g** | NET CARBS: **7.9g** | FIBER: **4.7g**

CHICKEN & SPINACH CARBONARA

SERVES 6

PREP TIME: 10 minutes

COOK TIME: 20 minutes

This 30-minute meal is a rich and satisfying dish featuring chunks of chicken, crispy bacon, garlic, and spinach, all tossed in a velvety cheese sauce. Made with eggs and Parmesan cheese, the sauce achieves its creamy texture naturally—no thickener or heavy cream needed. Pair it with my protein noodles or your favorite low-carb noodles.

1½ pounds boneless, skinless chicken thighs, cubed

1 teaspoon salt

1 teaspoon ground black pepper

6 slices regular-cut bacon, chopped

4 cloves garlic, minced

½ cup chicken broth, plus more if needed

3 large eggs

1½ cups grated Parmesan cheese

4 cups baby spinach

6 servings Protein Noodles (page 253) or your favorite low-carb, high-protein pasta, cooked and drained

Chopped fresh parsley, for garnish (optional)

1. Season the chicken with the salt and pepper. Set aside.
2. Cook the bacon in a large skillet over medium heat until crispy, about 5 minutes. Transfer the bacon to a paper towel–lined plate. Leave 2 tablespoons of the bacon grease in the skillet. Return the pan to medium heat.
3. Cook the chicken in the bacon grease until browned and cooked through, 5 to 6 minutes. (When done, the chicken will no longer be pink at the center.) Transfer the chicken to a bowl and set aside.
4. In the same skillet, cook the garlic over medium heat until fragrant, about 30 seconds. Stir in the broth and scrape up any brown bits. Simmer for 2 minutes, then turn the heat down to low.
5. Whisk together the eggs and Parmesan in a medium bowl.
6. Slowly stir the egg mixture into the skillet and cook, stirring continuously, until smooth. Add the spinach and stir until wilted. Stir in the bacon and chicken. Add more broth if the sauce is too thick.
7. Serve over protein noodles. Garnish with chopped parsley, if desired.

notes

For the best flavor, use freshly grated Parmesan cheese.

If using protein noodles prepared ahead of time and stored in the refrigerator, reheat them in the microwave for 20 to 30 seconds, until warmed.

(per serving)

CALORIES: **640** | PROTEIN: **52g** | FAT: **45g** | TOTAL CARBS: **10.1g** | NET CARBS: **3.3g** | FIBER: **6.8g**

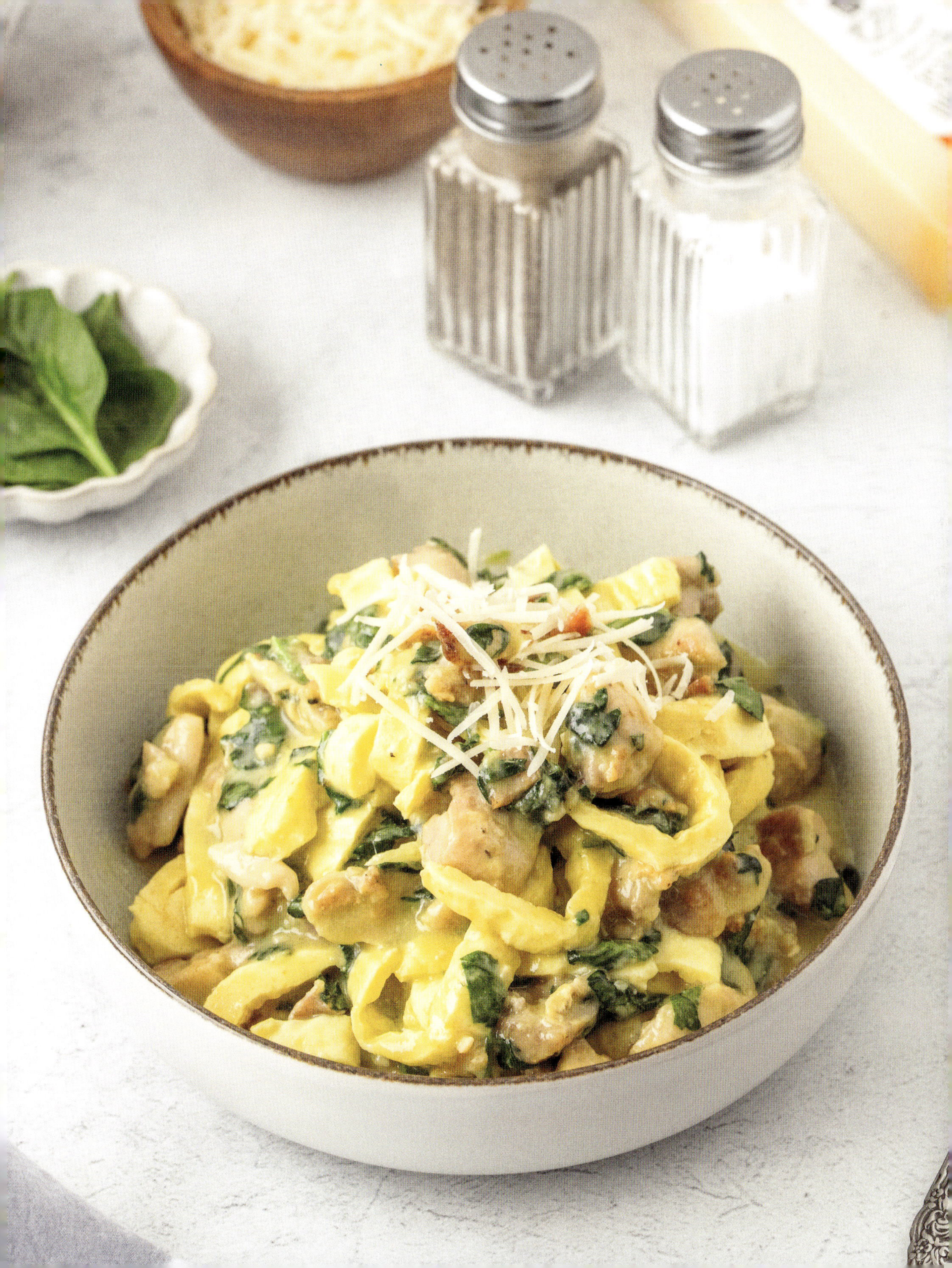

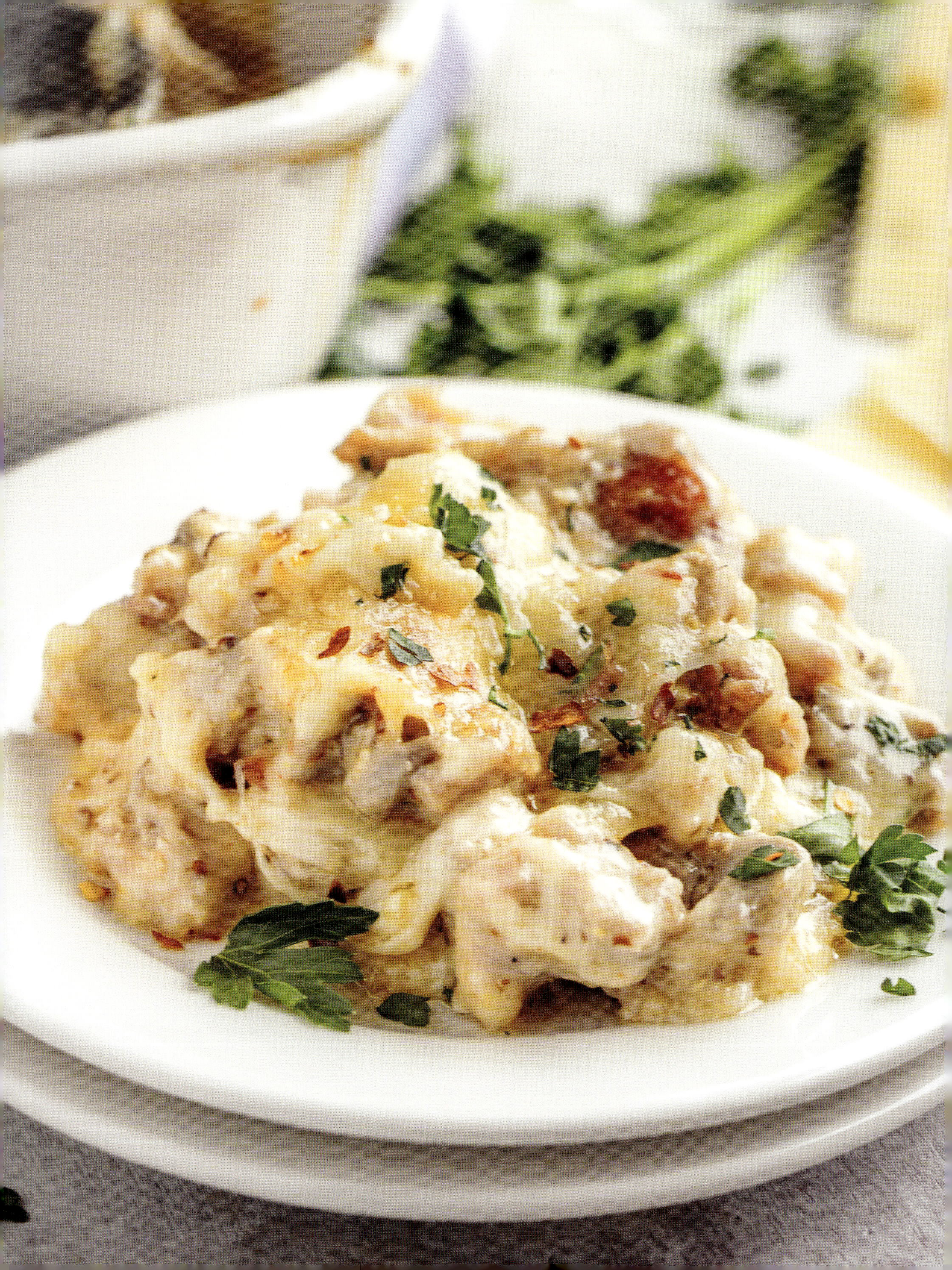

CHICKEN CORDON BLEU CASSEROLE

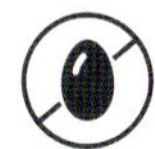

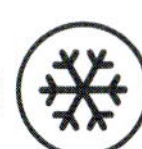
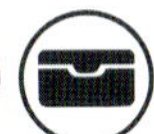

SERVES 6

PREP TIME: 15 minutes

COOK TIME: 45 minutes

A fuss-free way to enjoy the classic flavors of chicken cordon bleu is to turn it into a casserole! This deconstructed version combines the iconic taste of Dijon mustard and white wine sauce with layers of chicken, ham, and Swiss cheese—all baked together in one dish. By skipping the breading step of the original, you get the same rich, comforting flavors with less carbs and also less hassle and mess, making it a perfect recipe for busy weeknights.

1 tablespoon avocado oil

2 pounds boneless, skinless chicken breasts or thighs, cubed

8 ounces precooked ham, cut into bite-size pieces (see notes)

2 tablespoons salted butter

⅓ cup heavy cream

¼ cup chicken broth

¼ cup dry white wine (see notes)

1½ cups shredded Monterey Jack cheese

2 tablespoons Dijon mustard

½ teaspoon red pepper flakes (optional), plus more for garnish if desired

¼ teaspoon cayenne pepper (optional)

¼ teaspoon salt

¼ teaspoon ground black pepper

1½ cups shredded Swiss cheese

Chopped fresh parsley, for garnish (optional)

1. Preheat the oven to 350°F. Have on hand a 9-inch square or 10 by 8-inch rectangular baking dish.
2. Preheat a large skillet over medium-high heat and pour in the avocado oil. Working in batches, sear the chicken until golden brown on all sides, 3 to 4 minutes per batch. Transfer the chicken to a large bowl and set aside.
3. Put the ham in the skillet and cook for 2 to 3 minutes to heat through and lightly brown. Remove to the bowl with the chicken.
4. Lower the heat to medium. Melt the butter in the skillet. Slowly whisk the cream, broth, and wine into the melted butter. Scrape the bottom of the skillet to break up the brown bits stuck to the bottom. Simmer gently for 1 to 3 minutes, but don't allow it to boil. Add the Monterey Jack a handful at a time, stirring until melted after each addition.
5. Stir in the mustard, red pepper flakes (if using), cayenne (if using), salt, and black pepper. Remove the pan from the heat.
6. Stir the chicken and ham pieces to evenly distribute them, then transfer them to the baking dish. Pour on the cheese sauce and top with the Swiss. Bake for 20 to 25 minutes, until the cheese is melted and bubbly. Let rest for 3 to 5 minutes before serving. Garnish with parsley and/or red pepper flakes, if desired.

notes

Look for precooked ham that is low in sugar.

If you prefer to avoid alcohol, double the amount of chicken broth used to deglaze the pan in Step 4, using ½ cup broth total, and add 1 tablespoon lemon juice to brighten the flavor.

(per serving)

CALORIES: **558** | PROTEIN: **47.3g** | FAT: **39.1g** | TOTAL CARBS: **1.6g** | NET CARBS: **1.5g** | FIBER: **0.1g**

CHICKEN CRUST PIZZA

  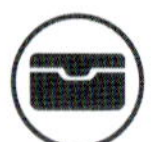

SERVES 4
PREP TIME: 10 minutes
COOK TIME: 20 minutes

This versatile pizza crust is a very low-carb, protein-packed base that is made without nut flours or coconut flour. Made from ground chicken, it can be kept thick or pressed out super thin for a crispier texture; just increase or decrease the bake time accordingly. Finish it with a classic red sauce and cheese and, if desired, your favorite pizza toppings.

FOR THE CHICKEN CRUST

1 pound ground chicken

1 large egg

½ cup shredded mozzarella cheese

¼ cup grated Parmesan cheese

1 teaspoon salt

1 teaspoon Italian seasoning

½ teaspoon garlic powder

FOR THE TOPPINGS

3 tablespoons low-carb marinara sauce

1 cup shredded mozzarella cheese

ADDITIONAL TOPPINGS (OPTIONAL)

Pepperoni

Salami

Sliced black olives

Sliced mushrooms

Torn fresh basil leaves

1. Preheat the oven to 450°F. Line a rimmed baking sheet or pizza pan with parchment paper.
2. In a medium bowl, combine all the ingredients for the crust using clean hands or a spoon. Form the mixture into a ball.
3. Place the ball in the center of the prepared pan, flatten with your palm, and press it out into a round pizza crust shape that is about ½ inch thick.
4. Bake for 15 minutes, or until the crust is golden brown on top and no longer pink in the center.
5. Top with the marinara sauce and cheese and, if desired, other toppings of your choice. Turn the oven to the high broil setting. Return the pizza to the oven to broil on the top rack until the cheese is melted.

(per serving)
CALORIES: **351** | PROTEIN: **38.7g** | FAT: **21.9g** | TOTAL CARBS: **2.6g** | NET CARBS: **2.3g** | FIBER: **0.3g**

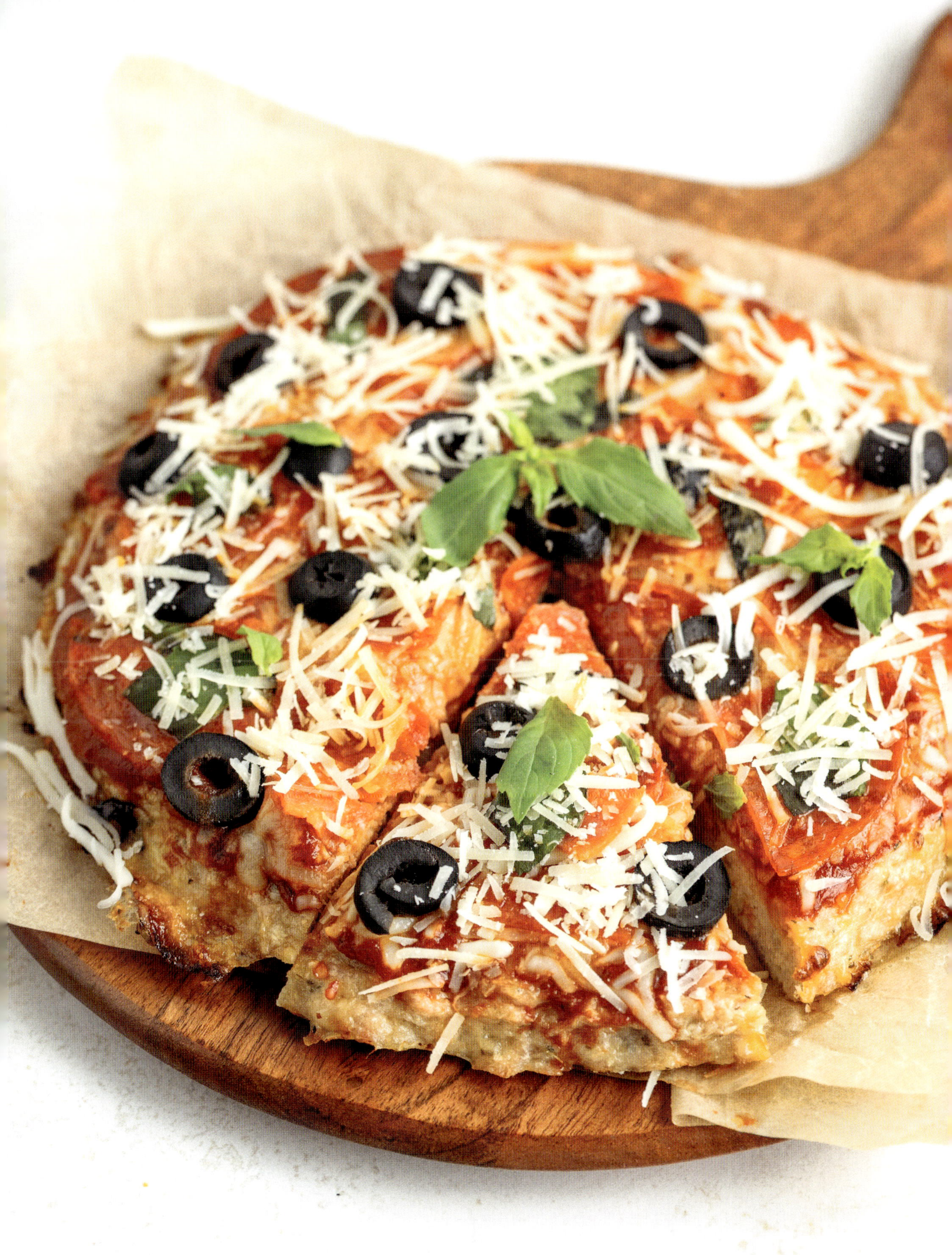

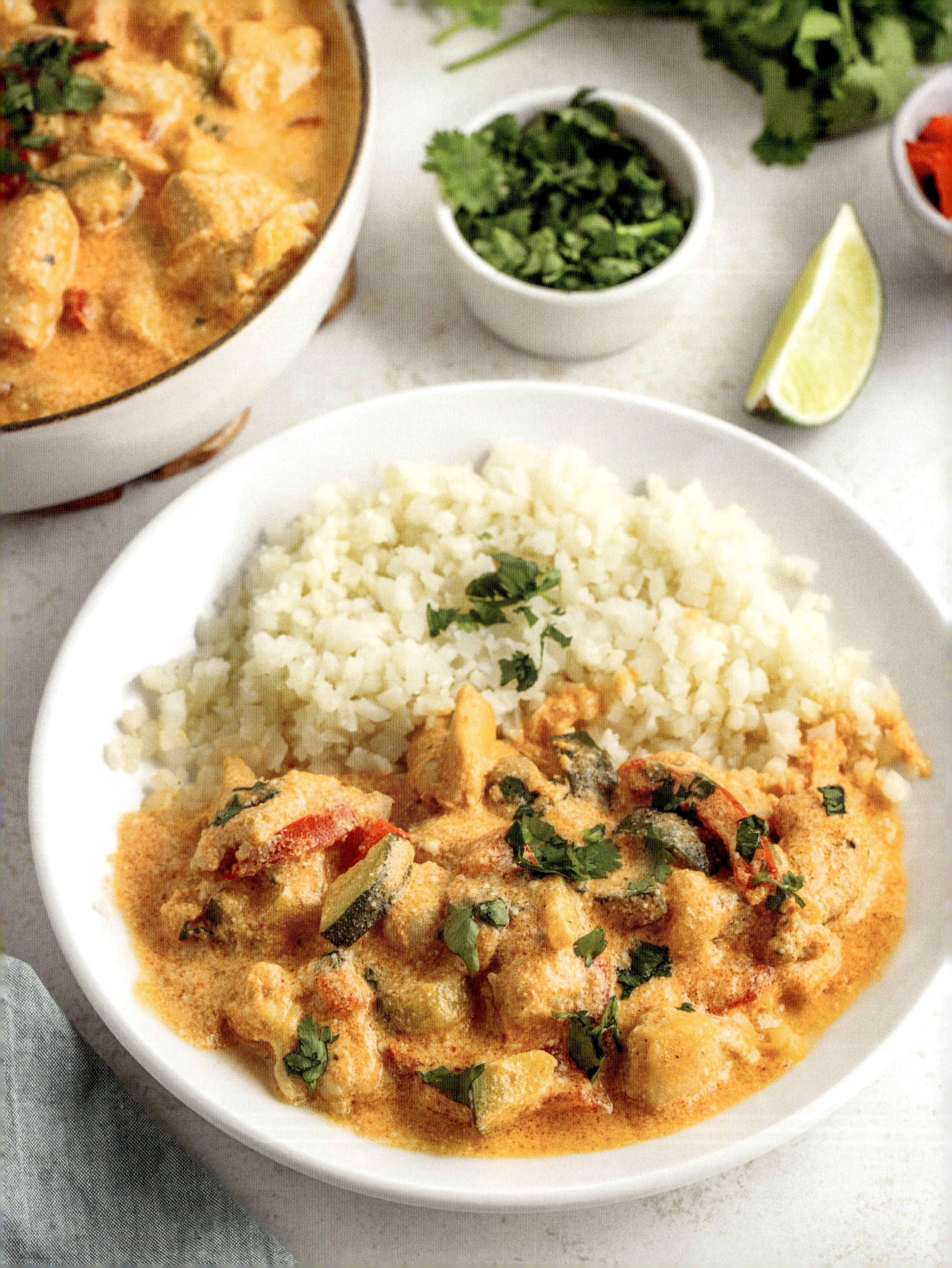

CHICKEN CURRY

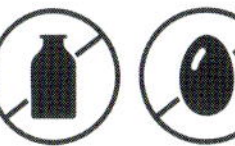
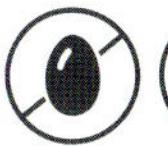
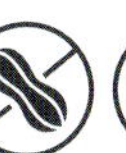
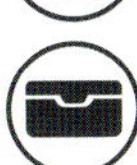

SERVES 4
PREP TIME: 15 minutes
COOK TIME: 30 minutes

This curry is a quick and easy dish made with a few simple ingredients. Red curry paste, fish sauce, lime juice, and coconut milk create a rich, flavorful base. Zucchini and red bell pepper add color, flavor, and fiber, but you can use other low-carb vegetables like snap peas, broccoli, and green bell pepper. I serve this curry with cauliflower rice for a complete meal that is full of good fats and protein and keeps you feeling full.

---

1 (10-ounce) bag frozen cauliflower rice

2 tablespoons coconut oil or avocado oil

1½ pounds boneless, skinless chicken thighs, cubed

Salt and pepper

2 (14-ounce) cans unsweetened full-fat coconut milk, divided

3 tablespoons red curry paste

2 teaspoons lime juice

1 teaspoon fish sauce

1 medium zucchini, diced

½ red bell pepper, julienned

Chopped fresh cilantro, for garnish

1. Preheat a large skillet over medium heat. Pour the frozen cauliflower rice into the dry skillet. Cook, stirring occasionally, until most of the moisture has evaporated and the rice is fluffy, 5 to 7 minutes. Transfer the rice to a bowl and set aside.
2. In the same skillet, heat the oil over medium-high heat. Add the cubed chicken, season generously with salt and pepper, and sauté, stirring occasionally, until lightly browned and cooked through (it will no longer be pink inside). Remove the pan from the heat and set aside.
3. Meanwhile, pour one can of coconut milk into a medium saucepan. Heat over medium-high heat until it boils. Lower the heat to medium and continue cooking at a medium boil until the milk has reduced by one-third to one-half.
4. Stir in the curry paste, then pour in the second can of coconut milk. Bring to a boil over medium heat and cook until the sauce has thickened, 5 to 10 minutes.
5. Stir in the lime juice, fish sauce, zucchini, and ½ teaspoon of salt. Cook for 2 minutes. Add the bell pepper and cooked chicken and cook for 1 minute.
6. Serve with the prepared cauliflower rice. Garnish with chopped cilantro.

(per serving)
CALORIES: **612** | PROTEIN: **37g** | FAT: **44g** | TOTAL CARBS: **13.5g** | NET CARBS: **11g** | FIBER: **2.5g**

CHICKEN POT PIE SOUP

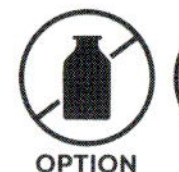
OPTION
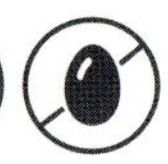
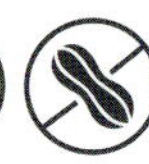
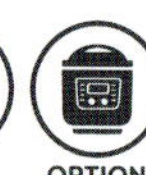
OPTION

OPTION
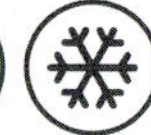
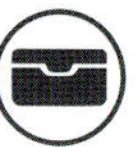

SERVES 4

PREP TIME: 10 minutes

COOK TIME: 35 minutes to 4 hours 15 minutes, depending on method

This soup has the comforting flavors of classic chicken pot pie, but without the crust or extra calories. Packed with tender chunks of chicken, veggies, and savory seasonings, it's hearty, filling, and gives over 40 grams of protein per 2-cup serving. Pair it with your favorite low-carb bread or stir in some of my protein noodles (page 253) if you need a little extra protein. When making this soup, you have the option of using the stovetop or a slow cooker or Instant Pot.

---

3 tablespoons salted butter

2 pounds boneless, skinless chicken breasts, cut into ½-inch cubes

8 ounces sliced mushrooms

2 cups chopped celery

½ cup chopped carrots

½ cup diced onions

½ cup fresh green beans, cut into 1-inch pieces

1 teaspoon salt

1 tablespoon fresh thyme leaves, or 1 teaspoon dried thyme leaves, plus more for garnish if desired

3 cloves garlic, minced

2 cups chicken broth

6 ounces frozen cauliflower rice

2 tablespoons chopped fresh parsley, plus more for garnish if desired

½ teaspoon ground black pepper

note

To make this dairy free, use avocado oil in place of the butter.

STOVETOP INSTRUCTIONS:

1. In a Dutch oven or other large heavy-bottomed pot, melt the butter over medium-high heat. Working in batches, sear the chicken in the butter until golden brown on all sides, 5 to 7 minutes. (It will not be cooked all the way through at this point, as it will continue to cook as the soup simmers.) Return all the chicken to the pot.
2. Lower the heat to medium. Add the mushrooms, celery, carrots, onions, green beans, salt, and thyme. Cook until the vegetables are softened, about 8 minutes. Stir in the garlic and cook for another minute, or until fragrant.
3. Stir in the broth and scrape the brown bits off the bottom of the pot to incorporate their flavor into the broth. Bring to a simmer, then stir in the frozen cauliflower rice. Simmer for 10 minutes, or until the rice is heated through.
4. Remove the pot from the heat and stir in the parsley and pepper. Add salt to taste if needed. Ladle into bowls and top with more parsley and/or thyme, if desired.

INSTANT POT INSTRUCTIONS:

1. Turn the Instant Pot to the Sauté function. Put the butter in the Instant Pot. Once melted, add half of the cubed chicken and sear until lightly browned on all sides, 5 to 7 minutes. Remove the seared chicken and repeat with the other half of the chicken.
2. Return all the chicken to the Instant Pot. Add the mushrooms, celery, carrots, onions, green beans, salt, thyme, garlic, and broth and stir to combine. Secure the lid and set the vent to sealing. Pressure-cook on high for 10 minutes. Allow the Instant Pot to vent naturally for 10 minutes before turning or pressing the vent to release the remaining pressure. Remove the lid and stir in the cauliflower rice. Set the Instant Pot to the Sauté function and simmer for 10 minutes, or until the rice is heated through.

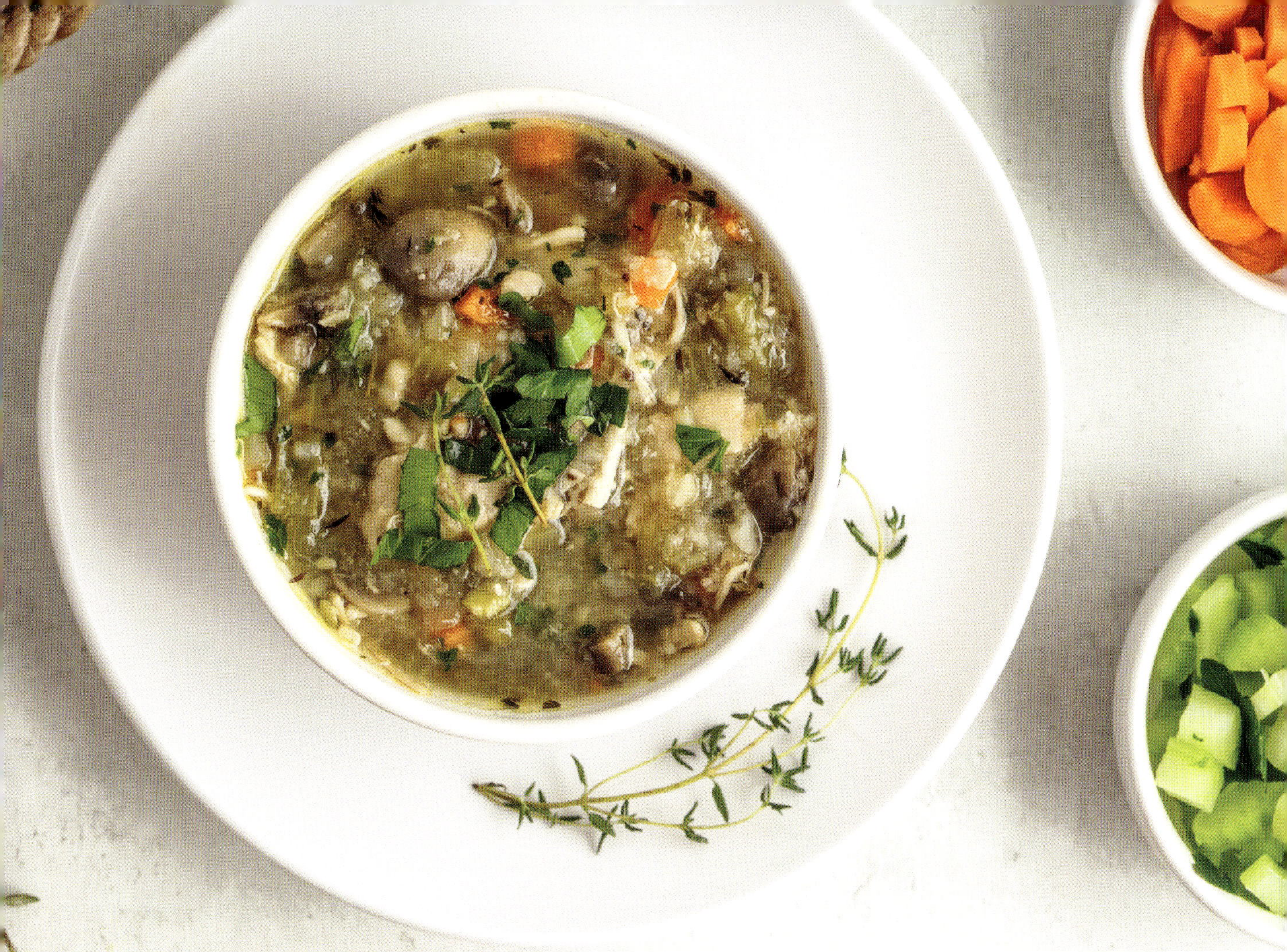

3. Turn off the Instant Pot and stir in the parsley and pepper before serving. Add more salt to taste if needed. Ladle into bowls and top with more parsley and/or thyme, if desired.

SLOW COOKER INSTRUCTIONS:

1. In a large skillet, melt the butter over medium-high heat. Working in batches, sear the chicken until browned on all sides, 5 to 7 minutes.
2. While the chicken is cooking, put the mushrooms, celery, carrots, onions, green beans, salt, thyme, garlic, broth, and pepper in the slow cooker. Once seared, add the chicken to the slow cooker and stir to combine.
3. Cover and cook on low for 3½ hours, or until the chicken is cooked through and the vegetables are tender. Pour in the cauliflower rice, cover, and continue cooking for 30 minutes, or until the rice is heated through. Right before serving, stir in the parsley and add more salt if needed. Ladle into bowls and top with more parsley and/or thyme, if desired.

note

You can skip Step 1 and add the raw chicken directly to the slow cooker along with the rest of the ingredients in Step 2. However, the texture and flavor of the chicken will be better if you pan-sear it first to lock in the flavor and juices.

(per serving)
CALORIES: **358** | PROTEIN: **48.8g** | FAT: **14.7g** | TOTAL CARBS: **11.1g** | NET CARBS: **7.4g** | FIBER: **3.7g**

CHICKEN TORTILLA SOUP

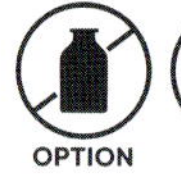

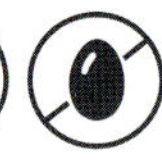
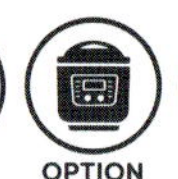

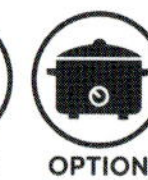

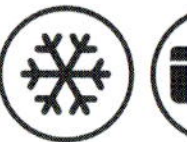

SERVES 6

PREP TIME: 15 minutes (not including time to make chips)

COOK TIME: 25 minutes to 4 hours, depending on method

Chicken tortilla soup is a must-have in this cookbook because it's my husband's favorite! This flavorful, easy-to-make soup can be cooked on the stovetop, in a slow cooker, or in an Instant Pot. It's loaded with bold flavors and ideal for customizing with toppings like shredded cheese, protein tortilla chips, sour cream, lime, and extra jalapeños if you need more spicy kick.

---

2 tablespoons avocado oil

½ medium onion, diced

½ green bell pepper, diced

3 cloves garlic, minced

1 jalapeño pepper, seeded, ribs removed, and finely diced

1 teaspoon ground cumin

1 teaspoon chili powder

1 teaspoon salt

½ teaspoon ground black pepper

¼ teaspoon cayenne pepper

1 (10-ounce) can diced tomatoes with green chiles

4 cups chicken broth

3 pounds boneless, skinless chicken thighs

¼ cup finely chopped fresh cilantro, plus more for garnish if desired

1 batch Low-Carb Tortilla Chips (page 312), for serving

SUGGESTED TOPPINGS

Shredded Mexican blend cheese

Lime wedges

Diced avocado

Sour cream

STOVETOP INSTRUCTIONS:

1. Heat the oil in a Dutch oven or other large heavy-bottomed pot over medium heat. Add the onion, bell pepper, garlic, and jalapeño. Sauté until the onion is translucent and the jalapeño is softened.
2. Stir in the cumin, chili powder, salt, black pepper, and cayenne. Cook for 1 to 2 more minutes, until the seasonings are fragrant.
3. Add the diced tomatoes with green chiles, broth, and chicken thighs. Bring to a boil, then lower the heat to medium-low. Let simmer for 25 to 30 minutes, until the chicken is cooked through. (It should no longer be pink in the center.)
4. Remove the chicken to a plate and shred using two forks.
5. Using an immersion blender or a countertop blender, puree the soup. (*Note:* If using a countertop blender, blend the soup in two batches if needed to avoid overfilling it.)
6. Return the pureed soup to the pot along with the shredded chicken. Stir in the cilantro. Adjust the seasoning if needed.
7. Ladle the soup into serving bowls and serve with the tortilla chips. Top with shredded cheese, additional cilantro, a squeeze of lime juice, diced avocado, and/or sour cream, if desired.

SLOW COOKER INSTRUCTIONS:

Place all the ingredients except the cilantro in the slow cooker and stir to distribute evenly. Cover with the lid and cook on high for 4 hours or on low for 8 hours. Continue with Steps 4 through 7.

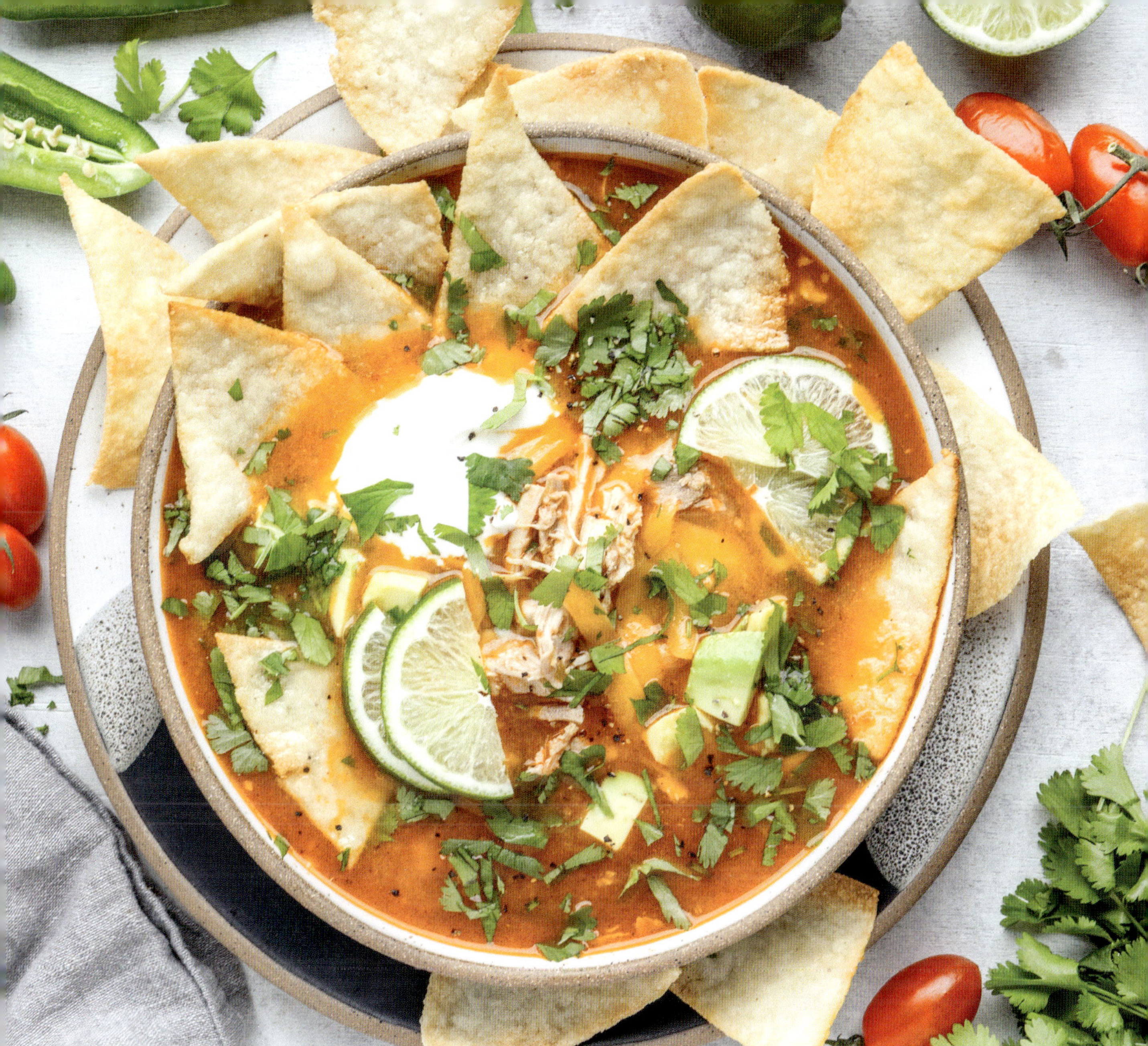

note

To make this dairy free, omit the cheese and sour cream toppings.

INSTANT POT INSTRUCTIONS:

1. Turn the Instant Pot to the Sauté function. Pour the oil into the Instant Pot. Add the onion, bell pepper, garlic, and jalapeño. Sauté until the onion is translucent and the jalapeño has softened. Stir in the cumin, chili powder, salt, black pepper, and cayenne. Cook for 1 to 2 more minutes, until fragrant. Add the tomatoes with green chiles, broth, and chicken.
2. Stir to combine. Secure the lid on the Instant Pot and pressure-cook on high for 15 minutes. Allow the pressure to vent naturally for 10 minutes before turning or pressing the vent to release the remaining pressure. Continue with Steps 4 through 7.

(per serving)
CALORIES: **475** | PROTEIN: **43.8g** | FAT: **31.5g** | TOTAL CARBS: **8.2g** | NET CARBS: **4.7g** | FIBER: **3.5g**

CRISPY "DOUBLE PROTEIN" FRIED CHICKEN 

SERVES 8

PREP TIME: 35 minutes, plus 30 minutes to dry chicken skin

COOK TIME: 35 minutes

This recipe is a game changer, combining the natural protein from the chicken with a crispy, flaky crust made from protein powder that is reminiscent of Southern fried chicken. Making your own low-carb buttermilk is key to tenderizing the chicken and achieving an ultra-crispy crust, while egg whites help the coating adhere without adding excess moisture that would come if you used the whole egg. A splash of vodka (optional) helps create even flakier layers in the crust, and baking powder adds puffiness and enhances the browning. This recipe may be a labor of love, but it is 100 percent worth the effort.

---

8 pieces bone-in, skin-on chicken thighs and/or drumsticks (about 4 pounds)

2 tablespoons salt

Avocado oil, for frying

FOR THE BUTTERMILK WASH

2 teaspoons distilled white vinegar

1 cup heavy cream

2 large egg whites

2 tablespoons vodka (optional)

1 teaspoon baking powder

FOR THE SEASONING BLEND

3 tablespoons smoked paprika

1 tablespoon garlic salt

1 tablespoon ginger powder

1 tablespoon ground black pepper

1 tablespoon ground mustard

2 teaspoons dried thyme leaves

1 teaspoon celery seed

1 teaspoon dried oregano leaves

FOR THE BREADING

2 cups unflavored protein powder

1 teaspoon baking powder

1 teaspoon salt

Remaining seasoning blend (from above)

1. Place the chicken on a rimmed baking sheet lined with a paper towel. Sprinkle the salt all over the chicken. Set aside at room temperature for 30 minutes or refrigerate overnight. (If refrigerating overnight, allow the chicken to come to room temperature for 30 minutes before frying.)
2. Meanwhile, make a low-carb buttermilk for the buttermilk wash by stirring the vinegar into the cream. Let sit until the mixture has curdled slightly, 15 to 30 minutes.
3. Make the seasoning blend by combining all the ingredients in a small bowl.
4. Pat the chicken pieces dry and coat them all over with about half of the seasoning blend.
5. Pour enough avocado oil into a Dutch oven or large saucepan to cover the chicken completely (a depth of 2 to 3 inches should do it). Heat the oil over medium heat until it is about 350°F. Create a cooling station for the fried chicken by lining a rimmed baking sheet with paper towels and placing a wire rack on top.
6. Make the buttermilk wash by combining the homemade buttermilk, egg whites, vodka (if using), and baking powder in a medium bowl.
7. Make the breading mixture by combining the protein powder, baking powder, salt, and remaining seasoning blend in a shallow bowl or plate.

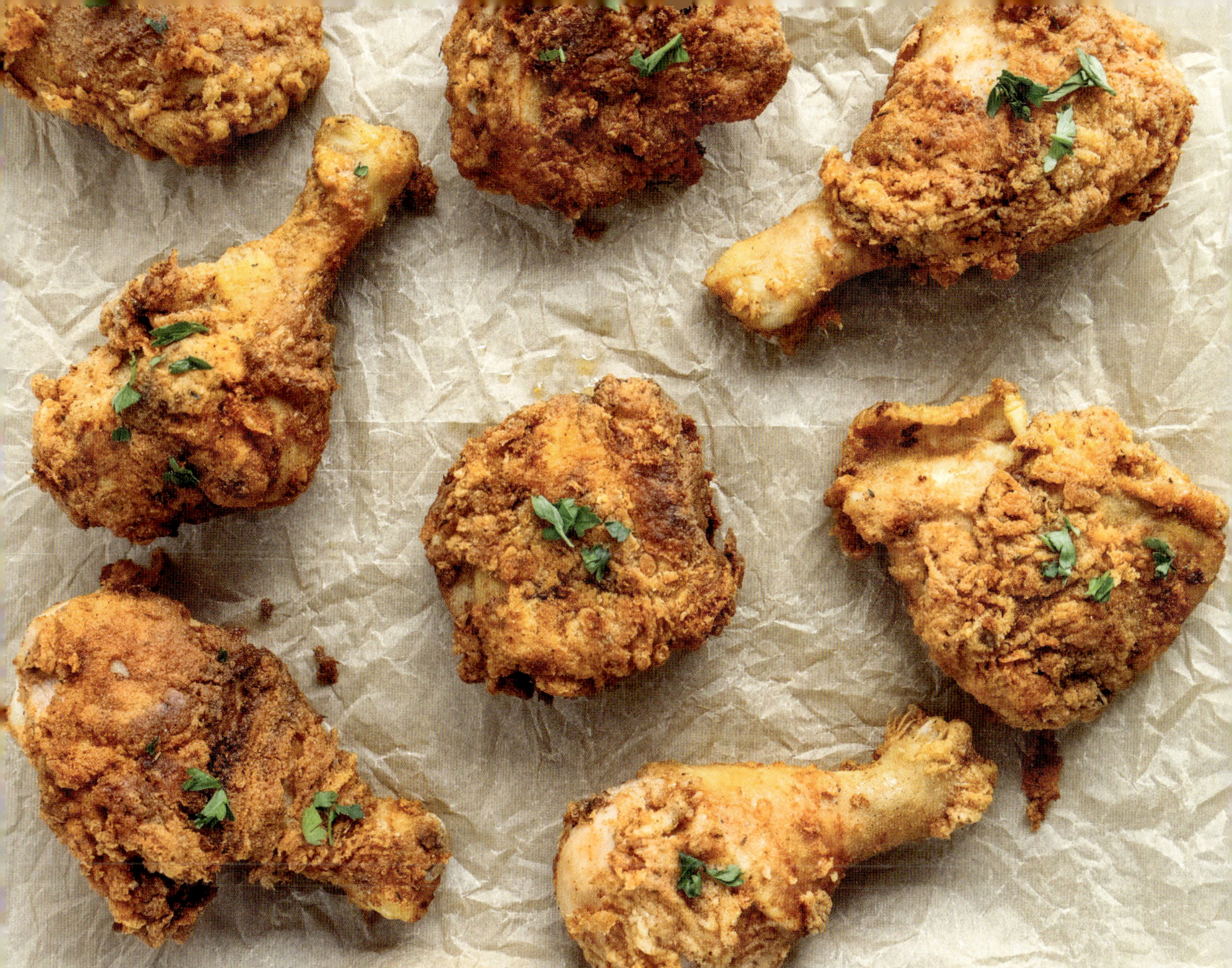

STORAGE INSTRUCTIONS: Store leftovers in the refrigerator for up to 4 days. The breading will become soft; however, you can get it crispy again by reheating the chicken in the air fryer at 350°F for 3 to 5 minutes.

8. Work with only enough chicken pieces that will fit in the pot or pan at once. Dip a piece of chicken in the buttermilk wash to coat. Then place in the breading mixture. Turn the chicken in the mixture and press the breading in to create a thick layer that completely coats the chicken.
9. Immediately place the chicken in the hot oil. Repeat with more chicken, but only enough to fill the pot without overcrowding. If you coat the chicken and let it sit, the protein powder will absorb the moisture from the buttermilk wash and the coating will peel off.
10. Fry the chicken, turning it in the oil occasionally to cook all sides evenly, until the internal temperature reaches 165°F, 12 to 15 minutes.
11. Transfer the chicken to the cooling station and place in a low oven to keep warm. Repeat with the remaining chicken pieces, buttermilk wash, and breading. Check the temperature of the oil periodically to make sure it doesn't get too hot.

(per serving)
CALORIES: **417** | PROTEIN: **40.7g** | FAT: **26.6g** | TOTAL CARBS: **3g** | NET CARBS: **1.9g** | FIBER: **1.1g**

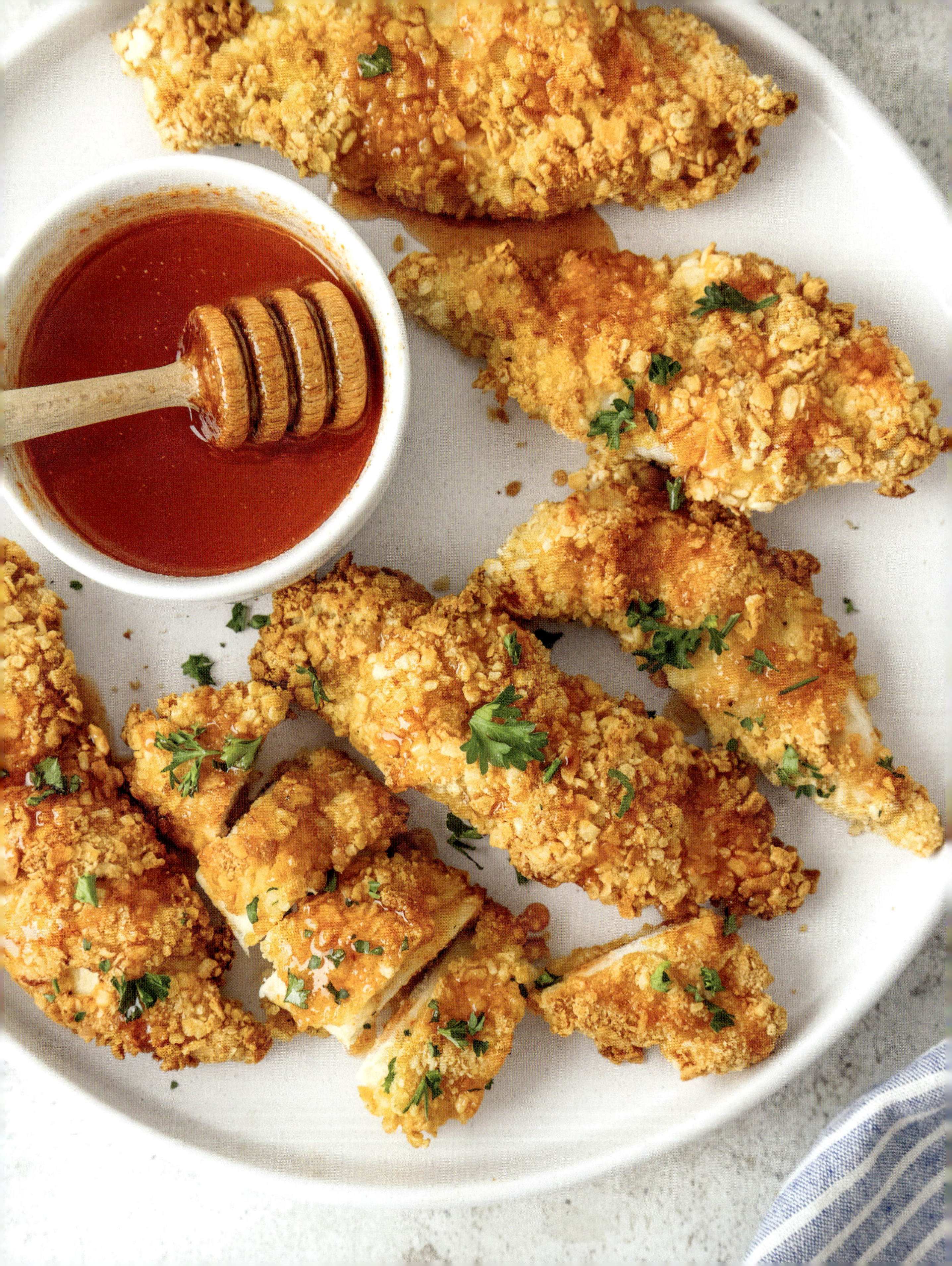

HOT HONEY CHICKEN TENDERS

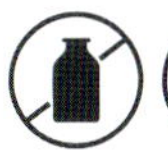
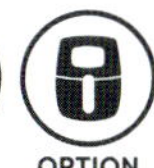

SERVES 6

PREP TIME: 15 minutes

COOK TIME: 12 to 20 minutes, depending on method

Chicken tenders are a family favorite. But the star of this recipe is the hot honey sauce—a perfectly balanced blend of sweet and heat. A double layer of almond flour and pork panko creates extra-crispy chicken strips while boosting the protein. You can cook the tenders in the air fryer or fry them on the stove—either way will give them a crunchy coating ideal for soaking up the sweet and spicy sauce.

FOR THE CHICKEN TENDERS

2 pounds chicken tenderloins

Salt and pepper

3 cups pork panko

⅔ cup blanched, super-fine almond flour

2 teaspoons garlic powder

1 teaspoon onion powder

2 large eggs

2 tablespoons water

Avocado oil (if frying on the stovetop)

FOR THE HOT HONEY

½ cup sugar-free or regular honey

1 to 2 tablespoons sriracha, according to taste

1 teaspoon cayenne pepper

¾ teaspoon chili powder

½ teaspoon garlic powder

1. Pat dry the chicken with a paper towel to remove the excess moisture. Season lightly with salt and pepper. Set aside.
2. In a shallow bowl or plate, mix together the pork panko, almond flour, garlic powder, onion powder, ½ teaspoon salt, and ½ teaspoon pepper.
3. In a shallow bowl, whisk the eggs with the water.
4. Add a couple of chicken tenders to the bowl with the pork panko mixture. Dust until coated.
5. Dip each tender in the egg wash, then put back in the bowl with the pork panko mixture. Press the mixture into the tender to stick. Repeat with the remaining tenders, breading, and egg wash.
6. To cook in the air fryer: Arrange the chicken in a single layer in the air fryer basket or tray. Spray the tops of the chicken tenders with cooking spray. Air-fry at 350°F for 8 to 12 minutes, until the chicken is crispy, golden, and cooked all the way through. (Once cooked through, it will no longer be pink in the center.)

   To cook on the stovetop: Pour ¾ inch of avocado oil into a large skillet and heat over medium heat. Once the oil ripples as you turn the skillet, it is ready. Working in a couple of batches, add the breaded chicken to the hot oil and fry for 3 to 5 minutes on each side, until the chicken is crispy, golden, and cooked through. (Once cooked through, it will no longer be pink in the center.) Remove and set on a paper towel–lined plate.
7. While the chicken is cooking, prepare the hot honey. In a small bowl, stir together all the ingredients.
8. To serve, drizzle the hot honey over the chicken.

(per serving, using 1 tablespoon sriracha)

CALORIES: **449** | PROTEIN: **54.8g** | FAT: **21.1g** | TOTAL CARBS: **25.9g** | NET CARBS: **3.7g** | FIBER: **9.8g**
SUGAR ALCOHOLS: **13.3g**

PUMPKIN TURKEY CHILI

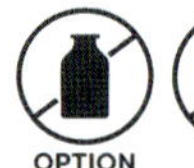

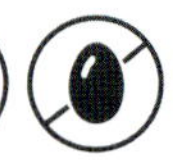
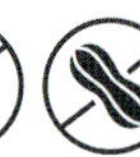
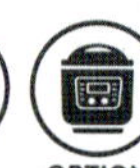

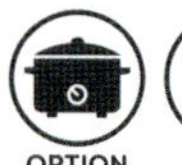

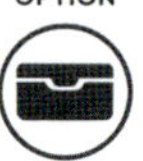

SERVES 6

PREP TIME: 10 minutes

COOK TIME: 30 minutes to 2 hours 40 minutes, depending on method

This boldly flavored chili is the perfect comfort food, full of nutritious ingredients from the colorful veggies. Plus, it's packed with over 40 grams of protein per serving! The pumpkin not only serves as a natural thickener but also adds a subtle sweetness to balance the spice blend. Using turkey instead of beef keeps the chili lean, but you can easily swap in ground beef or chicken if you prefer. You'll find three convenient options for cooking the chili below: stovetop, slow cooker, and Instant Pot.

---

1 tablespoon avocado oil

½ small onion, diced

1 orange bell pepper, diced

1 jalapeño pepper, seeded, ribs removed, and finely diced

3 cloves garlic, minced

3 pounds ground turkey (85/15)

2 teaspoons salt

½ teaspoon ground black pepper

1 medium zucchini, cut into quarter-moons

3 tablespoons chili powder

1 tablespoon ground cumin

2 teaspoons dried oregano leaves

1 (14.5-ounce) can diced tomatoes

1 tablespoon tomato paste

1 cup chicken broth

1 cup pumpkin puree

FOR SERVING (OPTIONAL)

Avocado slices

Jalapeño slices

Sour cream

Chopped fresh cilantro

Keto chips

STOVETOP INSTRUCTIONS:

1. Preheat a Dutch oven or other large heavy-bottomed pot over medium-high heat. Pour in the avocado oil and add the onion, bell pepper, jalapeño, and garlic. Sauté for 2 to 3 minutes, until almost softened.
2. Stir in the ground turkey, salt, and pepper. Cook, stirring occasionally, until the turkey is cooked three-quarters of the way through, leaving a few pink spots in the meat.
3. Stir in the zucchini, chili powder, cumin, and oregano. Cook for 1 to 2 minutes, until the zucchini has softened slightly and the spices are fragrant.
4. Add the diced tomatoes, tomato paste, chicken broth, and pumpkin puree. Lower the heat to medium and simmer for 10 to 15 minutes.

SLOW COOKER INSTRUCTIONS:

1. Heat the avocado oil in a large skillet over medium-high heat. Add the ground turkey and cook until the meat is three-quarters of the way done (with just a few pink spots), breaking it up while it cooks.
2. Transfer the turkey to the slow cooker. Add the rest of the ingredients, except the zucchini. Stir well, cover, and cook on high for 2 hours or on low for 4 hours. Carefully remove the lid and stir in the zucchini, then cover and cook for 30 more minutes, or until the zucchini is tender.

INSTANT POT INSTRUCTIONS:

1. Turn the Instant Pot to the Sauté function and pour in the avocado oil. Add the ground turkey, salt, and pepper and cook until the meat is three-quarters of the way done (with just a few pink spots), breaking it up while it cooks. Add the onion, bell pepper, and jalapeño and cook for another 3 minutes, stirring often. Add the garlic, chili powder, cumin, oregano, diced tomatoes, tomato paste, chicken broth, and pumpkin puree and stir well.

(per serving)
CALORIES: **528** | PROTEIN: **40.5g** | FAT: **37.1g** | TOTAL CARBS: **13.7g** | NET CARBS: **8.8g** | FIBER: **4.9g**

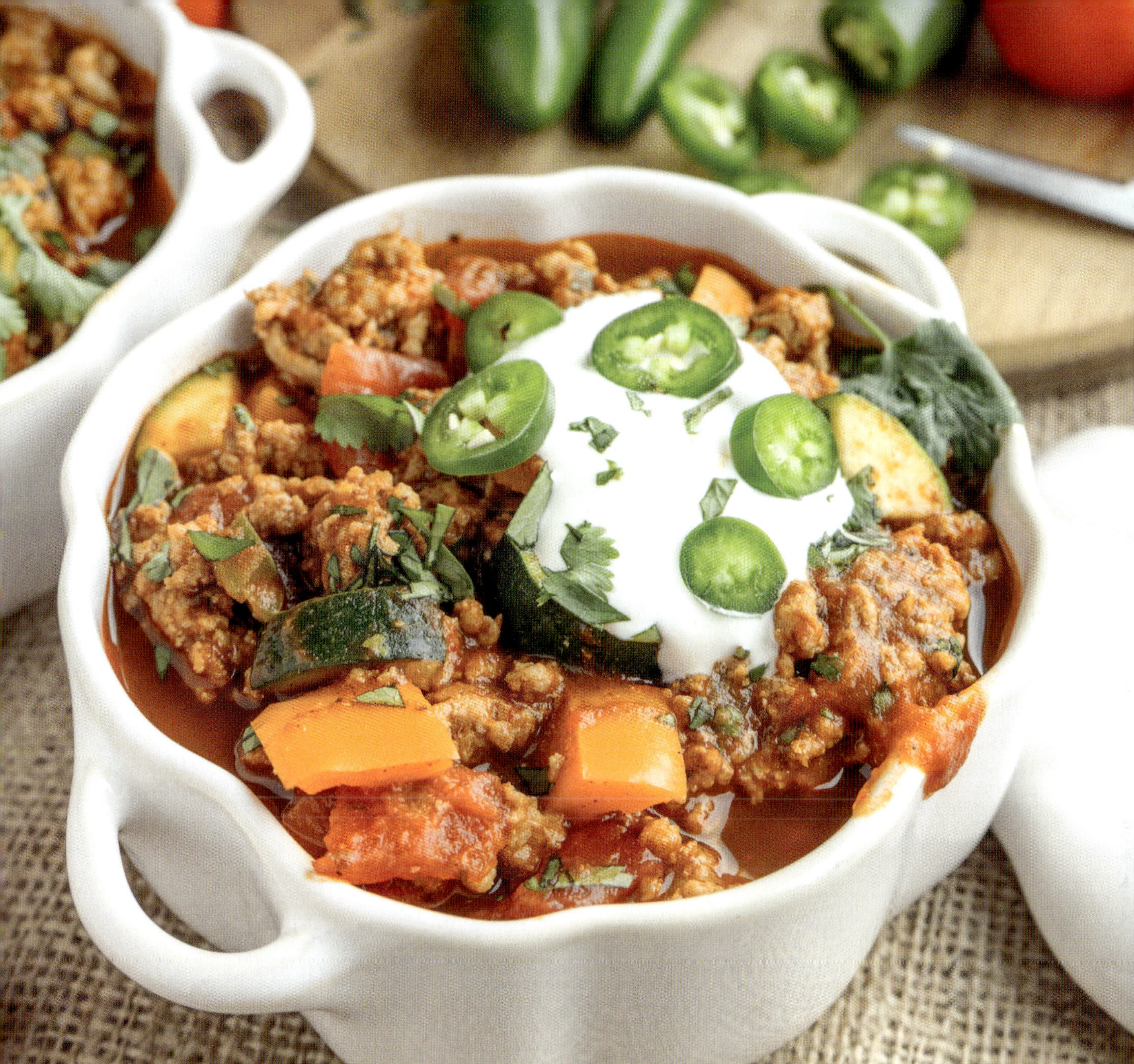

note

I recommend cooking the turkey in a skillet prior to adding it to the slow cooker or Instant Pot for the best texture and to keep it from losing moisture.

2. Secure the lid and pressure-cook on high for 15 minutes. Allow the pressure to vent naturally for 15 minutes before turning or pressing the vent to release the remaining pressure.
3. Remove the lid and turn the Instant Pot to the Sauté function. Add the zucchini, stir, and cook for 5 minutes. Then turn the Instant Pot to the Warm function and allow the chili to rest for 10 minutes before serving.

FOR ALL METHODS:

Serve with avocado slices, jalapeño slices, sour cream, cilantro, and/or chips, if desired.

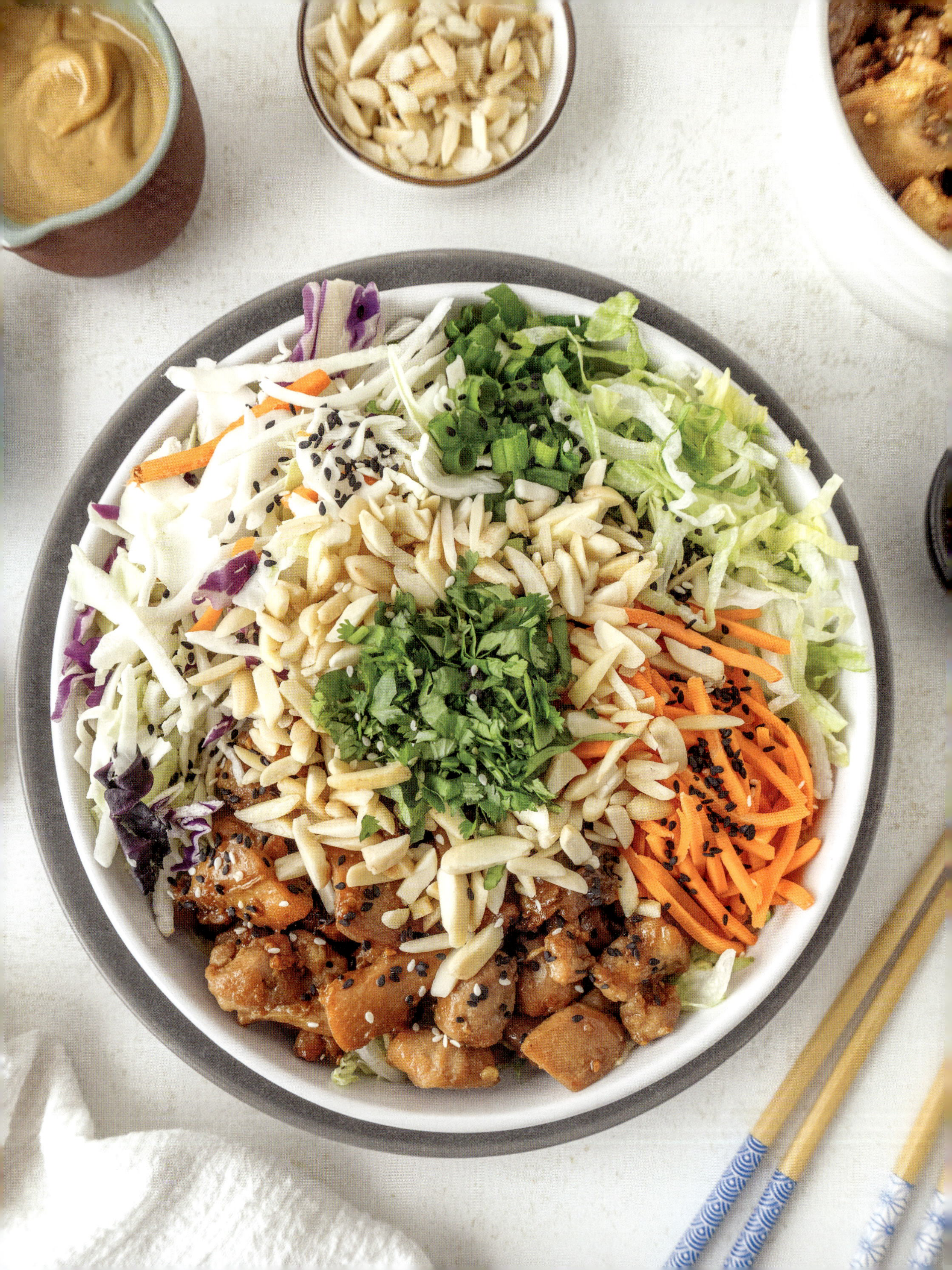

SESAME CHICKEN SALAD

 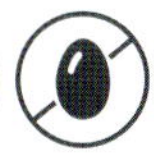 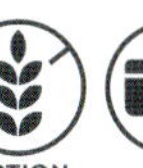 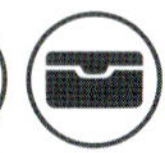

OPTION

SERVES 4

PREP TIME: 20 minutes, plus 15 minutes to marinate chicken

COOK TIME: 15 minutes

This Asian-inspired salad is easy to make and perfect for meal prep. With 47 grams of protein per serving, it will keep you full. The chicken is marinated in a sweet sesame garlic sauce and served over a colorful salad of coleslaw mix, lettuce, carrots, cilantro, almonds, and sesame seeds. Tossed with a sweet tahini dressing, it is a delicious high-protein option that's simple enough for a weekday family dinner when you feel like salad but want a whole meal.

---

2 pounds boneless, skinless chicken thighs

1 to 2 tablespoons avocado oil, for the pan

FOR THE MARINADE

⅓ cup soy sauce or tamari

1 tablespoon brown sugar substitute

1 teaspoon toasted sesame oil

2 cloves garlic, grated or minced

½ teaspoon ground black pepper

FOR THE DRESSING

3 tablespoons tahini

2 tablespoons unseasoned rice vinegar

1 tablespoon soy sauce or tamari

1 teaspoon brown sugar substitute

¼ teaspoon salt

¼ teaspoon ground black pepper

FOR THE SALAD

1 (14-ounce) bag coleslaw mix

1 (8-ounce) bag shredded iceberg lettuce

2 green onions, sliced

¼ cup julienned carrots

¼ cup chopped fresh cilantro

¼ cup slivered almonds

1 tablespoon black and/or white sesame seeds

1. Cut the chicken into bite-size cubes.
2. In a large bowl, whisk together all the ingredients for the marinade. Add the cubed chicken and mix to evenly coat. Cover the bowl with plastic wrap and let marinate for 15 to 30 minutes.
3. While the chicken is marinating, whisk together all the ingredients for the dressing in a small bowl. Set aside.
4. Preheat a large wok or skillet over medium-high heat. Pour in 1 tablespoon of the avocado oil and heat until it ripples. Working in batches to avoid crowding, add the chicken and remaining marinade to the hot pan. Cook, stirring occasionally, until the liquid has cooked off and the chicken is no longer pink in the center and has a nice sear. Remove the cooked chicken to a plate or bowl and repeat with the remaining chicken, adding more oil to the pan if necessary. Let the chicken cool before assembling the salad.
5. To assemble the salad, put all the salad components in a large bowl. Top with the chicken, then pour on the dressing and toss to coat.

notes

For meal prep, portion out the salad, chicken, and dressing separately. Combine them just before eating.

To make this gluten free, use coconut aminos or liquid aminos in place of soy sauce or tamari.

(per serving)

CALORIES: **573** | PROTEIN: **47.1g** | FAT: **39.2g** | TOTAL CARBS: **18.6g** | NET CARBS: **8.9g** | FIBER: **5.7g**
SUGAR ALCOHOLS: **4g**

SMOKY CHIPOTLE CHICKEN SALAD WRAP

SERVES 2

PREP TIME: 10 minutes (not including time to cook chicken or flatbread)

This is an easy meal to make for lunch or dinner, and the chicken salad can be prepped ahead for even more convenience. Wrapped in a high-protein flatbread, the salad features shredded chicken mixed with a creamy, smoky sauce made from Greek yogurt, chipotle peppers, smoked paprika, and other flavorful ingredients. Crunchy bell peppers and onions add freshness and texture to each bite. If you don't want to make homemade flatbread, you can swap it for a store-bought low-carb tortilla or egg wrap.

FOR THE CHICKEN SALAD

1½ cups shredded cooked chicken

¼ cup finely diced red bell peppers

¼ cup finely diced red onions

¼ cup plain Greek or low-carb yogurt

2 tablespoons chopped fresh cilantro

1½ tablespoons diced chipotle peppers (see note, page 81)

1½ teaspoons lime juice

½ teaspoon smoked paprika

½ teaspoon salt

¼ teaspoon ground black pepper

1 serving Cottage Cheese Flatbread (page 241)

1. In a large bowl, combine all the ingredients for the chicken salad.
2. Lay the flatbread on a flat work surface, with a long side facing you. Place the chicken salad along the long end nearest you. Roll up tightly and slice in half.

(per serving)
CALORIES: **365** | PROTEIN: **48.8g** | FAT: **16g** | TOTAL CARBS: **8.1g** | NET CARBS: **7.1g** | FIBER: **1g**

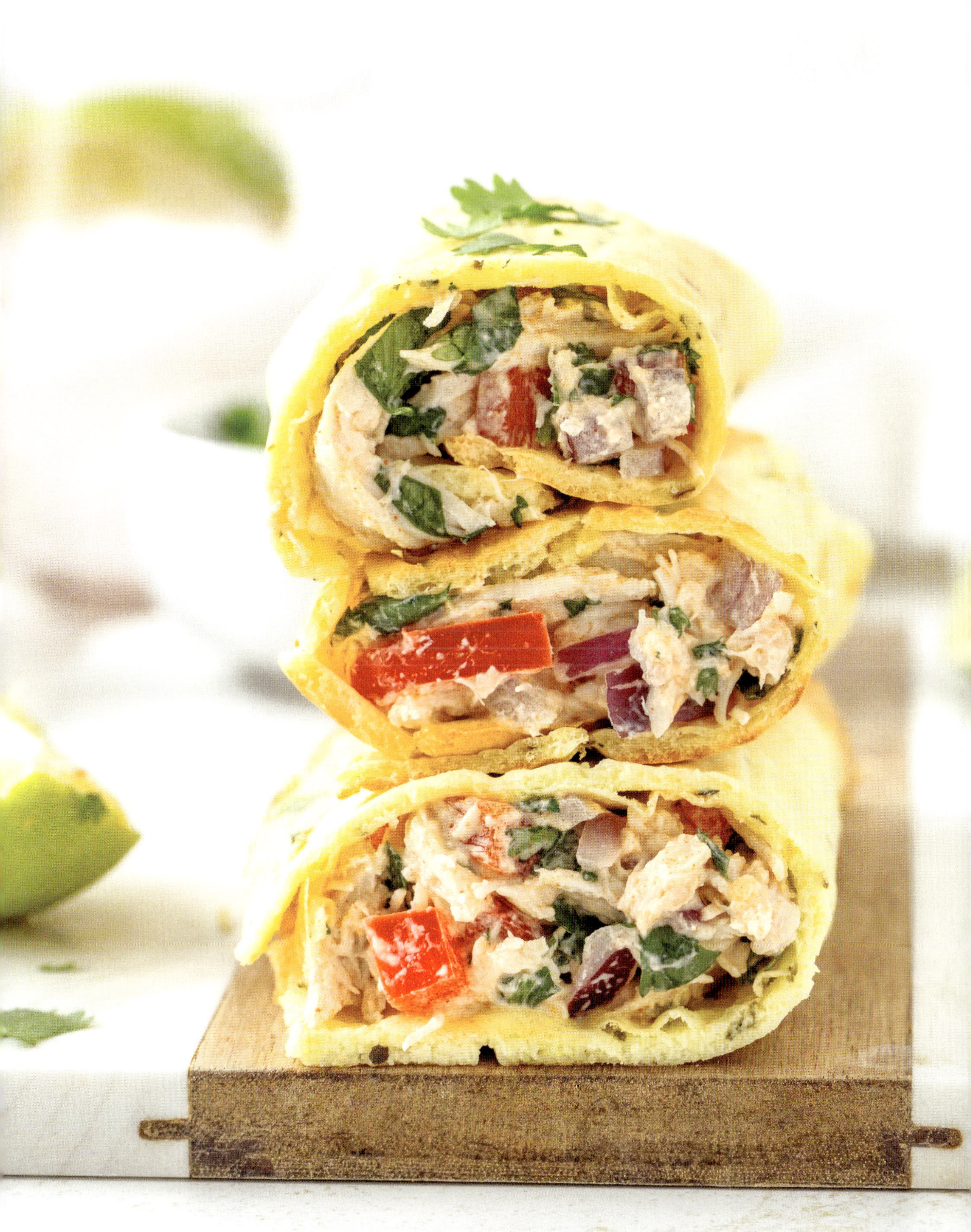

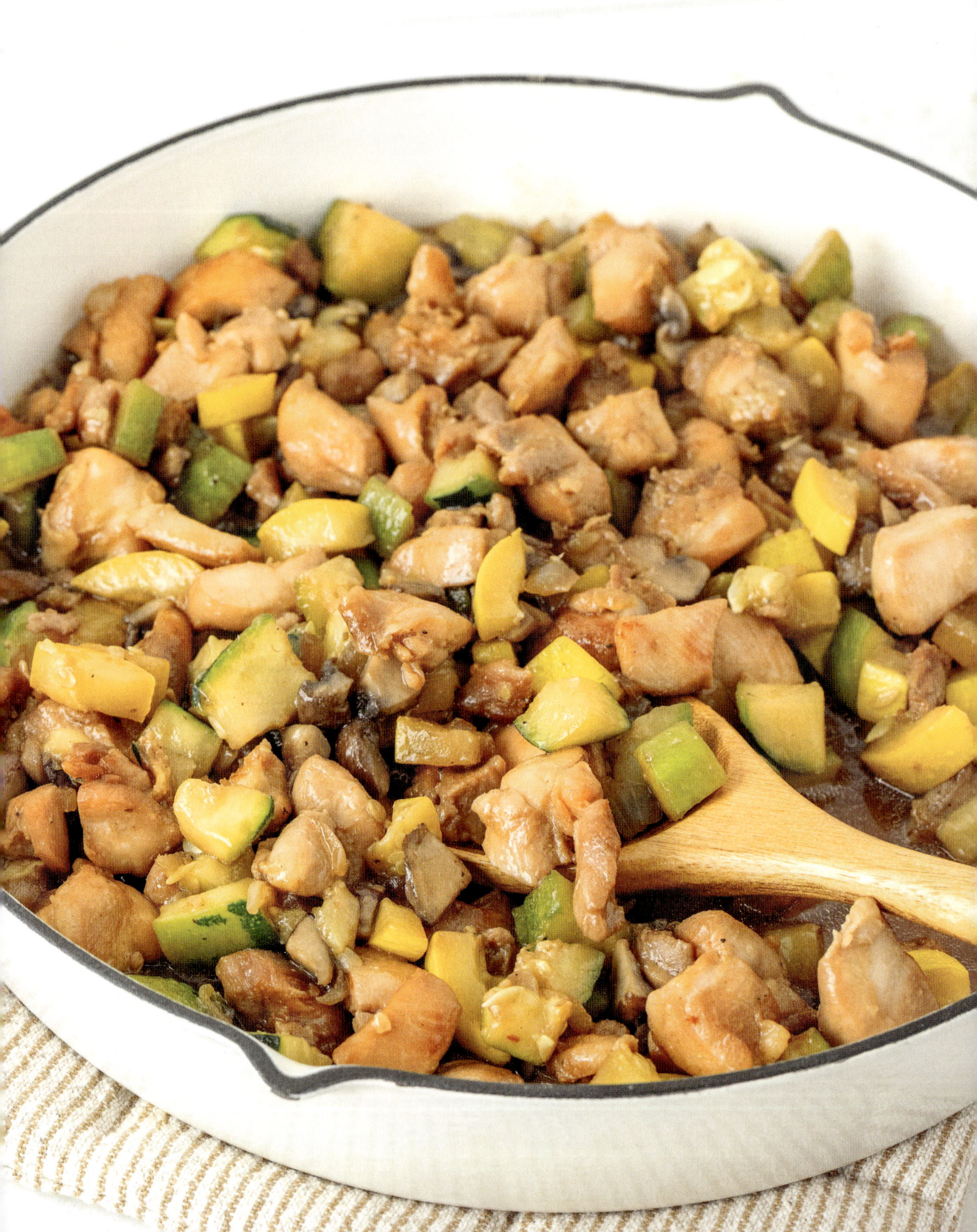

SUMMER CHICKEN STIR-FRY

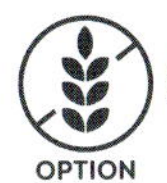
OPTION

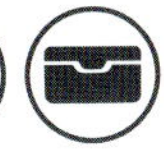

SERVES 4

PREP TIME: 10 minutes, plus 30 minutes to marinate chicken

COOK TIME: 4 minutes

This easy stir-fry features tender chunks of marinated chicken, summer squash, and mushrooms. It celebrates the flavors of tender-skinned squash harvested in summer, but you can enjoy this dish year-round. The stir-fry has sweet and savory flavors of ginger, garlic, and soy sauce (which you can swap for tamari, liquid aminos, or coconut aminos if you prefer). Topped with a creamy protein-rich sriracha mayo, this simple weeknight meal is delicious on its own or served over cauliflower rice.

FOR THE STIR-FRY

¼ cup soy sauce or tamari

1 tablespoon chili garlic sauce

1 tablespoon brown sugar substitute or sugar-free or regular honey

2 cloves garlic, minced

½ teaspoon ginger powder

2 pounds boneless, skinless chicken thighs, cubed

2 tablespoons avocado oil, divided, for the pan, plus more if needed

1 medium zucchini, sliced into quarter-moons

1 medium yellow summer squash, sliced into quarter-moons

8 ounces sliced cremini mushrooms

½ medium onion, diced

1 teaspoon salt

½ teaspoon ground black pepper

FOR THE SRIRACHA MAYO

¼ cup mayonnaise

2 tablespoons plain Greek or low-carb yogurt

1 to 2 tablespoons sriracha, according to taste

1 teaspoon sugar-free or regular honey

1. In a large bowl, stir together the soy sauce, chili garlic sauce, brown sugar substitute, garlic, and ginger powder. Add the cubed chicken and mix to evenly coat. Cover with plastic wrap and place in the refrigerator to marinate for 30 to 60 minutes.
2. While the chicken is marinating, prepare the sriracha mayo by combining all the ingredients in small bowl. Set aside until ready to serve.
3. Preheat a large wok or skillet over medium-high heat. Pour in 1 tablespoon of the avocado oil and heat until it ripples. Working in batches to avoid crowding, add the chicken and remaining marinade to the hot pan. Cook the chicken, stirring occasionally, until it is no longer pink in the center and has a nice sear. Remove the cooked chicken to a plate or bowl and repeat with the remaining chicken, adding more oil to the pan if necessary.
4. In the now-empty pan, heat the remaining tablespoon of avocado oil over medium heat. Add the zucchini, yellow squash, mushrooms, onion, salt, and pepper. Cook the vegetables until softened and the mushrooms have released their juices, 7 to 10 minutes.
5. Return the chicken to the pan and stir to combine with the vegetables. Serve topped with a drizzle of the sriracha mayo.

note

To make this gluten free, use coconut aminos or liquid aminos in place of soy sauce or tamari.

(per serving)
CALORIES: **467** | PROTEIN: **43.8g** | FAT: **25.6g** | TOTAL CARBS: **16.4g** | NET CARBS: **9.6g** | FIBER: **3g**
SUGAR ALCOHOLS: **3.8g**

THAI TURKEY BOWLS

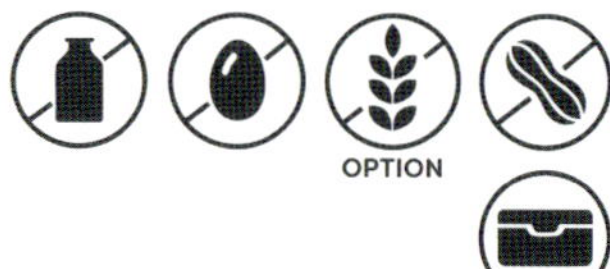

SERVES 4
PREP TIME: 12 minutes
COOK TIME: 10 minutes

This quick and colorful meal comes together in 20 minutes and is perfect for meal prep. The colorful salad features bagged coleslaw mix (saving you from hand-shredding cabbage), red bell pepper, and cucumber. Each bowl is topped with a savory-sweet ground turkey mix.

FOR THE SALAD

1 (14-ounce) bag tricolor coleslaw mix

1 red bell pepper, thinly sliced

1 medium cucumber, sliced into matchsticks

2 green onions, sliced

½ cup chopped fresh cilantro, plus more for garnish if desired

3 tablespoons toasted sesame oil

1½ tablespoons lime juice

1½ tablespoons sugar-free or regular honey

1 tablespoon fish sauce

FOR THE STIR-FRIED TURKEY

1 tablespoon avocado oil or coconut oil

1½ pounds ground turkey (85/15)

4 cloves garlic, minced

1 tablespoon ginger powder

¼ cup sweet chili sauce

2 tablespoons soy sauce or tamari

FOR GARNISH (OPTIONAL)

Black sesame seeds

1. In a large bowl, combine the coleslaw mix, bell pepper, cucumber, green onions, and cilantro.
2. Make the dressing: In a small bowl, stir together the sesame oil, lime juice, honey, and fish sauce.
3. Pour the dressing over the salad and toss to coat. Set aside.
4. Prepare the turkey: In a large wok or skillet, heat the oil over medium-high heat. Add the ground turkey, break it up into crumbles, and cook until only touches of pink remain and the meat is beginning to brown, about 10 minutes.
5. Stir in the garlic and ginger powder and continue cooking the turkey until cooked through and no longer pink. Remove the pan from the heat.
6. Stir in the sweet chili sauce and soy sauce.
7. Divide the salad evenly among four bowls. Top with the turkey mixture. Garnish with chopped cilantro and sesame seeds, if desired.

notes

Yai's Thai makes a low-carb sweet chili sauce; however, if you can't find this brand, use the one that is the lowest in sugar and carbs.

To make this gluten free, use coconut aminos or liquid aminos in place of soy sauce or tamari.

For meal prep, store the salad, dressing, and cooked turkey separately until ready to serve.

(per bowl)
CALORIES: **486** | PROTEIN: **31.9g** | FAT: **32.7g** | TOTAL CARBS: **20.5g** | NET CARBS: **11.1g** | FIBER: **5.6g**
SUGAR ALCOHOLS: **3.8g**

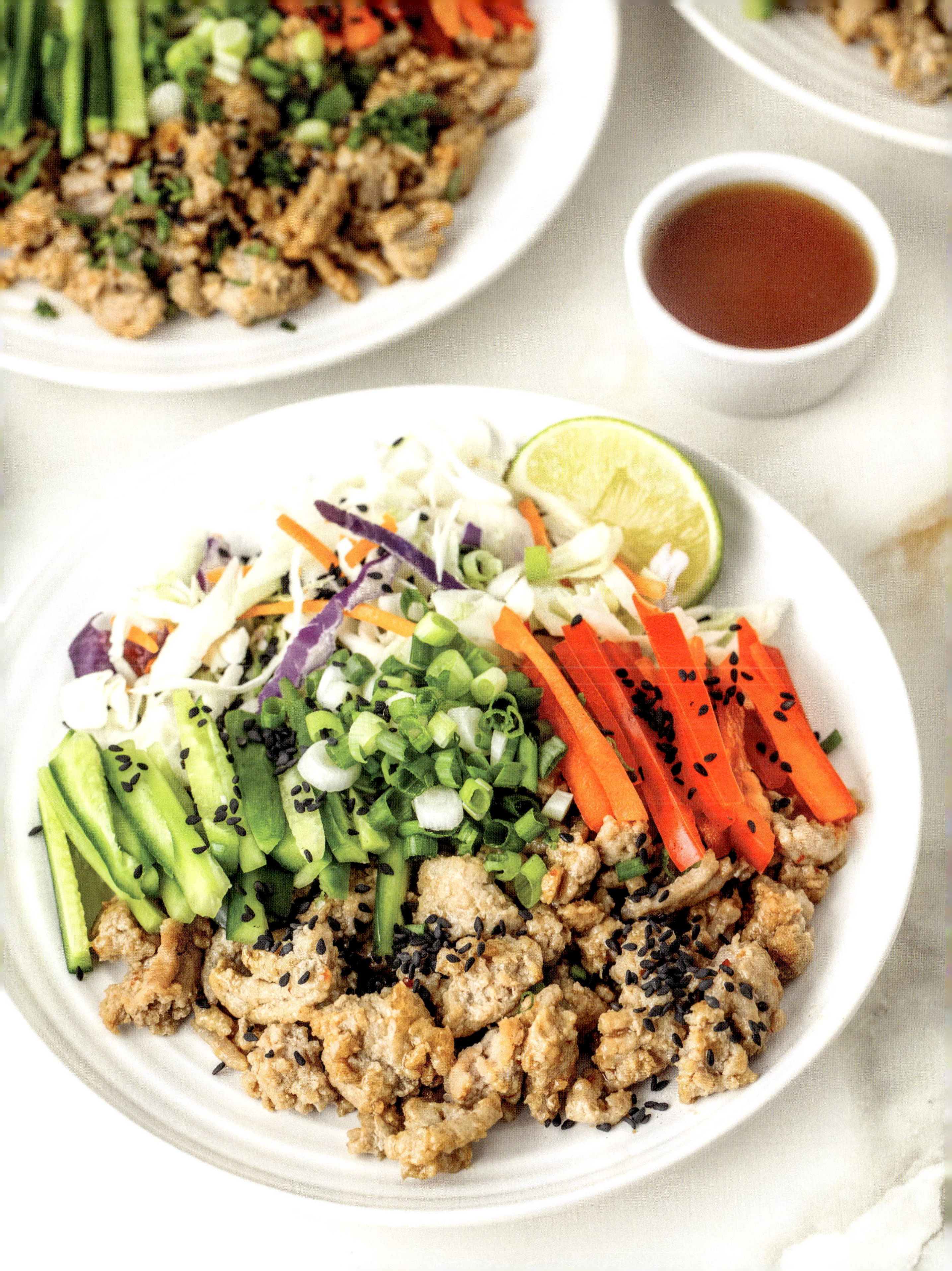

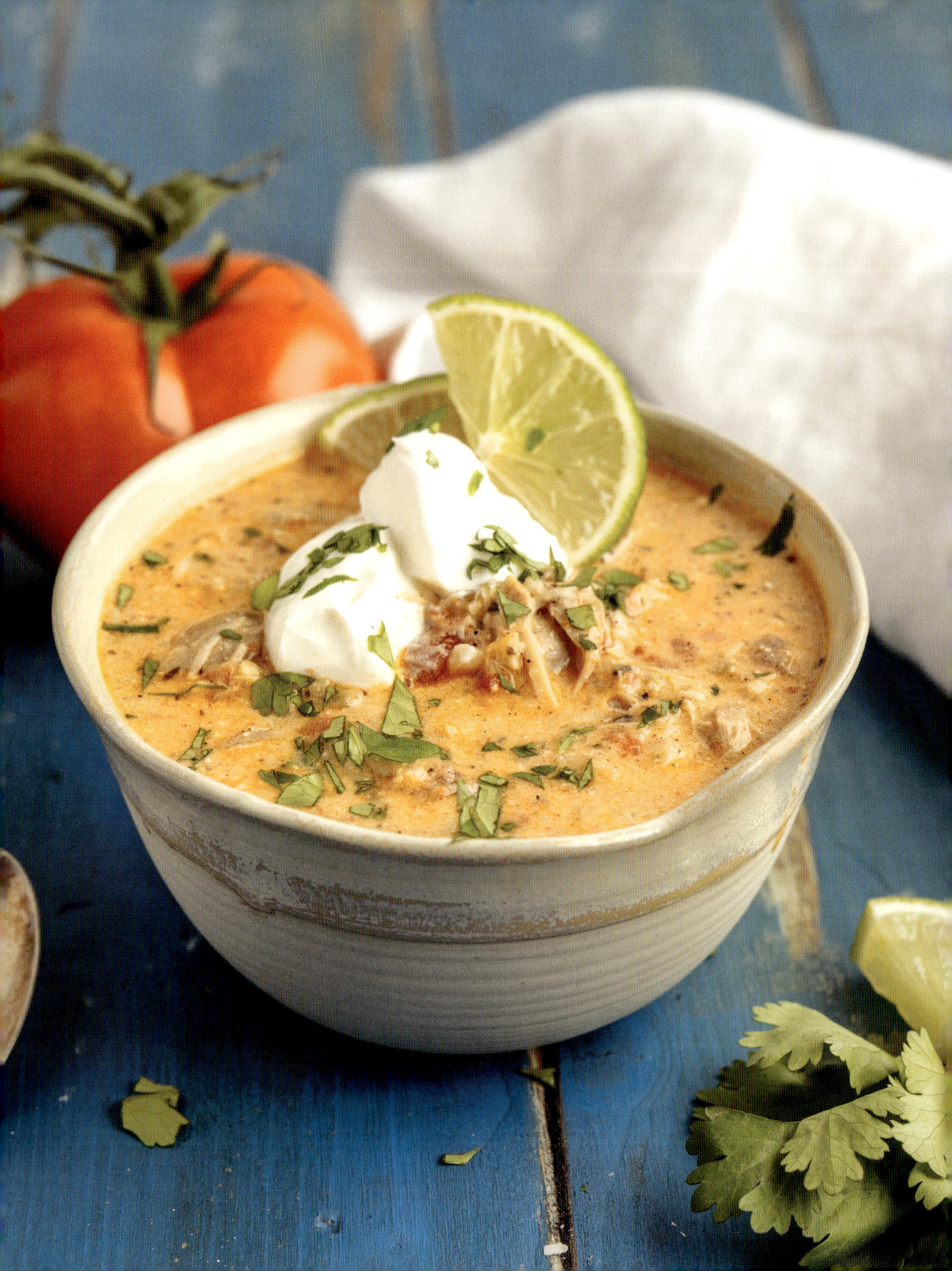

WHITE CHICKEN CHILI

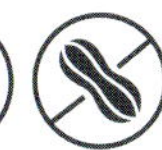
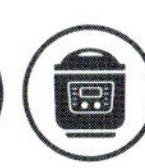
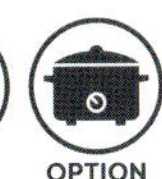

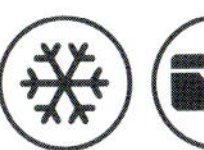

SERVES 4

PREP TIME: 10 minutes

COOK TIME: 20 minutes or 4 hours 20 minutes, depending on method

This creamy chili is the ultimate comfort food for a chilly fall or winter day when you don't want to fuss around in the kitchen too long. Made in an Instant Pot or slow cooker, this beanless chili features shredded chicken thighs and cauliflower rice mixed into a spicy broth for a hearty, protein-rich meal.

1½ pounds boneless, skinless chicken thighs

1½ cups chicken broth

1 (14.5-ounce) can diced tomatoes

1 (4.5-ounce) can diced green chiles

2 tablespoons heavy cream

1½ teaspoons chili powder

1 teaspoon salt

1 teaspoon dried parsley

1 teaspoon ground cumin

½ teaspoon garlic powder

½ teaspoon onion powder

½ teaspoon dried oregano leaves

½ teaspoon ground black pepper

1 (8-ounce) package cream cheese, cubed

1 (10-ounce) bag frozen cauliflower rice

SUGGESTED TOPPINGS

Sour cream

Avocado slices

Lime wedges

Shredded cheese of choice

Chopped fresh cilantro

INSTANT POT INSTRUCTIONS:

1. Put the chicken thighs, broth, tomatoes, green chiles, heavy cream, and seasonings in the Instant Pot. Stir to combine.
2. Top the chicken mixture with the cream cheese cubes, spreading them out evenly. Secure the lid and pressure-cook on high for 15 minutes. Let the pressure release naturally for 10 minutes before turning or pressing the vent to release the remaining pressure.
3. Shred the chicken in the Instant Pot using an electric hand mixer or two forks.
4. Add the cauliflower rice and let sit for 2 minutes, or until the rice is heated through.
5. Serve with the toppings of your choice.

SLOW COOKER INSTRUCTIONS:

1. Put the broth, tomatoes, green chiles, heavy cream, and seasonings in the slow cooker. Stir to combine. Add the chicken thighs and cream cheese. Cover and cook on high for 3 to 4 hours or on low for 6 to 8 hours, until the chicken is cooked through.
2. Twenty minutes before serving, stir in the cauliflower rice and cook, covered, until the rice is heated through.
3. Serve with the toppings of your choice.

(per serving)
CALORIES: **614** | PROTEIN: **45.6g** | FAT: **43.2g** | TOTAL CARBS: **14g** | NET CARBS: **10.2g** | FIBER: **3.8g**

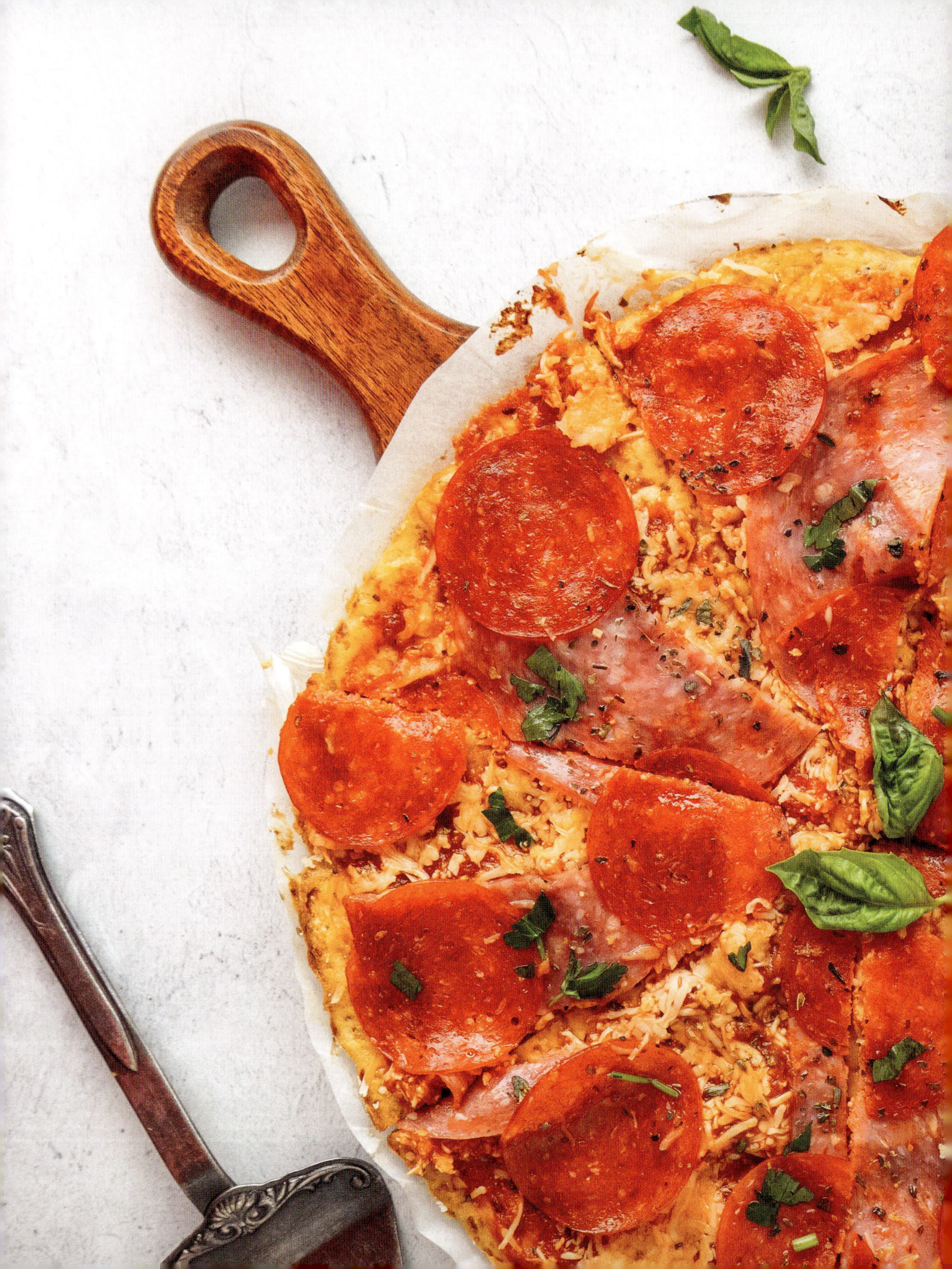

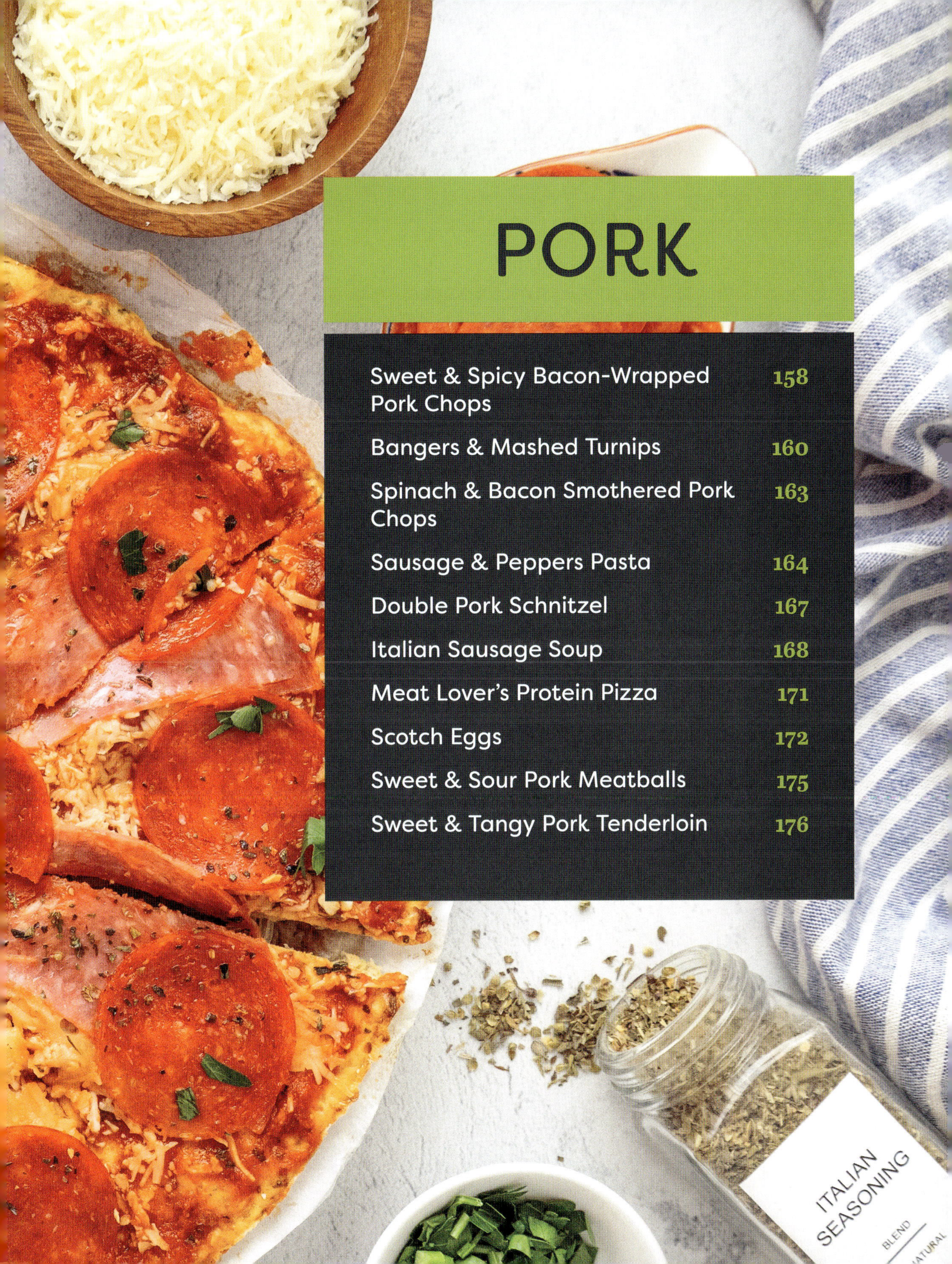

PORK

SWEET & SPICY BACON-WRAPPED PORK CHOPS

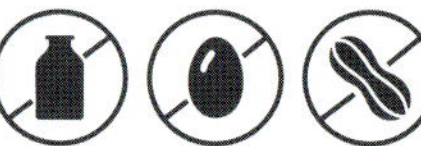

SERVES 4

PREP TIME: 5 minutes

COOK TIME: 22 minutes

These juicy chops are the ultimate weeknight dinner. Wrapping the chops in smoky bacon not only adds incredible flavor but also keeps them moist and tender during cooking. Each pork chop is dusted with a sweet and spicy seasoning blend, creating a flavor harmony with the smoky bacon.

---

4 (4-ounce) boneless pork chops (about 1 inch thick)

8 slices regular-cut bacon

FOR THE SEASONING MIX

1½ tablespoons chili powder

1 tablespoon brown sugar substitute

½ teaspoon salt

½ teaspoon paprika

½ teaspoon ground black pepper

½ teaspoon cayenne pepper

½ teaspoon garlic powder

Chopped fresh parsley, for garnish (optional)

1. Place one rack in the bottom third of the oven and another in the top position. Preheat the oven to 400°F. Line a rimmed baking sheet with foil and fit it with a wire rack.
2. Pat the pork chops dry with a paper towel.
3. Tightly wrap two slices of bacon around each pork chop. Tuck the ends of the bacon under the weave on the bottom so the top looks nice and the ends of the bacon are secured.
4. In a small bowl, whisk the ingredients for the seasoning mix.
5. Sprinkle the seasoning all over the bacon-wrapped pork chops (top, sides, and bottom) until evenly coated. Press or rub the seasoning in to get it to stick.
6. Place the chops on the rack in the prepared pan, seam side down and spaced at least an inch apart.
7. Bake for 15 to 18 minutes, until a thermometer reads 140°F when inserted in the thickest part of the chop. Move the pan to the top rack and turn on the broiler to high; broil the chops for 2 to 4 minutes, until they reach 145°F. Let rest for 5 minutes before serving. Garnish with chopped parsley, if desired.

(per serving)
CALORIES: **225** | PROTEIN: **29.5g** | FAT: **11g** | TOTAL CARBS: **5.1g** | NET CARBS: **0.9g** | FIBER: **1.2g**
SUGAR ALCOHOLS: **3g**

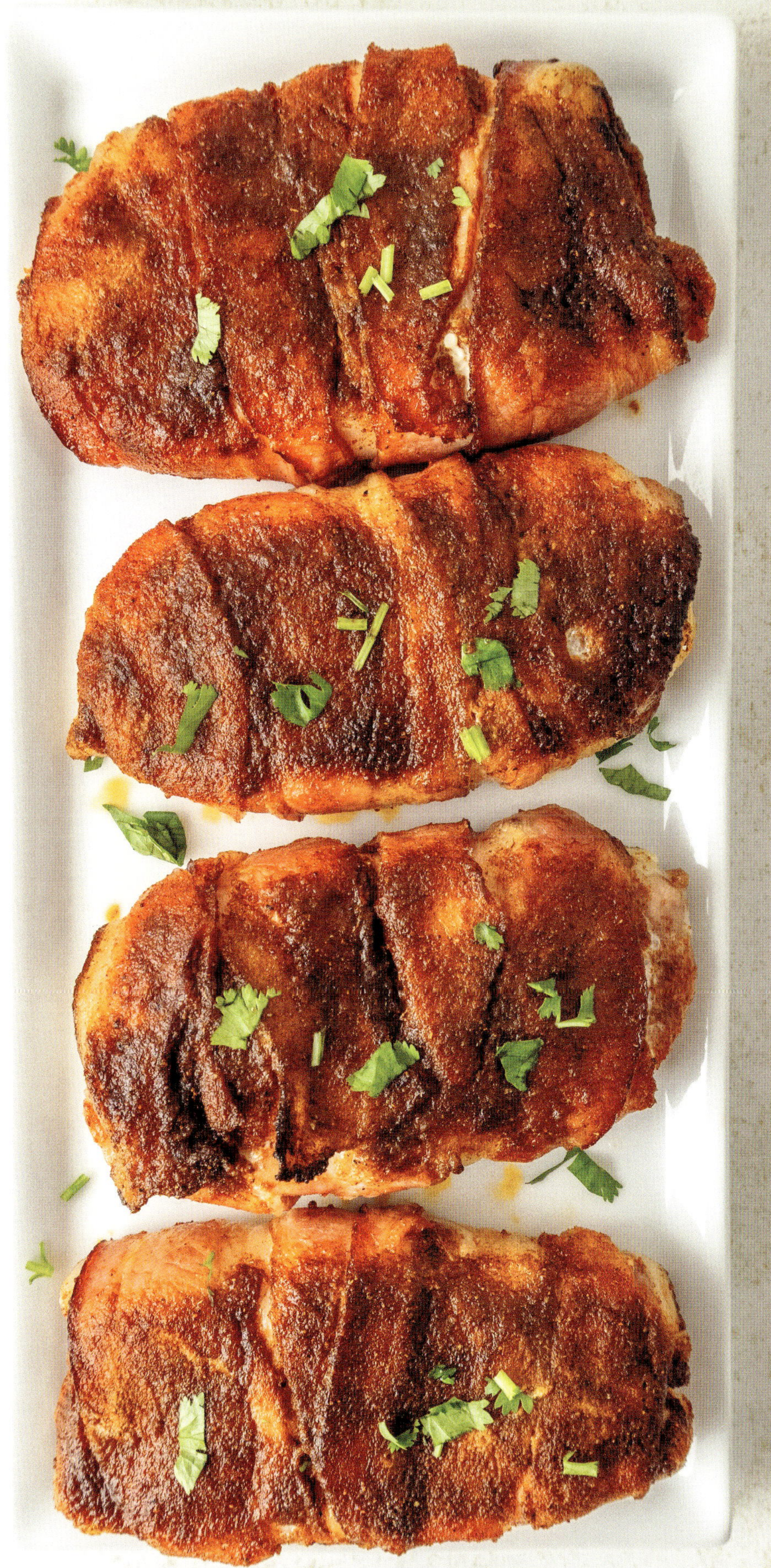

BANGERS & MASHED TURNIPS

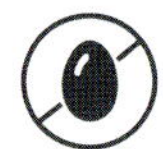 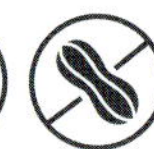 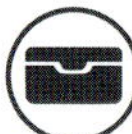

SERVES 4

PREP TIME: 20 minutes

COOK TIME: 40 minutes

This twist on classic bangers and mash swaps traditional mashed potatoes for mashed turnips, creating a low-carb version of the popular dish. To reduce the bitterness of the turnips, I use a few clever techniques: selecting smaller turnips since they tend to be sweeter, boiling them with half a potato to absorb bitter compounds, and cooking off excess moisture after softening. The creamy mashed turnips are then topped with pork sausages cooked in a rich, savory onion gravy.

FOR THE MASHED TURNIPS

1½ pounds small turnips

1 small russet potato

1 cup beef broth

1 teaspoon salt

3 tablespoons salted butter

¼ cup plain Greek or low-carb yogurt

¼ teaspoon ground black pepper

FOR THE BANGERS

2 tablespoons avocado oil, plus more if needed

1 pound large fresh pork sausage links

2 tablespoons salted butter, divided

1 large onion, cut in half and very thinly sliced crosswise

4 cloves garlic, minced

½ teaspoon dried thyme leaves

2 teaspoons arrowroot powder

2 cups beef broth

¼ cup dry red wine

¼ cup heavy cream

1 tablespoon apple cider vinegar

Chopped fresh parsley, for garnish (optional)

1. Peel the turnips, then cut them into ¾-inch cubes.
2. Put the cubed turnips in a large saucepan. Cut the potato in half and place the halves on top of the turnips. Pour in the broth, then add enough water to cover the turnips and potato. Add the salt.
3. Bring to a boil and cook until the turnips have softened enough for a fork to easily pierce them, about 20 minutes.
4. While the turnips are cooking, cook the sausages. Heat the oil in a large skillet over medium-high heat. Prick the sausages a few times using a fork. Add the sausages to the hot skillet and sear, turning occasionally, until browned all over, 3 to 4 minutes. Lower the heat to medium, cover, and cook until the sausages are fully cooked and the internal temperature reads 155°F. This will take 4 to 6 minutes. Transfer to a plate, leaving any drippings in the skillet. Add 1 tablespoon of the butter to the skillet.
5. Cook the sliced onion in the drippings and butter over medium heat, stirring occasionally, until caramelized, 10 to 12 minutes. (Add 1 to 2 tablespoons of avocado oil if the pan is dry.) Stir in the garlic and thyme and cook until fragrant, 30 to 60 seconds.
6. Stir in the arrowroot powder, then gradually pour in the broth, scraping up any brown bits that are stuck to the skillet. Add the wine and cream. Bring to a simmer and cook, stirring occasionally, until the gravy has reduced by half and thickened.
7. Stir in the vinegar and remaining tablespoon of butter. Return the sausages to the skillet. Toss to coat them in the gravy and cook until heated through. Meanwhile, complete the mash.
8. When the turnips are done, drain the water and discard the potato. Return the cooked turnips to the pan and put back on the stovetop over medium heat. Dry cook the turnips until most of the remaining moisture is gone.

(per serving)
CALORIES: **661** | PROTEIN: **22g** | FAT: **53.4g** | TOTAL CARBS: **20.8g** | NET CARBS: **17.1g** | FIBER: **3.7g**

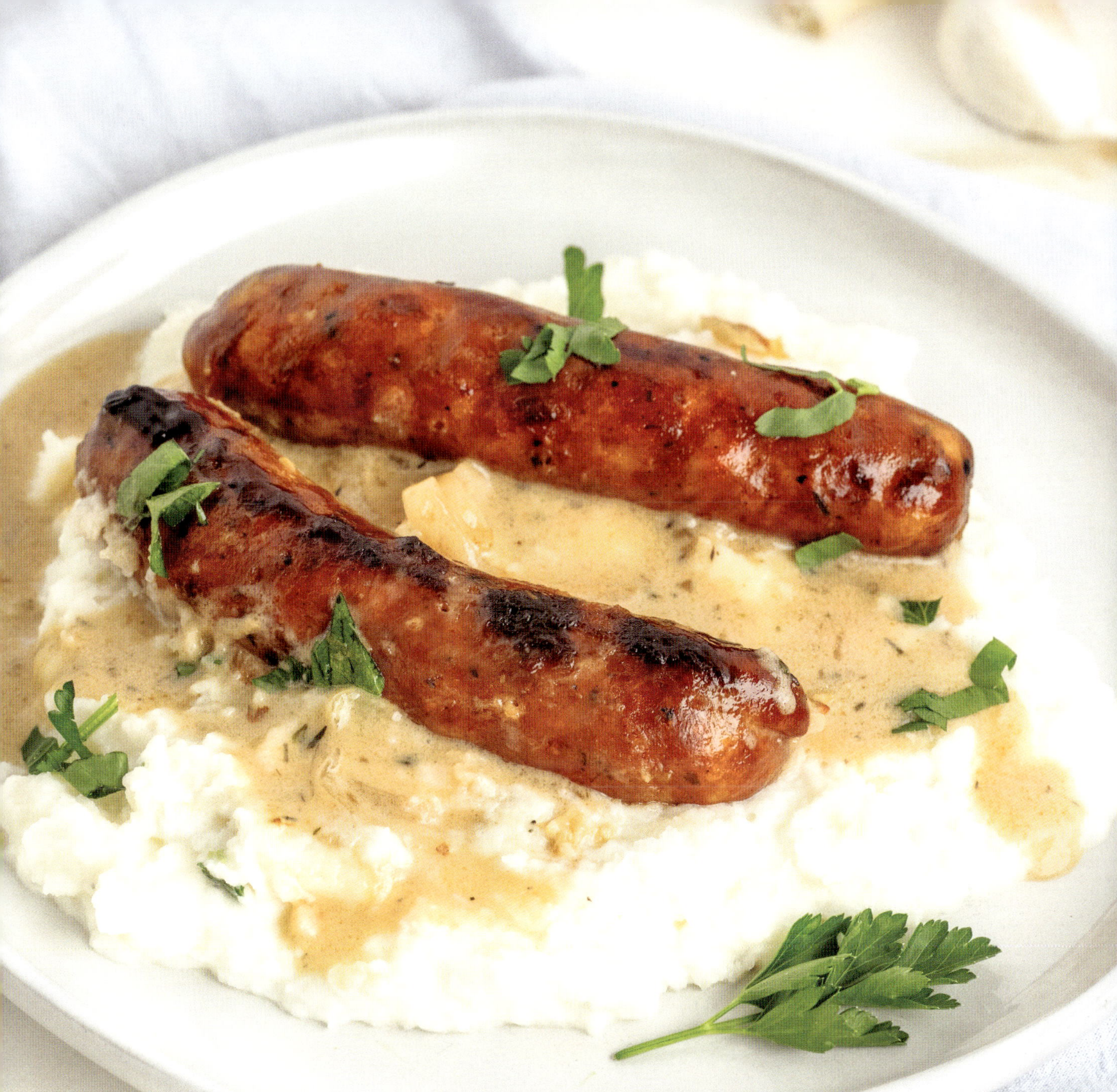

9. Transfer the turnips to a food processor or blender. Add the butter, yogurt, and pepper. Pulse until pureed into a mashed "potato" texture. Season with more salt if needed.
10. To serve, evenly heap the mash onto four plates, then divide the sausages among the plates. Pour the gravy on top. Garnish with chopped parsley, if desired.

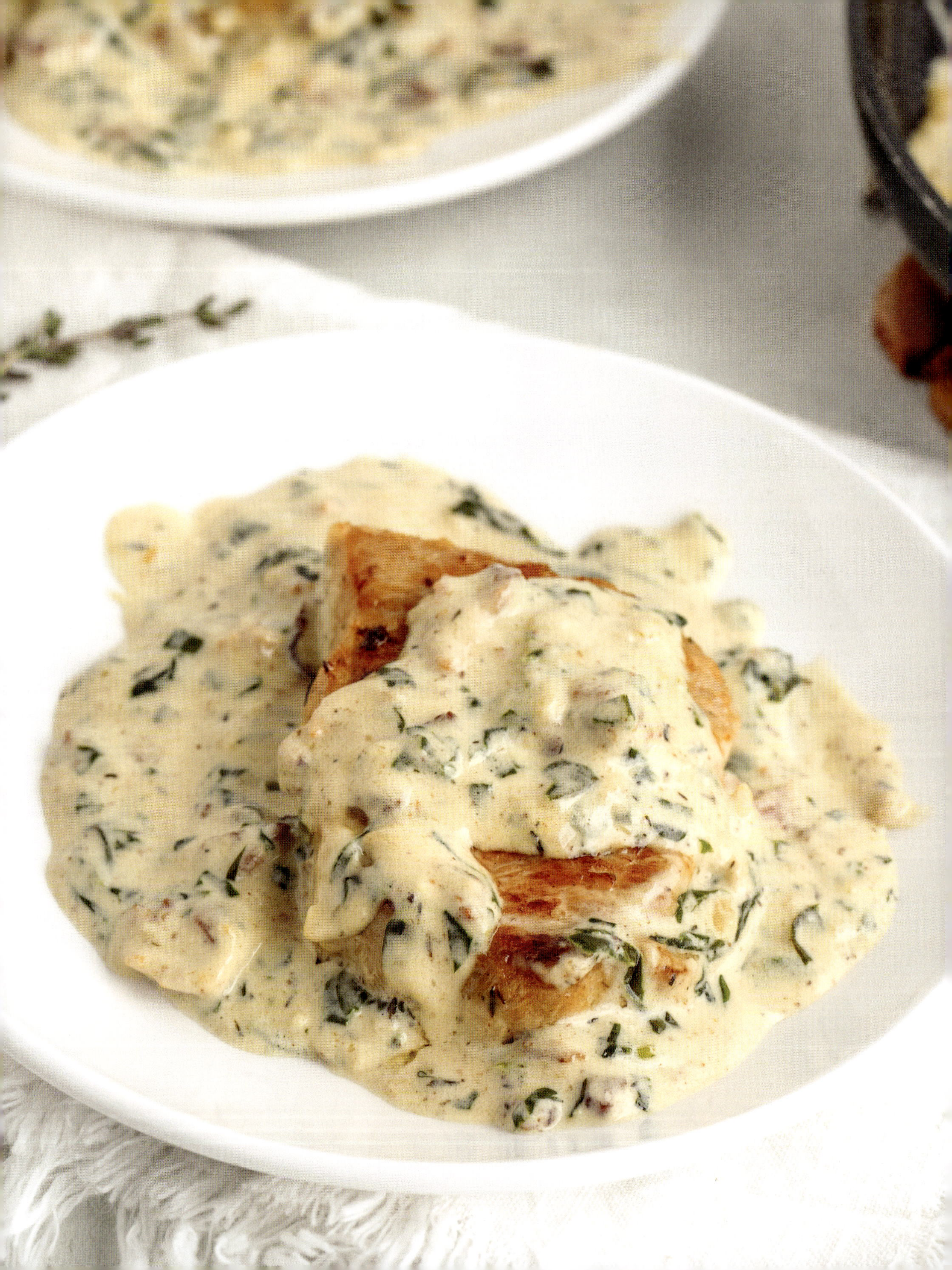

SPINACH & BACON SMOTHERED PORK CHOPS

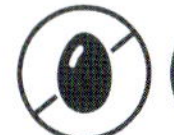
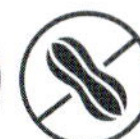
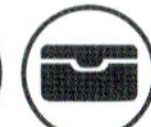

SERVES 4

PREP TIME: 10 minutes

COOK TIME: 30 minutes

This hearty, quick-to-prepare one-pan recipe will have your family coming back for seconds like mine did. Juicy pan-seared pork chops are nestled in a creamy, tangy Dijon sauce with spinach and crispy bacon.

---

4 (6-ounce) boneless pork chops (about 1 inch thick) (see note)

Salt and pepper

2 tablespoons avocado oil

4 slices regular-cut bacon, chopped

1 tablespoon salted butter

4 cloves garlic, minced

1 teaspoon dried thyme leaves

1 cup heavy cream

¼ cup Dijon mustard

¼ cup grated Parmesan cheese

2 cups baby spinach

1. Pat the pork chops dry with a paper towel. Season both sides generously with salt and pepper.
2. Preheat a large skillet over medium heat. Pour in the avocado oil and heat until it ripples. Evenly space the pork chops in the skillet, leaving at least 1 inch of space between them. Cook for 4 to 6 minutes per side, until the internal temperature reaches 140°F. You may need to cover the skillet if the chops are greater than 1 inch thick. Remove the pork chops from the pan and set aside. Leave the drippings in the skillet.
3. Using the same skillet, cook the chopped bacon over medium heat until crispy. Remove the bacon from the skillet but leave behind the bacon grease.
4. Melt the butter in the pan with the bacon grease over medium heat, then add the garlic and thyme. Cook for 1 minute, or until fragrant.
5. Stir in the cream and mustard, scraping the bottom of the pan to deglaze and mix any delicious brown bits stuck to the pan into the sauce. Continue to cook until the sauce has thickened slightly.
6. Stir in the Parmesan cheese and spinach. Cook until the spinach wilts. Return the cooked pork chops and bacon to the sauce. Coat the chops with the sauce. Serve immediately.

note

You can use 12-ounce bone-in pork chops; however, they will take longer to cook.

(per serving)
CALORIES: **617** | PROTEIN: **41g** | FAT: **49g** | TOTAL CARBS: **2g** | NET CARBS: **2g** | FIBER: **0g**

SAUSAGE & PEPPERS PASTA

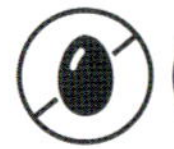   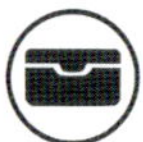

SERVES 4

PREP TIME: 10 minutes

COOK TIME: 20 minutes

This dish features fusilli pasta, sausage or ground pork, two colors of bell peppers, and spinach tossed in a creamy garlic sauce. It uses a low-carb, high-protein pasta made from lupin flour, a gluten-free ingredient derived from the lupini bean that's also high in fiber and low in net carbs. This easy meal is perfect for when you want the comfort of pasta or you want to meal prep.

---

8 ounces lupini fusilli (aka rotini) pasta (see note)

1 teaspoon avocado oil

1 pound bulk Italian sausage or ground pork

½ small onion, diced

1 red bell pepper, diced

1 yellow or orange bell pepper, diced

4 cloves garlic, minced

½ cup heavy cream

3 to 4 handfuls baby spinach

Salt and pepper

1. Prepare the pasta according to the package directions, then drain. (This pasta has a shorter cook time than traditional pasta, so make sure you don't overcook it, or the pasta will fall apart when you combine it with the remaining ingredients.)
2. While the pasta is cooking, prepare the rest of the ingredients. Heat the avocado oil in a large skillet over medium-high heat. Add the sausage and cook, crumbling it with a spatula, until fully browned, 5 to 7 minutes. Remove from the skillet and set aside, leaving any drippings in the pan.
3. Lower the heat to medium. To the skillet, add the onion and bell peppers. Cook until softened. Add the garlic and cook for 1 minute, or until fragrant.
4. Stir in the cream and cook for 1 to 2 minutes, until slightly thickened. Return the sausage and add the spinach. Stir until the spinach is wilted. Gently stir in the pasta until coated, season with salt and pepper, and serve.

note

Kaizen makes a lupin flour pasta that looks and tastes similar to wheat-based pasta. It's my favorite pasta alternative to conventional pasta.

(per serving)
CALORIES: **585** | PROTEIN: **38.5g** | FAT: **39.9g** | TOTAL CARBS: **28.4g** | NET CARBS: **12.1g** | FIBER: **16.3g**

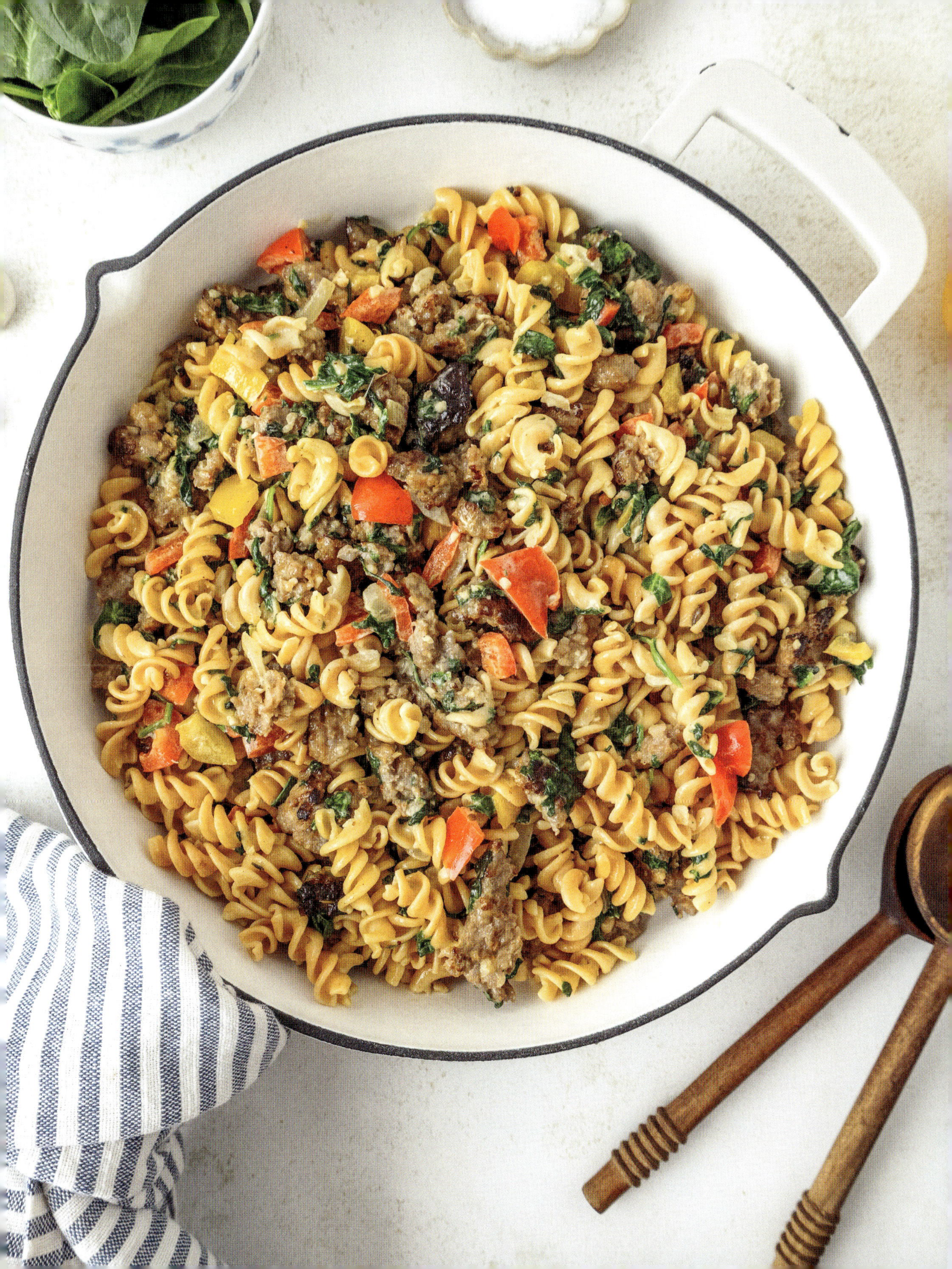

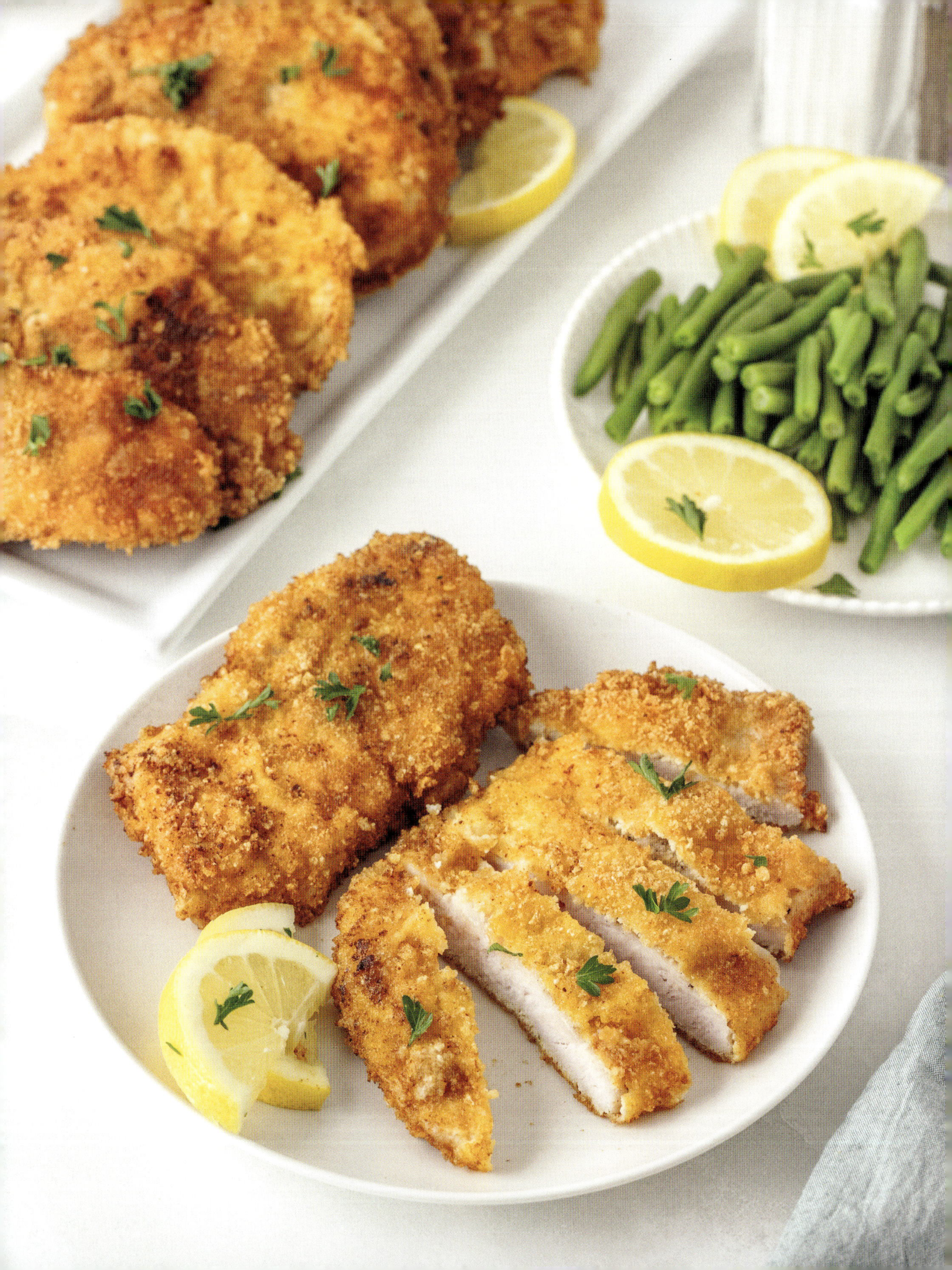

DOUBLE PORK SCHNITZEL

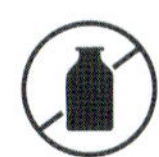

SERVES 4

PREP TIME: 10 minutes

COOK TIME: 20 minutes

This crispy, protein-packed dish requires minimal ingredients and is ready in just 30 minutes. For a low-carb breading, I use almond flour and pork panko. The panko adds a crunchy texture while boosting the protein. For a comforting addition, top it with creamy country gravy, like the one from my Chicken-Fried Venison recipe (page 208). Serve with green beans or your favorite vegetables.

---

4 thin-cut boneless center-cut pork chops (aka cutlets) (4 to 5 ounces each)

1 teaspoon salt

1 teaspoon ground black pepper

⅓ cup blanched, super-fine almond flour

2 large eggs

1¾ cups pork panko

Avocado oil, for the pan

FOR GARNISH/SERVING (OPTIONAL)

Chopped fresh parsley

Lemon wedges

1. Trim any excess fat from the pork chops. Line a cutting board with plastic wrap, place the cutlets in a single layer on the prepared cutting board, and cover with plastic wrap (this prevents splatter). Pound the cutlets with a meat mallet or a rolling pin until they are ¼ to ⅛ inch thick.
2. Season the pork on both sides with the salt and pepper.
3. Grab three shallow bowls and put the almond flour in one bowl. Whisk the eggs in the second bowl and put the pork panko in the third bowl.
4. Working with one pork cutlet at a time, place the cutlet in the almond flour bowl first and turn to coat all over. Gently shake off any excess flour, dip in the egg mixture, and then dredge in the pork panko. Press the panko into the pork to create an evenly thick layer. Transfer to a clean plate and set aside. Repeat with the remaining pork chops and breading. Do not stack the breaded chops; keep them in a single layer to prevent the breading from falling off.
5. Pour ½ inch of avocado oil into a large skillet and place over medium heat. The oil is hot enough to cook the breaded chops when a small piece of breading mixture sizzles in the skillet.
6. Working in batches to avoid crowding, place two breaded pork chops in the skillet, making sure to leave about ½ inch of space around each. Gently shake the pan back and forth over the stovetop to allow the hot oil to slide over the edges and tops of the breaded chops. This makes the edges crispy.
7. Cook for 3 to 4 minutes on each side, until the breading is golden brown and the internal temperature of each chop reaches 145°F. Transfer to a wire rack to cool for up to 5 minutes before serving. Repeat with the remaining pork chops. Garnish with parsley and serve with lemon wedges, if desired.

(per serving)
CALORIES: **385** | PROTEIN: **45.7g** | FAT: **22.5g** | TOTAL CARBS: **2.3g** | NET CARBS: **1.2g** | FIBER: **1.1g**

ITALIAN SAUSAGE SOUP

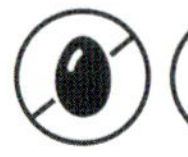

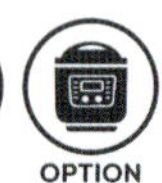
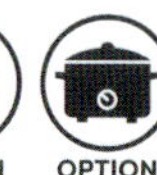

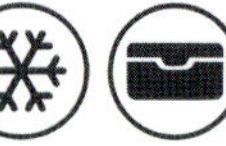

SERVES 4

PREP TIME: 15 minutes

COOK TIME: 35 minutes to 4 hours 35 minutes, depending on method

This hearty, easy-to-make soup is perfect for any night of the week. Made with Italian sausage, carrots, tomatoes, zucchini, spinach, and Parmesan cheese, it's packed with wholesome ingredients and bold flavors. Whether you cook it on the stovetop, in a slow cooker, or in an Instant Pot, it comes together effortlessly. Each 3-cup serving delivers nearly 40 grams of protein.

---

2 pounds bulk Italian sausage

3 cloves garlic, minced

1 cup sliced carrots

½ medium onion, diced

2 teaspoons Italian seasoning

¼ teaspoon salt

¼ teaspoon ground black pepper

4 cups beef broth

1 (14.5-ounce) can diced tomatoes

2 small zucchini, sliced into quarter-moons

2 cups baby spinach

½ cup preshredded Parmesan cheese, plus more for garnish if desired

¼ cup chopped fresh parsley, plus more for garnish if desired

STOVETOP INSTRUCTIONS:

1. Preheat a Dutch oven or other large heavy-bottomed pot over medium-high heat. Put the sausage in the pot and cook, breaking the meat into crumbles, until browned, 5 to 7 minutes. Add the garlic and cook for 1 minute, or until fragrant.
2. Stir in the carrots, onion, Italian seasoning, salt, and pepper. Cook for 1 to 2 more minutes.
3. Stir in the broth and diced tomatoes with juices. Reduce the heat to medium-low, cover, and simmer for 15 minutes, or until the carrots begin to soften.
4. Stir in the zucchini, cover, and cook for 15 more minutes, or until the zucchini is tender.
5. Remove the pot from the heat, then stir in the spinach, Parmesan, and parsley. Continue stirring until the spinach is wilted. Serve topped with more Parmesan and parsley, if desired.

SLOW COOKER INSTRUCTIONS:

1. Preheat a large skillet over medium-high heat. Put the sausage and garlic in the pan and cook, breaking the meat into crumbles, until browned, 5 to 7 minutes.
2. While the sausage is cooking, put the carrots, onion, Italian seasoning, salt, pepper, broth, and diced tomatoes with juices in the slow cooker. Add the cooked sausage and any cooking fat to the slow cooker and stir to combine. Cover and cook on low for 4 hours.
3. Stir in the zucchini, cover, and cook for 20 more minutes, or until the zucchini is tender. Turn the slow cooker to warm, then stir in the spinach, Parmesan, and parsley. Continue stirring until the spinach is wilted. Serve topped with more Parmesan and parsley, if desired.

(per serving)
CALORIES: **647** | PROTEIN: **39.8g** | FAT: **43.5g** | TOTAL CARBS: **25g** | NET CARBS: **20.2g** | FIBER: **4.8g**

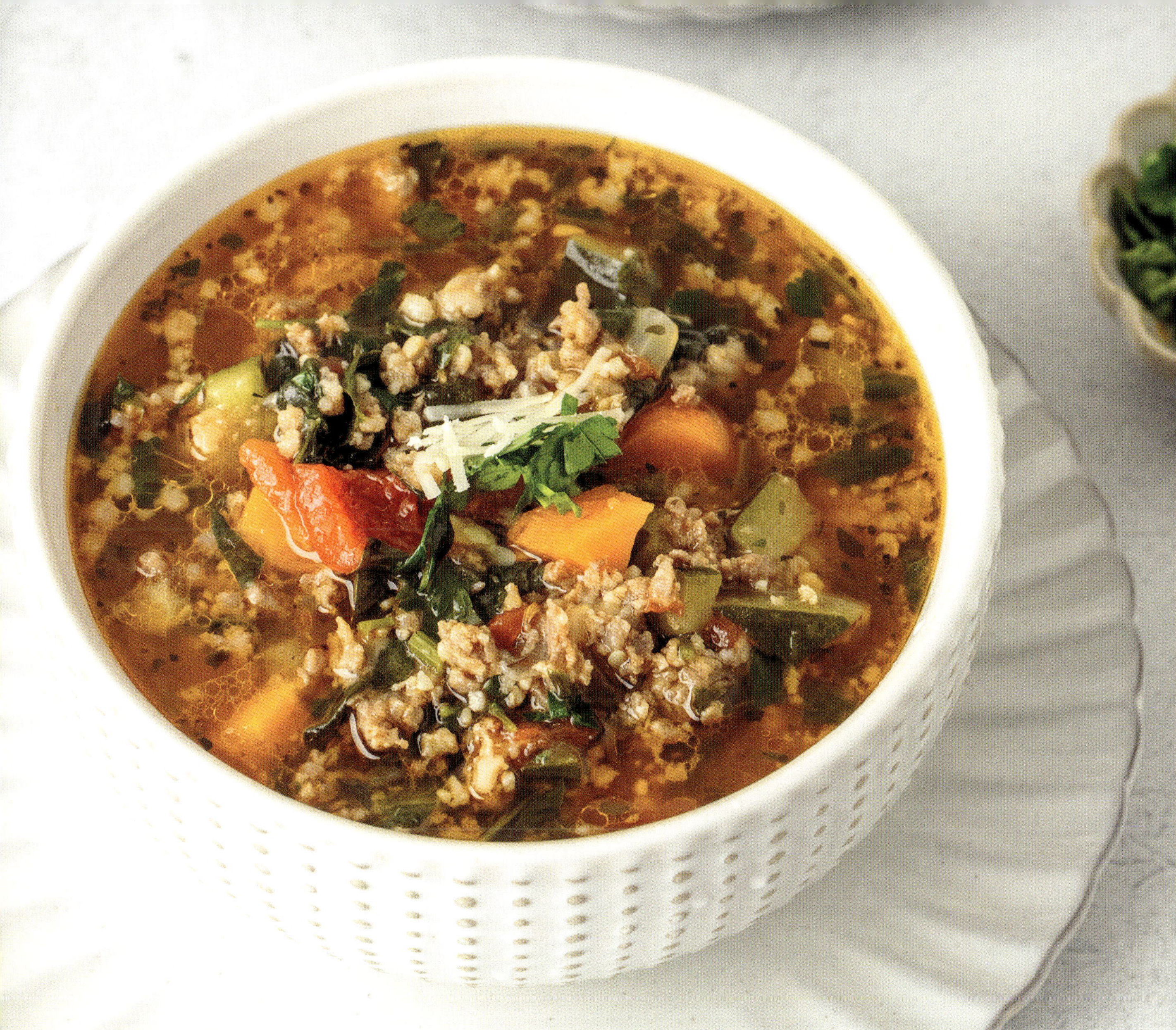

INSTANT POT INSTRUCTIONS:

1. Set the Instant Pot to the Sauté function. Once heated, put the sausage and garlic in the pot and cook, breaking the meat into crumbles, until browned, 5 to 7 minutes. Stir in the carrots, onion, Italian seasoning, salt, and pepper. Cook for 2 more minutes. Add the beef broth and diced tomatoes with juices and stir to combine.
2. Secure the lid and pressure-cook on high for 8 minutes. Allow the Instant Pot to vent naturally for 4 minutes before turning or pressing the vent to release the remaining pressure.
3. Remove the lid and turn the Instant Pot back to Sauté mode. Stir in the zucchini and cook for 10 minutes, or until the zucchini is tender. Turn off the Instant Pot. Stir in the spinach, Parmesan, and parsley. Continue stirring until the spinach is wilted. Serve topped with more Parmesan and parsley, if desired.

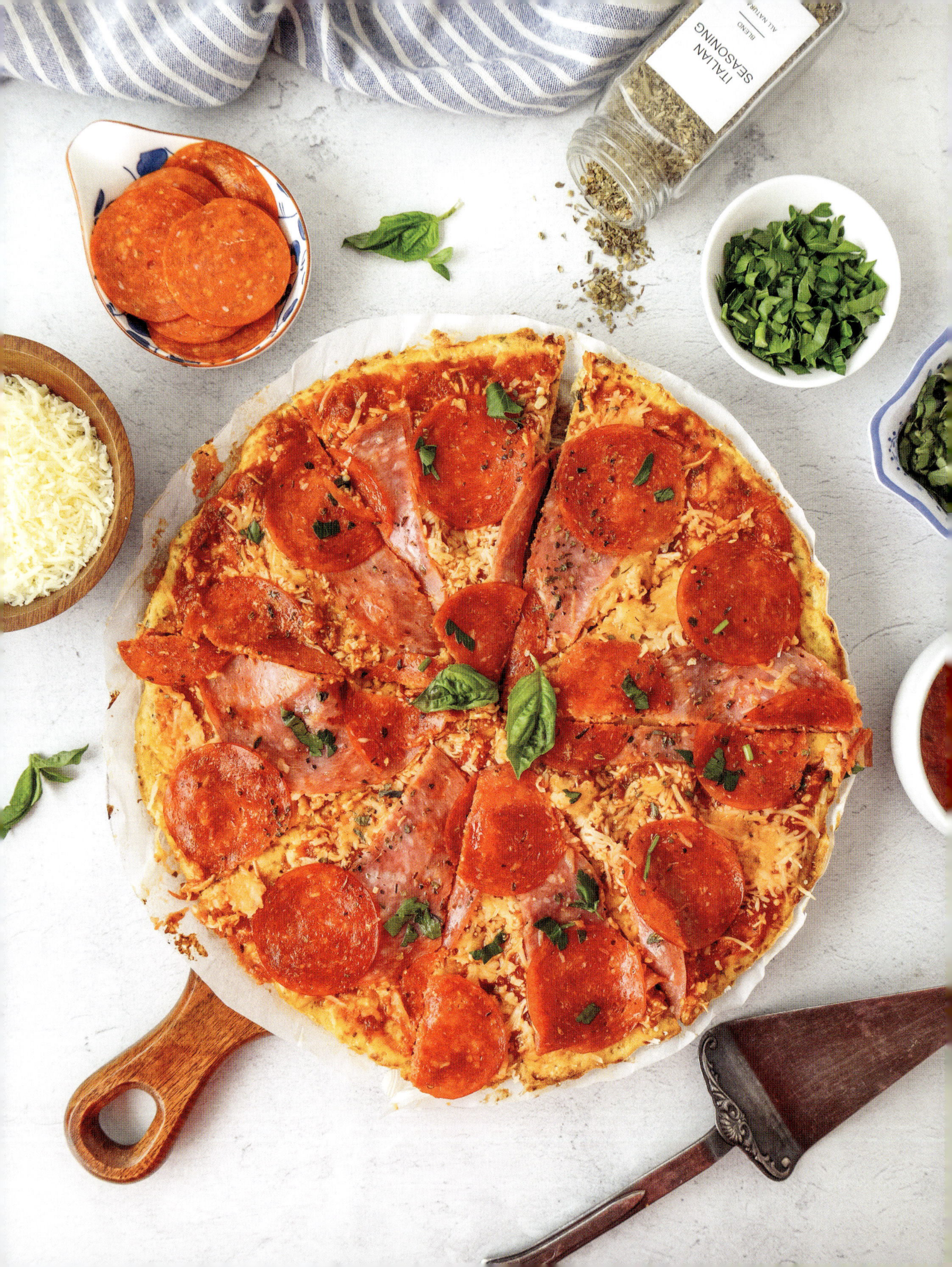
ITALIAN
SEASONING
BLEND

MEAT LOVER'S PROTEIN PIZZA

SERVES 2
PREP TIME: 20 minutes
COOK TIME: 45 minutes

This pizza features a high-protein crust made from cottage cheese, egg, and oat fiber for a sturdy, flavorful base. The cottage cheese and egg act as a glue to hold the crust together, while the oat fiber adds texture and a subtle boost of flavor to taste like pizza crust! Salami and pepperoni are perfect toppings for meat lovers, but it's just as versatile for adding veggies or other favorites.

FOR THE CRUST

1 cup cottage cheese (4% milkfat)

3 tablespoons oat fiber

2 large eggs

1 teaspoon Italian seasoning, plus more for garnish

½ teaspoon garlic powder

FOR THE TOPPINGS

3 tablespoons low-carb marinara sauce

¾ cup shredded mozzarella cheese

1 ounce pepperoni (about 16 slices)

1¼ ounces salami (about 8 slices)

Fresh basil leaves (optional)

1. Preheat the oven to 350°F. Line a rimmed baking sheet or 12-inch round pizza pan with parchment paper.
2. In a medium bowl, mix together the crust ingredients. Pour the mixture into the center of the prepared pan and spread into a circle that is 9 to 9½ inches in diameter. Bake for 40 minutes, or until cooked through and golden brown.
3. Remove the crust from the oven and let rest for 10 to 15 minutes. It will firm up as it cools.
4. Spread the marinara sauce on top of the crust, leaving a ½-inch border around the edge.
5. Sprinkle on the cheese. Top with the pepperoni and salami. Sprinkle on a bit more Italian seasoning.
6. Bake for 5 more minutes, or until the cheese is melted. Let rest for a few minutes before slicing. Top with basil, if desired.

(per serving)
CALORIES: **483** | PROTEIN: **39.3g** | FAT: **33.9g** | TOTAL CARBS: **7.2g** | NET CARBS: **5.1g** | FIBER: **2.1g**

SCOTCH EGGS

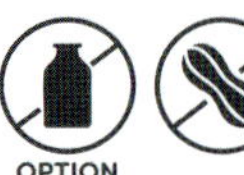

SERVES 4

PREP TIME: 30 minutes (not including time to hard-boil eggs)

COOK TIME: 20 minutes

These high-protein Scotch eggs feature a crunchy breading made from pork panko and protein powder. The panko provides a savory crunch, while the protein powder creates a crispy, Southern-fried texture when cooked. Perfect as a snack, meal, or appetizer, these eggs are great dipped in my homemade sriracha mayo or your favorite sauce.

---

4 large hard-boiled eggs, peeled

1 pound bulk sausage of choice

2 cloves garlic, grated

¼ cup unflavored protein powder

1 large egg

1 cup pork panko

Avocado oil, for the pan

FOR THE SRIRACHA DIPPING SAUCE

¼ cup mayonnaise

2 tablespoons plain Greek or low-carb yogurt

1 to 2 tablespoons sriracha, according to taste

1 teaspoon sugar-free or regular honey

Chopped fresh parsley, for garnish (optional)

note

To make these dairy free, omit the sauce.

1. Let the eggs sit at room temperature for 15 to 30 minutes.
2. Put the sausage and grated garlic in a large bowl. Mix with a spoon or your hands. Divide the meat mixture into four equal portions and form into balls. Set aside.
3. Grab three medium bowls. Put the protein powder in the first bowl. Beat the egg in the second bowl. Put the pork panko in the third bowl.
4. Pour enough oil in a large saucepan to cover the bottom by at least 2 inches. Heat the oil over medium-low heat until it is between 325°F and 350°F. Don't let the oil go past 350°F or the breading will burn.
5. While the oil is heating, form the Scotch eggs. Place a sausage ball on a piece of parchment paper and press into a flat oval (about 6 inches long) that will completely wrap around an egg. Place an egg in the center of the sausage oval, then use the parchment to wrap the sausage around the egg until it's fully enclosed. Carefully peel back the parchment and use it to gently shape and seal the sausage around the egg. Repeat with the remaining sausage balls and eggs.
6. Working in batches, grab two sausage-covered eggs and dust them with the protein powder. Then dip in the egg wash. Then dredge in the pork panko, pressing the breading gently to adhere.
7. Carefully lower the Scotch eggs into the hot oil. Fry for 7 to 10 minutes, flipping halfway through, until golden brown and the internal temperature of the sausage portion reaches 160°F. Remove from the oil and place on a paper towel–lined plate.
8. Repeat Steps 6 and 7 to bread and fry the remaining two sausage-covered eggs.
9. To make the dipping sauce, combine the sauce ingredients in a small bowl. Serve with the Scotch eggs, garnished with parsley, if desired.

(per serving)

CALORIES: **564** | PROTEIN: **38.5g** | FAT: **42.4g** | TOTAL CARBS: **3.3g** | NET CARBS: **1.9g** | FIBER: **0.6g**
SUGAR ALCOHOLS: **0.8g**

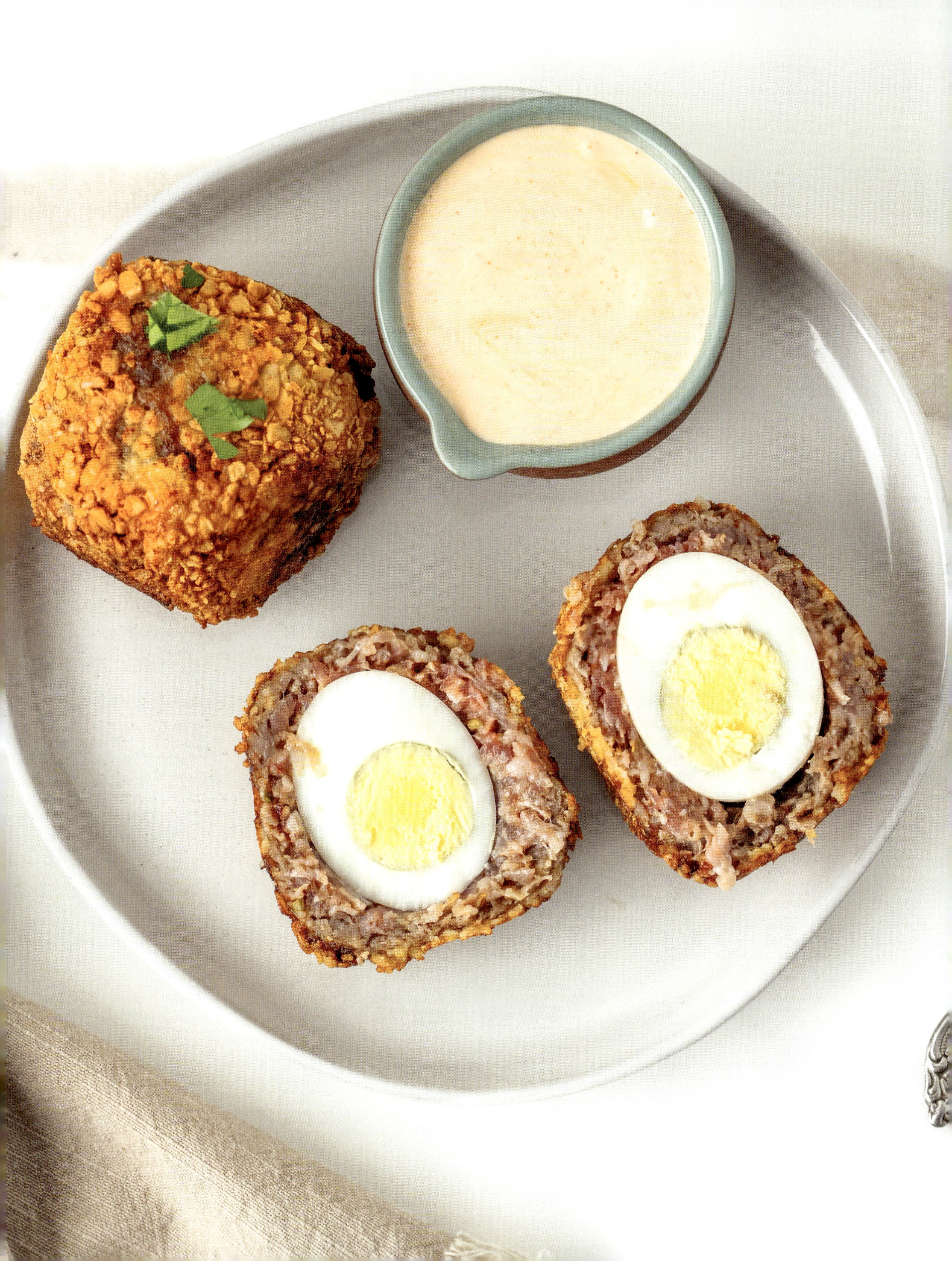

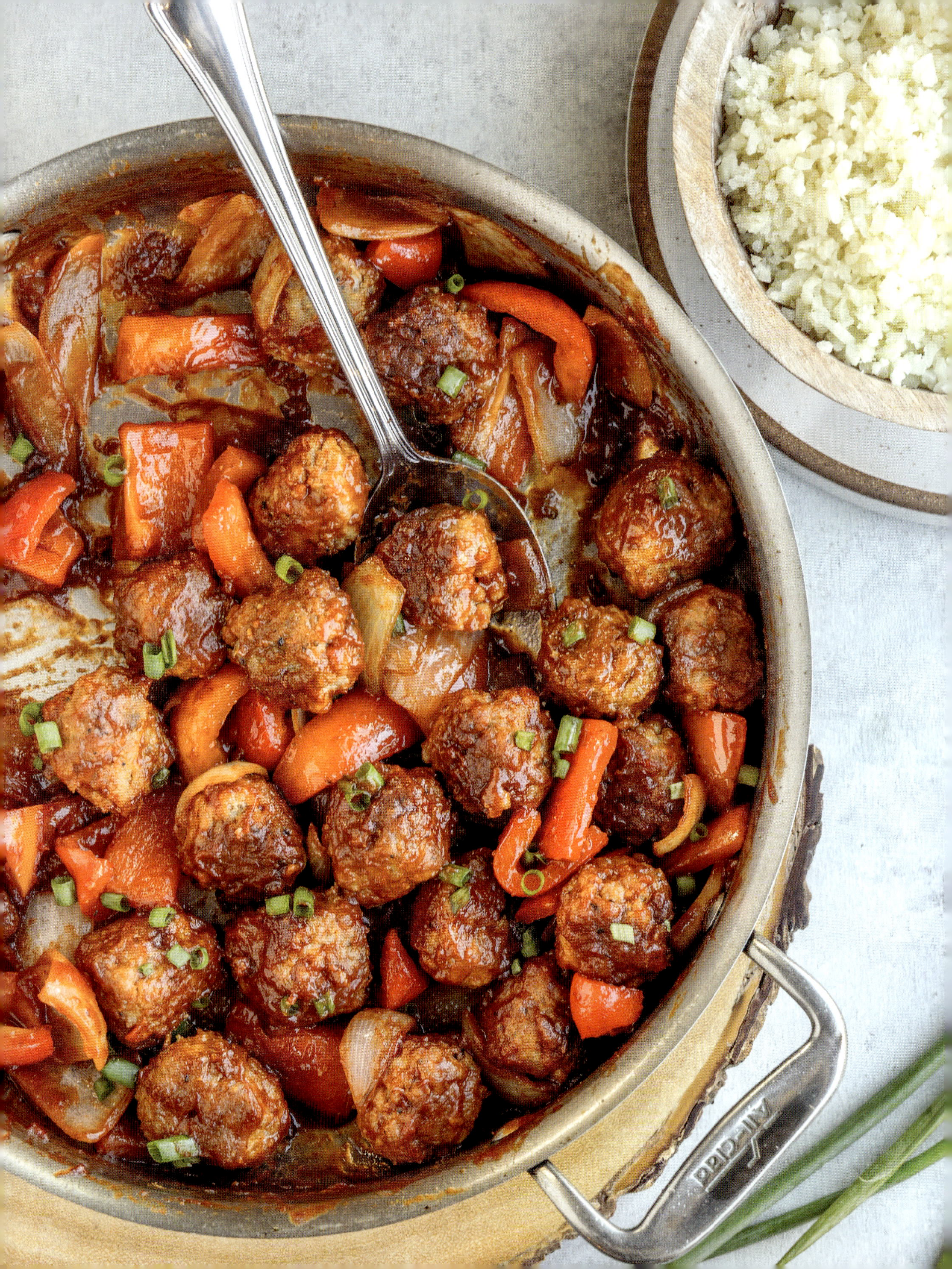
All-Clad

SWEET & SOUR PORK MEATBALLS

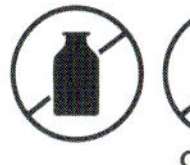
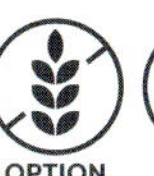

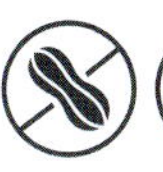
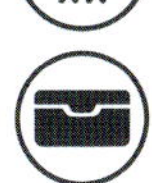

SERVES 4

PREP TIME: 15 minutes

COOK TIME: 20 minutes

These meatballs are an easy one-skillet dinner that's ready in just over 30 minutes. Inspired by Chinese meatballs, they are made with ground pork and pork panko, which serves as the breading. The tangy, sweet, and savory sauce combines apple cider vinegar, brown sugar substitute, tomato paste, and soy sauce. Chunks of red bell pepper and onion provide texture and color. Serve these over cauliflower rice for a complete meal or enjoy them as is for an appetizer; if serving as an appetizer, 1 to 2 meatballs per person should be enough.

---

1 pound ground pork

1 large egg

½ cup pork panko

1 teaspoon salt

½ teaspoon ground black pepper

½ teaspoon garlic powder

2 tablespoons avocado oil, divided

½ medium onion, diced

1 red bell pepper, diced

¼ cup apple cider vinegar

¼ cup tomato paste

2 tablespoons soy sauce or tamari

2 tablespoons brown sugar substitute

½ teaspoon arrowroot powder

2 tablespoons chopped green onions, for garnish

1. Put the ground pork, egg, pork panko, salt, pepper, and garlic powder in a large bowl and use your hands to mix until evenly combined.
2. Pinch off some of the mixture and roll it between your palms to form a ball about 1 inch in diameter. Continue with the remaining mixture. You should get 20 meatballs.
3. Pour 1 tablespoon of the avocado oil into a large skillet and heat over medium heat. Working in batches, add the meatballs to the skillet, spacing them about 1 inch apart. Roll them around every 1 to 2 minutes to cook evenly on all sides. Continue cooking until the meatballs reach an internal temperature of 160°F. Remove from the skillet. Repeat until all the meatballs are cooked.
4. Pour the remaining tablespoon of avocado oil into the skillet and add the diced onion. Increase the heat to medium-high and cook for 2 to 3 minutes, until softened. Stir in the bell pepper and cook for another 2 minutes, stirring occasionally, until softened.
5. Add the vinegar, tomato paste, soy sauce, brown sugar substitute, and arrowroot powder. Stir well. Bring to a simmer and cook until thickened. Return the meatballs to the pan and stir to coat. Remove from the heat and top with the green onions.

note

To make this gluten free, use coconut aminos or liquid aminos in place of soy sauce or tamari.

(per serving)

CALORIES: **456** | PROTEIN: **29g** | FAT: **34.4g** | TOTAL CARBS: **14.6g** | NET CARBS: **6.8g** | FIBER: **1.8g**
SUGAR ALCOHOLS: **6g**

SWEET & TANGY PORK TENDERLOIN

  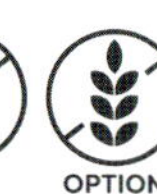 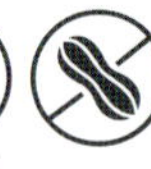

OPTION

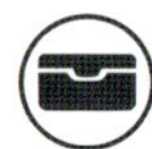

SERVES 6

PREP TIME: 10 minutes

COOK TIME: 1 hour

This pork tenderloin is oven-braised in a sweet and tangy sauce made with sugar-free honey, Dijon mustard, apple cider vinegar, and plenty of garlic, creating a meal that is full of flavor. With minimal prep time, this dish is perfect for a quick weeknight dinner or meal prepping lunches and dinners for the week. To make it extra tangy, serve with lemon wedges or Dijon mustard on the side.

⅓ cup chicken broth

⅓ cup sugar-free or regular honey

⅓ cup Dijon mustard

2 tablespoons minced garlic

1 tablespoon soy sauce or tamari

1 tablespoon Worcestershire sauce

1 tablespoon apple cider vinegar

1 teaspoon ground black pepper, divided

3 pounds pork tenderloins

2 teaspoons garlic powder

1 teaspoon paprika

1 teaspoon salt

Avocado oil, for the pan

Chopped fresh parsley, for garnish (optional)

1. Preheat the oven to 350°F.
2. In a medium bowl, combine the broth, honey, mustard, garlic, soy sauce, Worcestershire sauce, vinegar, and ½ teaspoon of the pepper. Set aside.
3. Pat the tenderloins dry with a paper towel. Mix together the garlic powder, paprika, salt, and remaining ½ teaspoon of pepper in a small bowl. Season all sides of the tenderloins with the seasoning mixture.
4. Preheat a large oven-safe skillet over medium-high heat. Pour in 1 tablespoon of avocado oil and swirl to coat the skillet. Add the pork tenderloins and sear on all sides until a golden-brown crust forms. Add more oil if the pan becomes dry.
5. Remove the pan from the heat. Pour the honey sauce over the seared tenderloins, then turn them in the sauce to coat.
6. Transfer the skillet, uncovered, to the oven and bake until the pork reaches an internal temperature of 145°F in the thickest part, 30 to 60 minutes depending on the thickness of the tenderloins. During cooking, baste the tenderloins every 15 minutes.
7. Let rest for 15 minutes before slicing. Garnish with parsley, if desired.

note

To make this gluten free, use coconut aminos or liquid aminos in place of soy sauce or tamari.

per serving, using sugar-free honey

CALORIES: **329** | PROTEIN: **48.3g** | FAT: **10.9g** | TOTAL CARBS: **17.7g** | NET CARBS: **2.5g** | FIBER: **6.3g**
SUGAR ALCOHOLS: **8.9g**

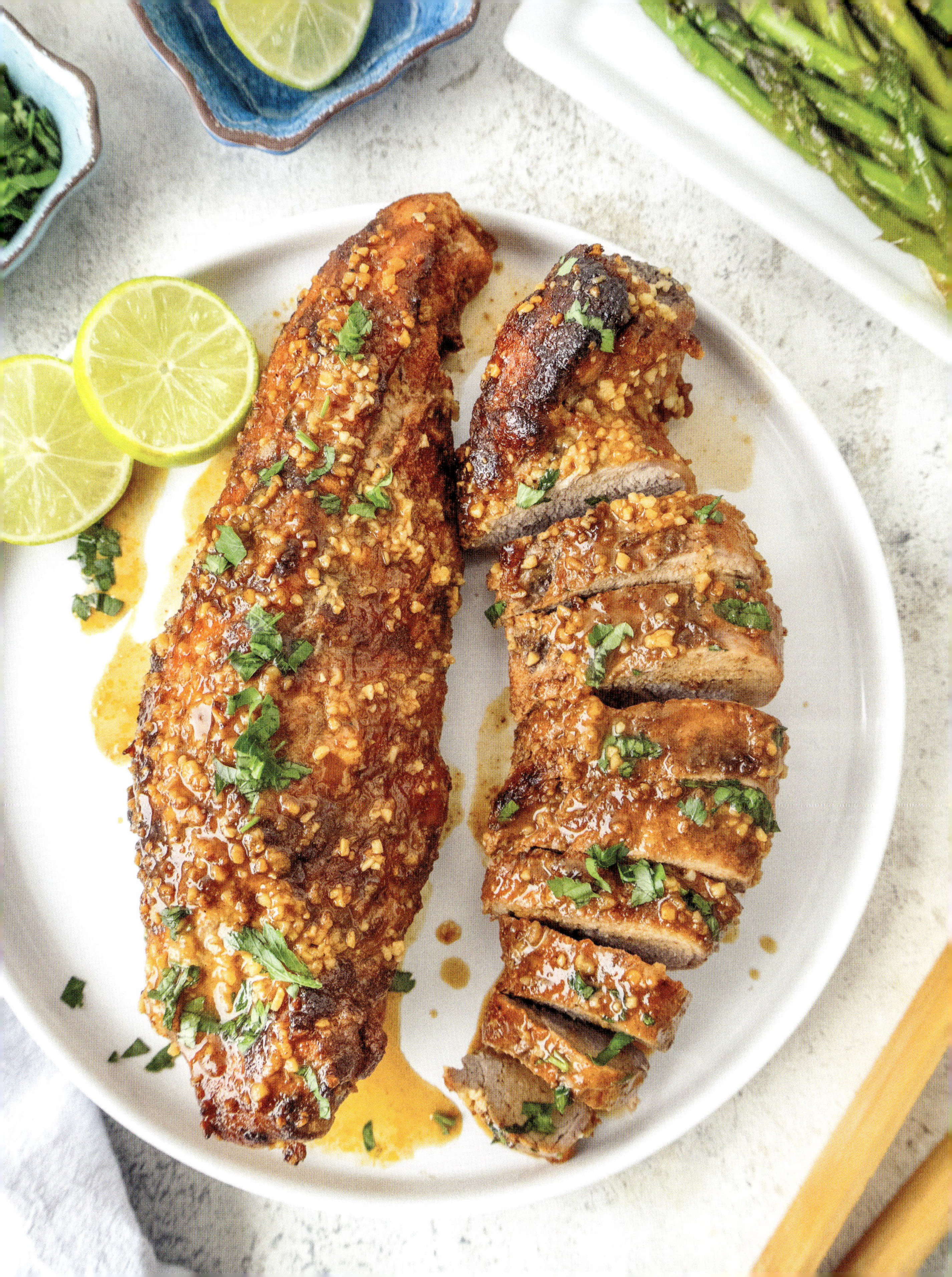

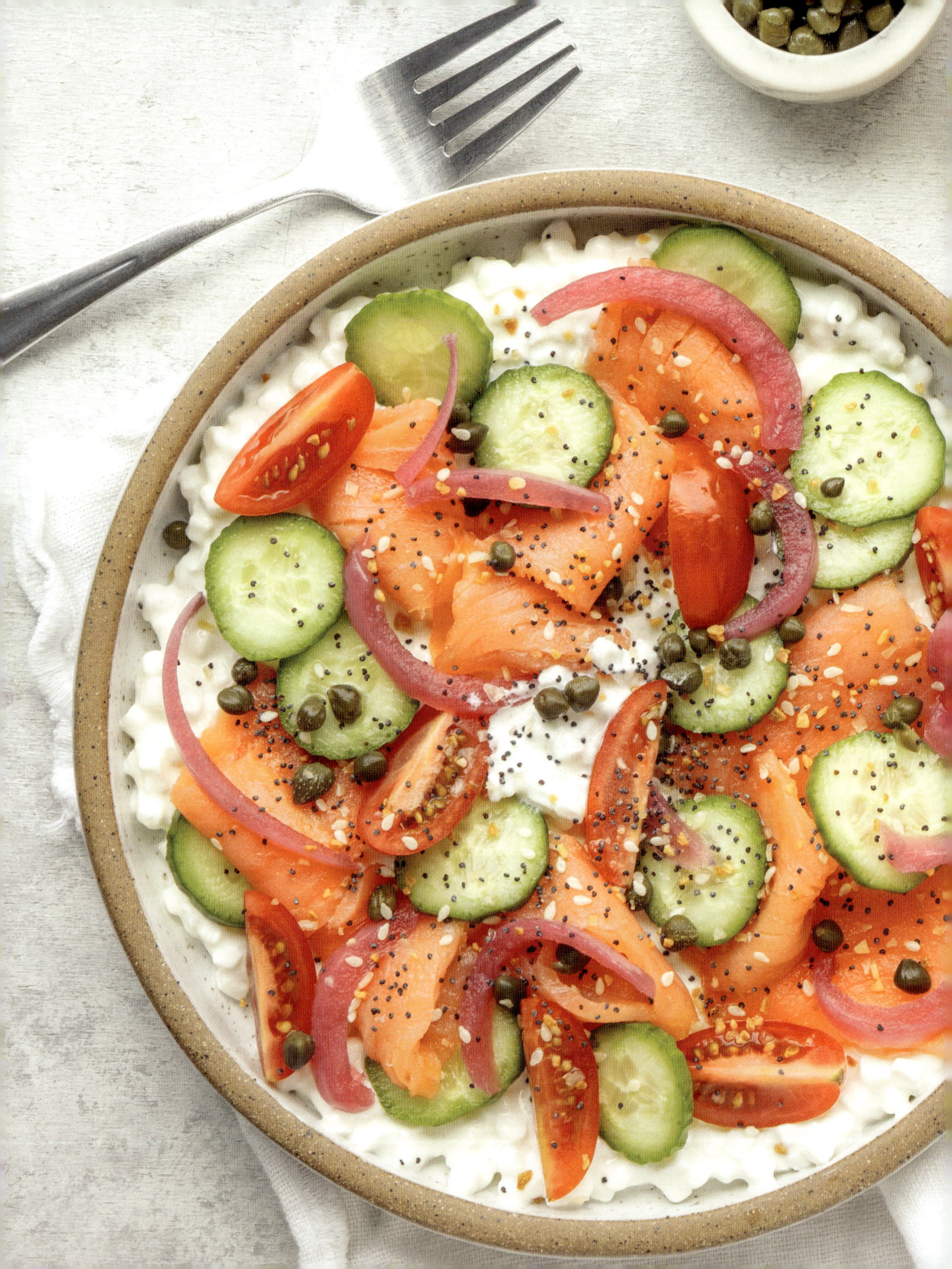

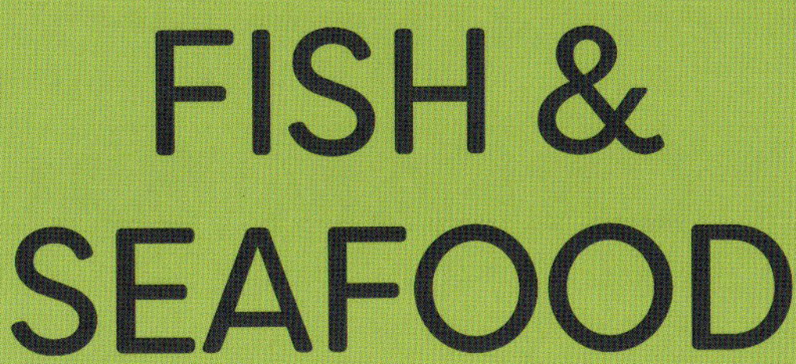

FISH & SEAFOOD

ALMOND FLOUR–CRUSTED ROCKFISH WITH TARRAGON LEMON CREAM SAUCE

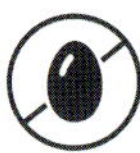

SERVES 4
PREP TIME: 10 minutes
COOK TIME: 30 minutes

This pan-fried fish is tender and flaky on the inside with a crusty exterior. No wonder this classic preparation is so popular, especially when paired with a creamy sauce, as here. When fried in olive oil, the combination of almond flour and protein powder creates a light, crunchy coating on the fillets. The sauce, enhanced with fresh tarragon and garlic, adds a bright and tangy finish. Since I live in the Pacific Northwest, rockfish is accessible at every grocery store. If it's not available where you live, you can substitute another mild white fish, like cod, halibut, or tilapia.

---

1 pound skinless rockfish fillets

Salt and pepper

½ cup blanched, super-fine almond flour

¼ cup unflavored protein powder

¼ cup avocado oil, for the pan

FOR THE CREAM SAUCE

1 tablespoon avocado oil

2 cloves garlic, minced

¼ cup dry white wine

¼ cup fresh lemon juice

½ cup heavy cream

4 tablespoons cold salted butter

1 teaspoon salt

2 tablespoons chopped fresh tarragon

FOR GARNISH/SERVING

Fresh tarragon sprigs

Freshly cracked black pepper

Lemon wedges (optional)

1. About 15 minutes prior to cooking, lightly season the fish with salt and pepper on both sides.
2. While the seasoned fish is resting, make the cream sauce. Heat the avocado oil in a medium saucepan over medium heat. Add the garlic and sauté for 30 seconds, or until fragrant. Pour in the wine and lemon juice. Cook until the liquid has reduced by half. Stir in the cream. Continue cooking until the mixture thickens, about 5 minutes. Stir in the butter until melted. Add the salt and tarragon. Continue cooking until the sauce coats the back of a spoon. Cover and set aside to stay warm.
3. In a shallow dish or plate, combine the almond flour and protein powder. Dredge each fish fillet in the flour mixture, pressing the mixture into both sides until fully coated.
4. Preheat a large skillet over medium heat, then pour in the avocado oil and allow it to heat up. The oil is hot enough when a crumb of breading sizzles in the skillet. Place each fillet in the hot oil, making sure not to overcrowd the pan and leaving about 1 inch between fillets. Fry until golden brown, 3 to 6 minutes, depending on the thickness. (For 1-inch-thick fillets, a cook time of 5 minutes per side is a good general guideline.) Flip the fillets over and cook for another 3 to 6 minutes, until both sides are golden brown, the interior is white and flaky, and the internal temperature of each fillet is 145°F. Transfer to a wire rack set over a paper towel–lined rimmed baking sheet to catch the excess oil.
5. To serve, pour the lemon cream sauce over the crusted fillets and top with tarragon sprigs and cracked pepper. Serve with lemon wedges, if desired.

(per serving)
CALORIES: **412** | PROTEIN: **28.5g** | FAT: **28.4g** | TOTAL CARBS: **4.2g** | NET CARBS: **2.7g** | FIBER: **1.5g**

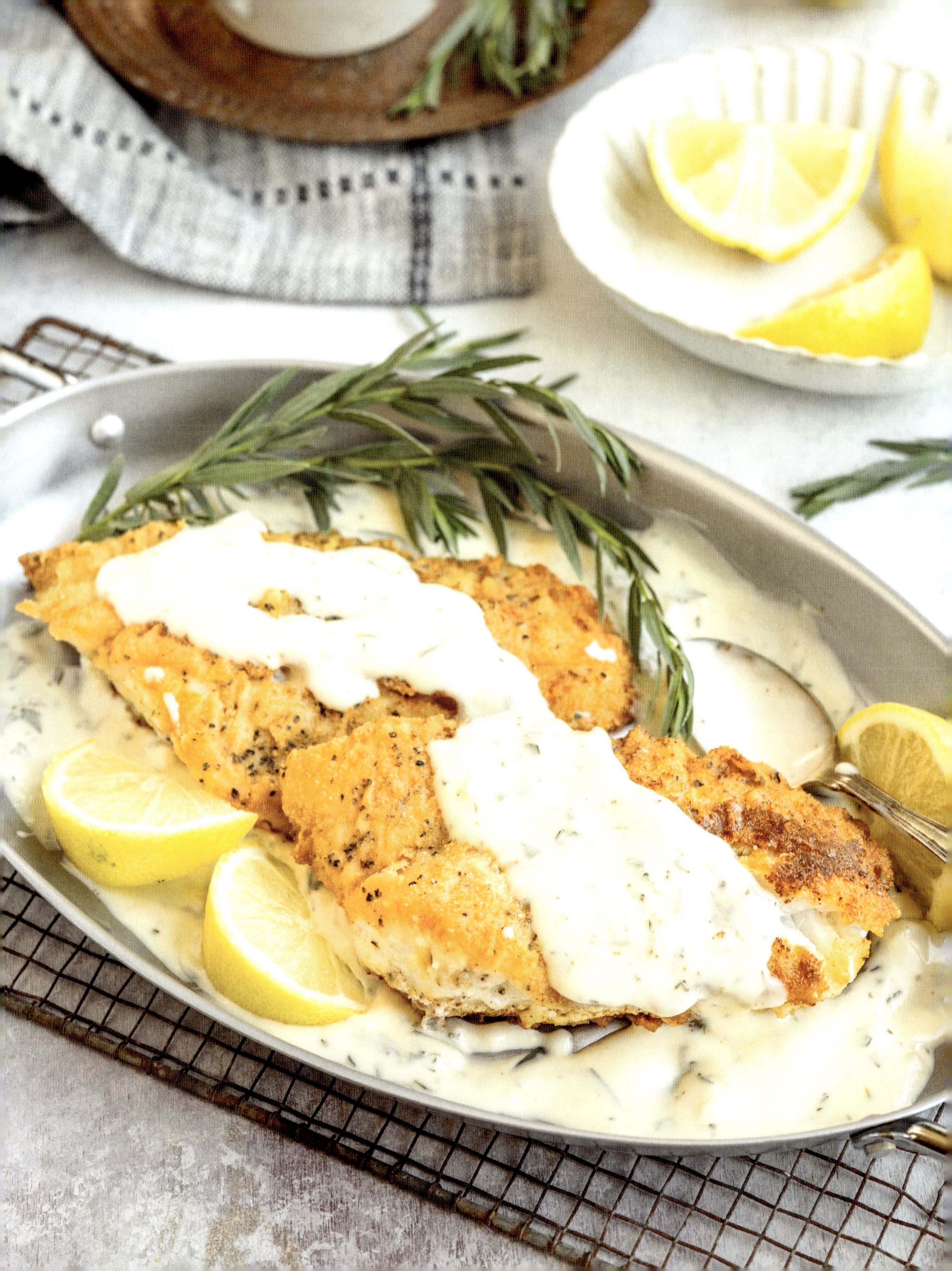

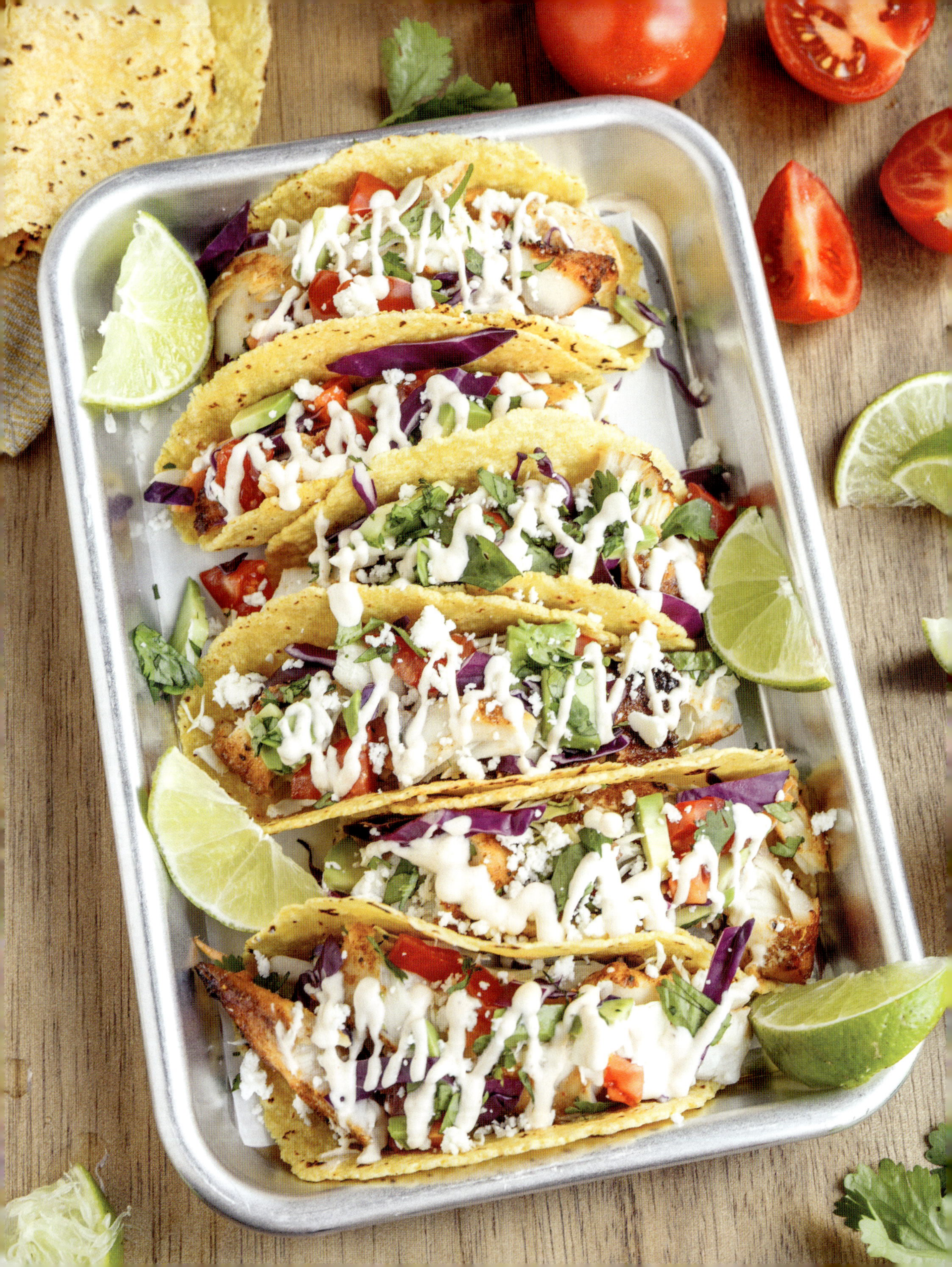

FISH TACOS

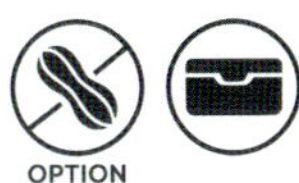

Makes 12 tacos (2 per serving)

PREP TIME: 15 minutes, plus 30 minutes to marinate fish

COOK TIME: 30 minutes

Making amazing fish tacos at home is quick and simple with this recipe. You start with tilapia—or any mild white fish, like cod, halibut, or rockfish—and bring it to life with a zesty marinade of lime juice, garlic powder, chili powder, and cumin. The star of the dish is the garlic lime cream sauce; it's so flavorful, you might want to eat it by the spoonful! Grab some low-carb tortillas and top with your favorite taco fixings.

---

2 pounds skinless tilapia fillets

12 (4-inch) low-carb flour tortillas, store-bought or homemade (page 249)

FOR THE MARINADE

¼ cup avocado oil

¼ cup lime juice

2 teaspoons chili powder

2 teaspoons ground cumin

1 teaspoon garlic powder

1 teaspoon salt

¼ teaspoon ground black pepper

FOR THE CREAM SAUCE

½ cup plain Greek or low-carb yogurt

⅓ cup mayonnaise

2 tablespoons lime juice

1 teaspoon garlic powder

1 teaspoon sriracha

SUGGESTED TOPPINGS

1 (14-ounce) bag coleslaw mix

1 avocado, sliced

1 Roma tomato, diced

¼ medium red onion, diced

½ bunch fresh cilantro, chopped

4 ounces Cotija cheese, crumbled

Lime wedges

1. Cut the tilapia fillets into 3- to 4-inch pieces.
2. In a small bowl, mix together the ingredients for the marinade. Put the tilapia pieces in a large baking dish and pour the marinade over them, gently turning to make sure each piece is coated. Cover and refrigerate for 30 to 45 minutes.
3. Meanwhile, prepare the cream sauce. In a small bowl, combine the ingredients for the sauce. Cover and refrigerate until ready to use.
4. Preheat the oven to 375°F. Line a rimmed baking sheet with foil.
5. Evenly space the marinated tilapia fillets on the prepared pan; discard the leftover marinade. Bake for 20 to 25 minutes, until the internal temperature reaches 140°F and the fish is flaky. To get the edges crispy, move an oven rack to the top position, turn the broiler to high, and broil for 3 to 5 minutes. Set aside for a few minutes to cool slightly.
6. To assemble the tacos, evenly distribute the fish pieces among the tortillas, then add the taco toppings of your choice. Drizzle the sauce on top, then fold and serve.

STORAGE INSTRUCTIONS: Cooked tilapia can be stored in a sealed container in the refrigerator for 3 to 4 days. Store the sauce and toppings separately. The cream sauce can be stored in a sealed container in the refrigerator for up to 5 days, and the toppings for 2 to 5 days.

note

To make this nut free, opt for store-bought nut-free tortillas; my tortilla recipe uses almond flour.

(per serving, using homemade tortillas)
CALORIES: **571** | PROTEIN: **40.8g** | FAT: **39.3g** | TOTAL CARBS: **18.3g** | NET CARBS: **9.1g** | FIBER: **9.2g**

HIGH-PROTEIN GUMBO

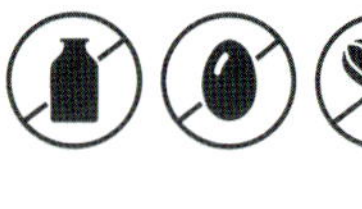

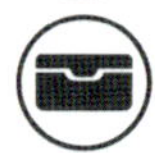

SERVES 4

PREP TIME: 15 minutes

COOK TIME: 30 minutes

This gluten-free gumbo is a flavorful take on the classic, made without flour and thickened with arrowroot powder. Packed with protein from the andouille sausage and shrimp, it features chunks of bell pepper, onion, celery, and tomatoes, along with bold Cajun flavor. Perfect as a hearty soup or served over cauliflower rice, this recipe is also freezer-safe, making it a great option for meal prepping.

---

1 tablespoon avocado oil

½ medium onion, diced

1 green bell pepper, chopped

4 celery stalks, sliced

3 cloves garlic, minced

12 ounces andouille sausage, thinly sliced

1½ teaspoons Cajun or blackening seasoning

¼ cup dry white wine (see note)

1½ cups chicken broth

1 (14.5-ounce) can diced tomatoes

1 to 2 tablespoons arrowroot powder

1 pound medium shrimp, peeled and deveined (tails off)

2 tablespoons chopped fresh parsley

Salt and pepper

1. Preheat a large Dutch oven or stockpot over medium-high heat. Pour in the avocado oil and heat until ripples form. Add the onion, bell pepper, celery, garlic, and sausage. Cook, stirring frequently, until the sausage is browned on the edges and the veggies are softened, 5 to 7 minutes.
2. Stir in the Cajun seasoning and cook until fragrant, about 1 minute. Pour in the wine and stir, scraping the brown bits from the bottom of the pot. These bits hold flavor, and you want to get that flavor into the liquid. Add the broth, tomatoes, and 1 tablespoon of arrowroot powder. Stir to combine. Bring to a boil, then reduce the heat to a simmer for 10 minutes, or until the liquid has thickened.
3. Stir in the shrimp and continue to simmer until the shrimp is pink and opaque, 3 to 4 minutes. If the gumbo isn't as thick as you'd like, stir in up to 1 tablespoon more arrowroot powder and simmer for 2 to 3 more minutes. Remove from the heat and stir in the parsley. Season with salt and pepper to taste.

note

If you prefer to avoid alcohol, use additional chicken broth in place of the wine.

(per serving)

CALORIES: **432** | PROTEIN: **41.3g** | FAT: **21.7g** | TOTAL CARBS: **16g** | NET CARBS: **12.5g** | FIBER: **3.5g**

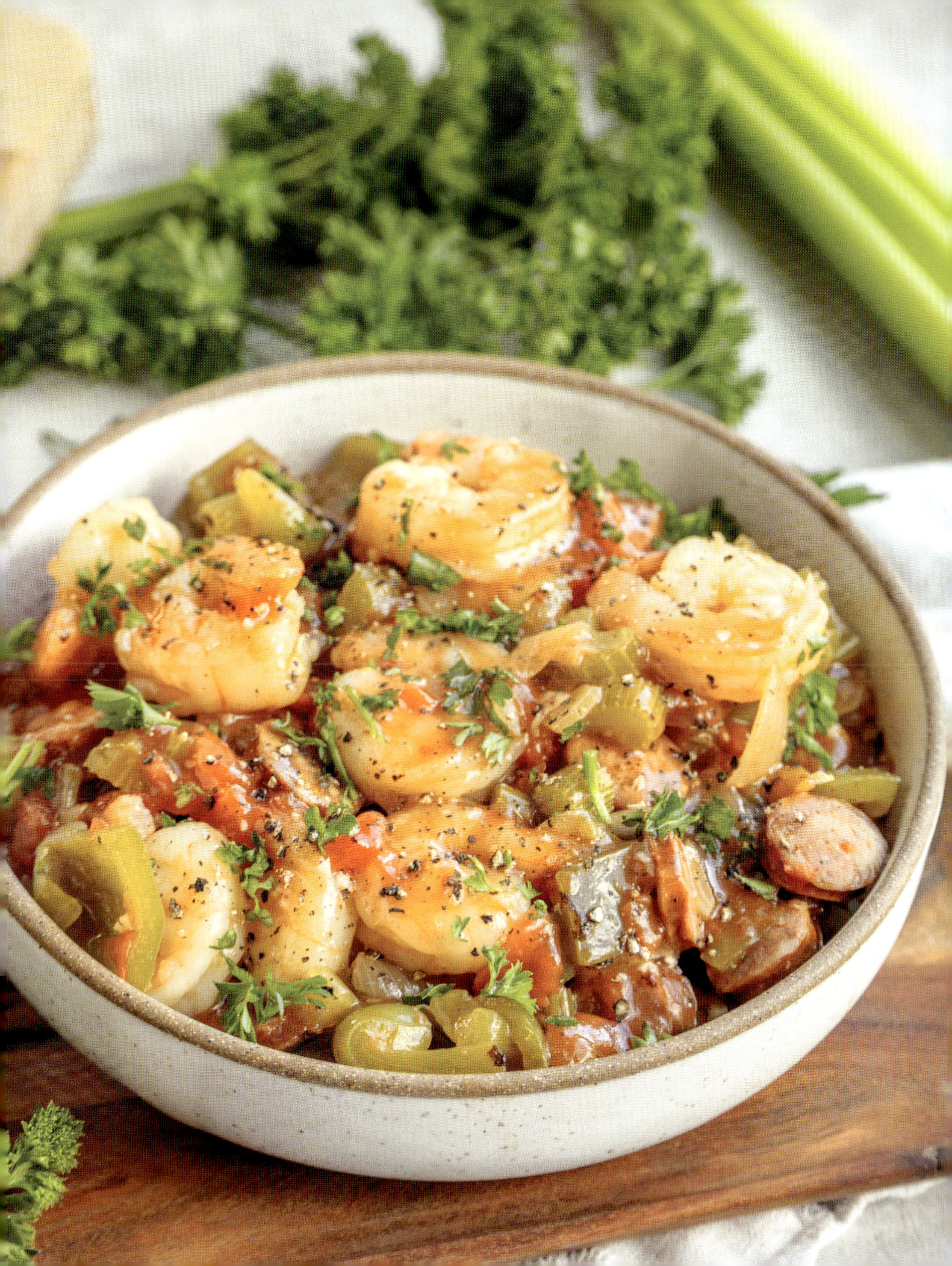

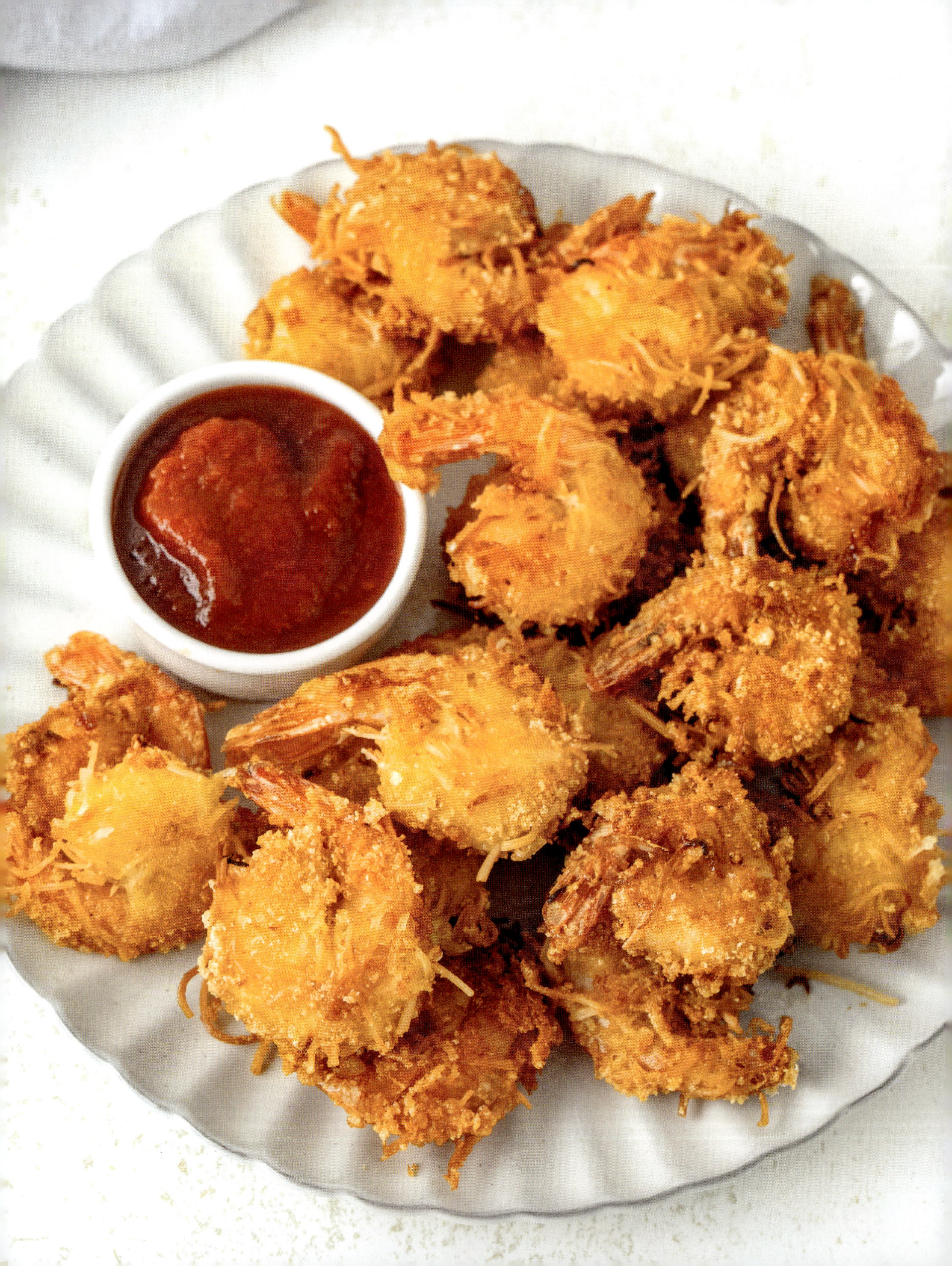

LOW-CARB COCONUT SHRIMP

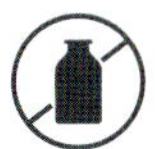

SERVES 4
PREP TIME: 15 minutes
COOK TIME: 30 minutes

This recipe is inspired by my in-laws, who can't resist ordering coconut shrimp whenever they see it on a menu. These shrimp are coated in a gluten-free, low-carb breading made from protein powder, pork panko, unsweetened coconut flakes, and, if desired, a powdered sugar-free sweetener for just the right touch of sweetness. The protein powder and panko create a perfect crispy layer surrounding the juicy shrimp. They're delicious on their own or paired with your favorite sweet chili sauce for dipping.

½ cup unflavored protein powder

½ teaspoon salt

½ teaspoon ground black pepper

2 large eggs

1 cup pork panko

1¼ cups unsweetened shredded coconut

2 tablespoons powdered sugar-free sweetener (optional)

Avocado oil, for frying

1 pound jumbo (21/25) shrimp, peeled and deveined (tails on)

Sweet chili sauce, for dipping (optional)

1. Start with three medium bowls. In the first bowl, combine the protein powder, salt, and pepper. Beat the eggs in the second bowl. Combine the pork panko, coconut, and sweetener (if using) in the third bowl.
2. Pour enough oil into a large saucepan to cover the bottom by at least 1 inch. Heat the oil over medium-low heat until it is between 325°F and 350°F. Don't let it go past 350°F or the breading will burn.
3. Working in batches, grab 3 or 4 shrimp and toss them in the protein powder mixture. Then dip in the egg wash. Then dredge the shrimp in the panko-coconut mixture, pressing the breading gently to adhere.
4. Gently drop the breaded shrimp into the hot oil. Fry for 2 minutes on each side, until golden brown and the internal temperature of the shrimp reaches 145°F. Using a slotted spoon, remove the shrimp from the oil and place on a rimmed baking sheet fitted with a wire rack. Repeat Steps 3 and 4 with the remaining shrimp.
5. If desired, serve with sweet chili sauce as a dip.

REHEATING INSTRUCTIONS: Leftover shrimp can be reheated in the air fryer to get them crispy again. Air-fry at 350°F for 2 to 3 minutes.

note

Don't bread the shrimp all at once, or the protein powder will absorb some of the moisture from the shrimp, which will prevent you from getting a puffy golden crust. It's better to bread each batch just before cooking.

(per serving)
CALORIES: **400** | PROTEIN: **49.3g** | FAT: **19.1g** | TOTAL CARBS: **10.7g** | NET CARBS: **2.9g** | FIBER: **3.8g**
SUGAR ALCOHOLS: **4g**

LOW-CARB FISH & CHIPS

OPTION

SERVES 4

PREP TIME: 15 minutes

COOK TIME: 30 minutes

To make this recipe gluten free and low carb, I coat the cod fillets in a breading made with protein powder and baking powder. Once fried, the coating develops a crispy texture reminiscent of beer-battered fried fish. Pair it with my high-protein tartar sauce, which is made lighter by swapping some of the mayo for Greek yogurt, or enjoy with a splash of malt vinegar. My Air-Fried Pickle Chips make the perfect side (assuming you are okay with the almond flour in the breading).

FOR THE PROTEIN TARTAR SAUCE

½ cup mayonnaise

½ cup plain Greek or low-carb yogurt

1 tablespoon chopped fresh dill

2 cloves garlic, grated

1 teaspoon lemon juice

1 teaspoon granulated sugar-free sweetener

¼ teaspoon ground black pepper

⅛ teaspoon salt

1½ pounds skinless cod fillets, cut into 8 equal-size pieces

Salt and pepper

Avocado oil, for frying

¼ cup Dijon mustard

2 large eggs

1⅔ cups unflavored protein powder

1 teaspoon baking powder

1 teaspoon salt

1 teaspoon dried thyme leaves

½ teaspoon garlic powder

Air-Fried Pickle Chips (page 309), for serving (optional)

1. Prepare the tartar sauce by putting all the ingredients in a small bowl and mixing until well combined. Refrigerate until ready to use.
2. Pat the cod fillets dry with a paper towel and season both sides lightly with salt and pepper. Set aside. Wrap a rimmed baking sheet in foil and place a wire rack on top. Set aside.
3. Pour enough avocado oil into a large saucepan or Dutch oven to double the thickness of the cod fillets. Heat the oil over medium-low heat until it is between 325°F and 350°F. Don't let it go past 350°F or the breading will burn.
4. Meanwhile, grab two shallow bowls. In the first bowl, whisk together the mustard and eggs. In the second bowl, mix together the protein powder, baking powder, salt, thyme, and garlic powder.
5. Once the oil is hot enough, begin coating the cod. Working in batches, dip two pieces of fish in the egg mixture and then dredge in the protein powder mixture, pressing the powder into each piece of fish to ensure it's completely coated on all sides. Only coat the number of fish pieces that you intend to fry right away because the breading tends to absorb moisture from the fish as it sits, which means you won't get that perfect crunchy crust on the outside when fried.
6. Carefully lower each piece of battered cod into the hot oil and fry for 3 to 5 minutes, flipping halfway through, until the fish is golden brown on the outside, white and flaky on the inside, and the internal temperature reaches 145°F. Remove using a fish spatula or slotted spatula and set on the wire rack.
7. Repeat with the remaining fish, egg wash, and breading mixture. Serve with the tartar sauce and pickle chips, if desired.

note

Fry in small batches (two fillets at a time) to help maintain the oil temperature and keep the oil from bubbling over. Monitor the temperature of the oil periodically to ensure it's not getting too hot.

(per serving, fish only)

CALORIES: **490** | PROTEIN: **57.8g** | FAT: **28.1g** | TOTAL CARBS: **4.2g** | NET CARBS: **2.7g** | FIBER: **0.5g**
SUGAR ALCOHOLS: **1g**

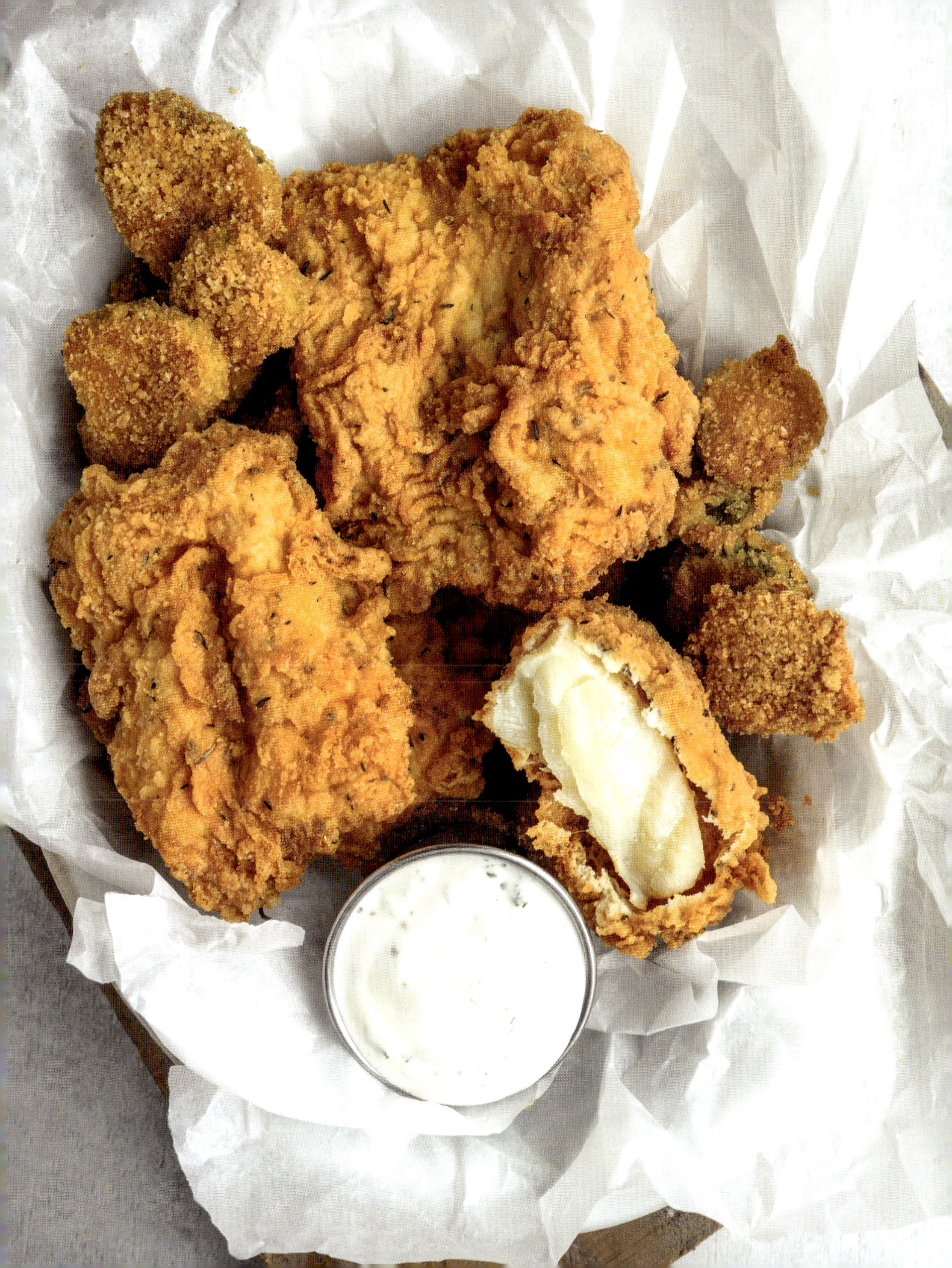

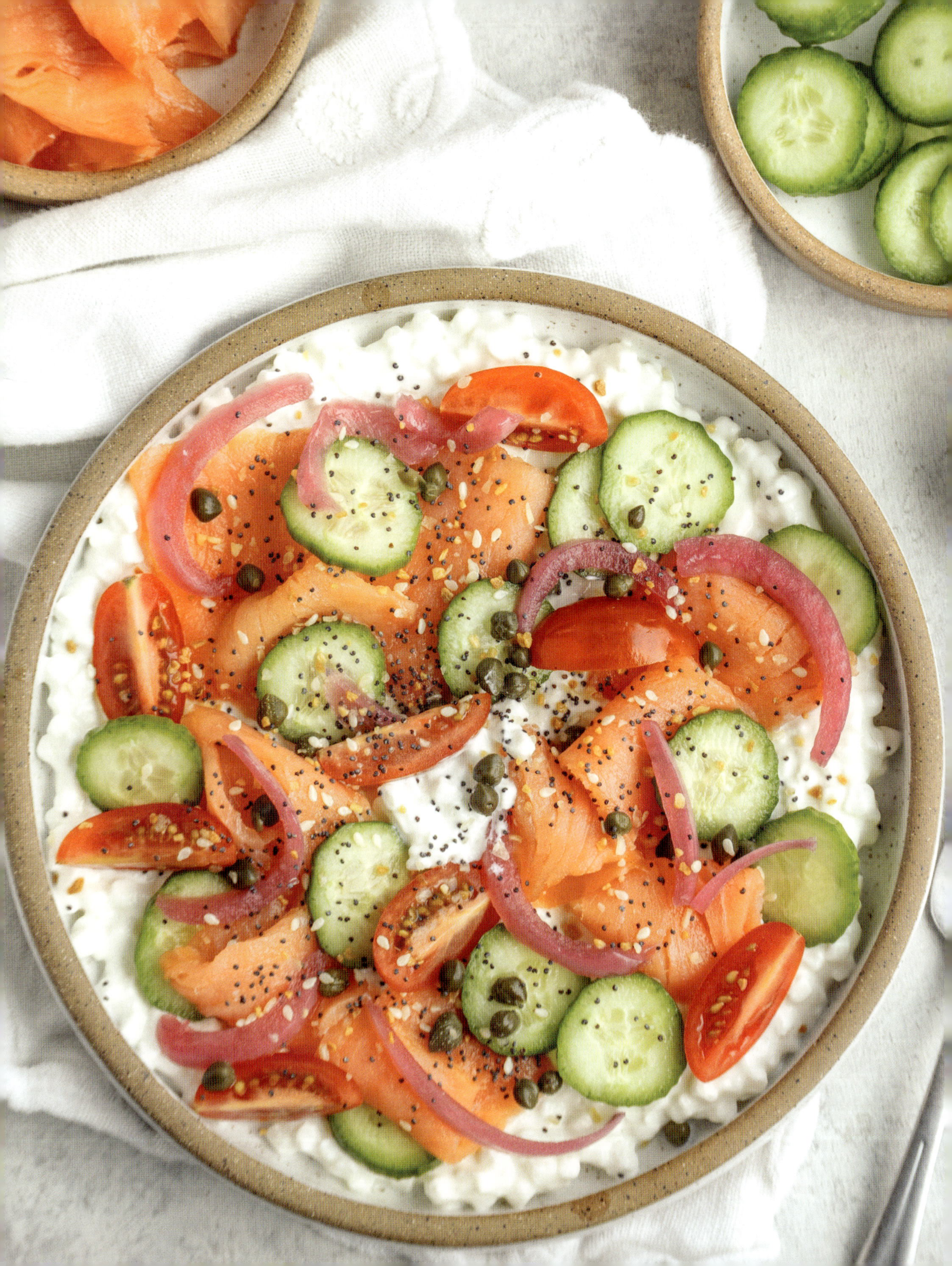

LOX COTTAGE CHEESE BOWL

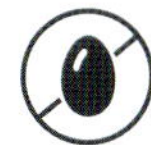

SERVES 1

PREP TIME: 5 minutes

This bowl combines all the flavors of a lox bagel—smoked salmon, capers, and pickled red onion—served over a bed of creamy cottage cheese. The fresh tomatoes and cucumber add brightness and crunch. It's a low-carb, high-protein meal that's ready in minutes, making it a perfect lunch or quick dinner.

¾ cup cottage cheese (4% milkfat)

2 ounces Nova lox, chopped

1 mini cucumber, sliced

3 grape tomatoes, quartered

¼ cup pickled red onions

1 teaspoon capers

½ teaspoon everything bagel seasoning

1. Spread the cottage cheese in a shallow serving bowl.
2. Top with the lox, cucumber, tomatoes, pickled onions, and capers.
3. Sprinkle the seasoning on top.

Pack It with Protein: Top with sliced hard-boiled eggs.

note

Want to lower the carbs? Omit the cucumber, tomatoes, and/or onions.

CALORIES: **344** | PROTEIN: **41.5g** | FAT: **10.4g** | TOTAL CARBS: **25.6g** | NET CARBS: **15.8g** | FIBER: **9.8g**

PESTO SALMON

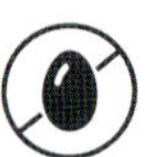

SERVES 4

PREP TIME: 5 minutes

COOK TIME: 20 minutes

Salmon fillets are generously coated with pesto and Parmesan cheese and baked until tender and flaky. This recipe is quick and easy, with minimal prep work, making it ideal as a light, wholesome meal for busy weeknights. Serve with some steamed broccoli or asparagus and a helping of Mashed Turnips (page 250).

---

4 (6-ounce) skin-on salmon fillets

¾ teaspoon salt

½ teaspoon ground black pepper

4 tablespoons pesto sauce

2 tablespoons preshredded Parmesan cheese

½ lemon

1. Preheat the oven to 350°F. Line a rimmed baking sheet with foil.
2. Season the salmon fillets with the salt and pepper and place skin side down on the prepared pan. Cover loosely with foil and bake for 10 minutes.
3. Remove from the oven and spread 1 tablespoon of pesto over each fillet. Evenly sprinkle the fillets with the Parmesan cheese. Return the pan to the oven, uncovered, and bake until the cheese is melted; the fish is moist, tender, and flaky; and the internal temperature of each fillet is 130°F, about 10 minutes more. Salmon is safe to eat when cooked to this temperature, which keeps it tender and juicy, while higher temperatures can cause it to dry out.
4. Remove from the oven and squeeze the lemon over the fillets.

(per serving)
CALORIES: **319** | PROTEIN: **39.9g** | FAT: **15.9g** | TOTAL CARBS: **1.1g** | NET CARBS: **0.8g** | FIBER: **0.3g**

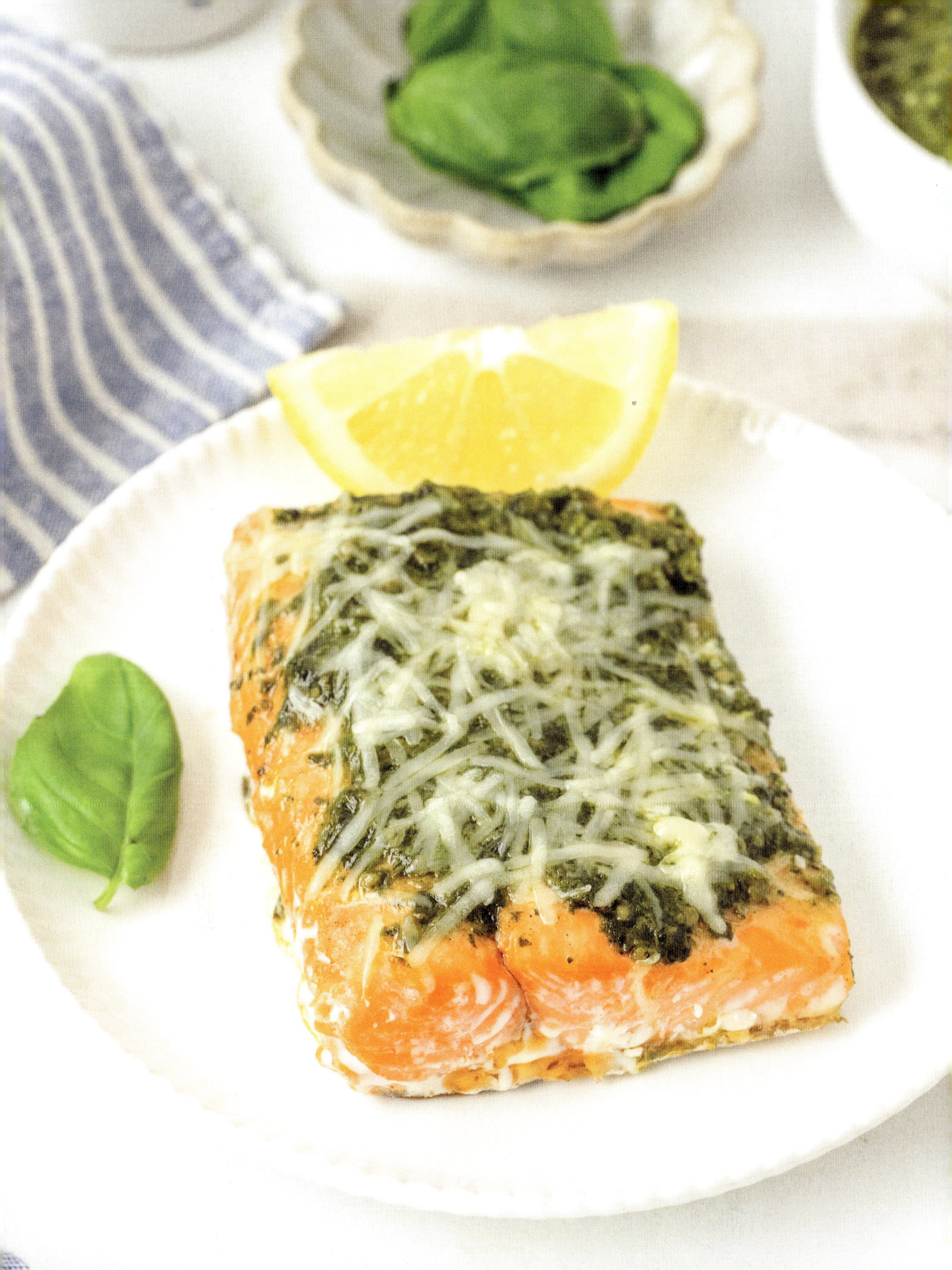

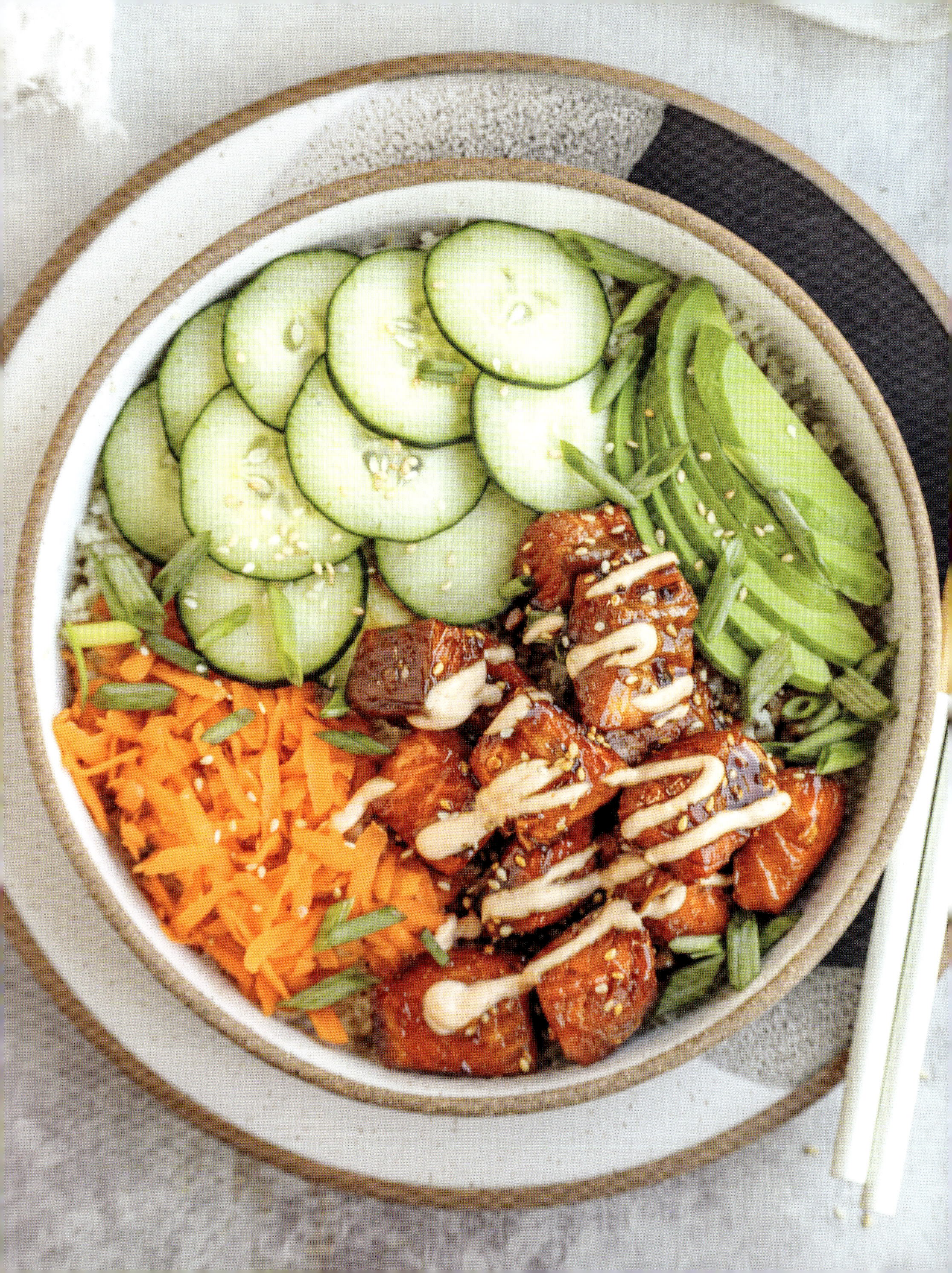

SWEET & SPICY SALMON BOWL

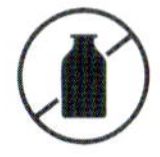

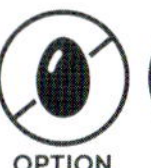

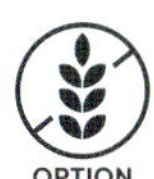

SERVES 1

PREP TIME: 10 minutes (not including time to cook cauliflower rice)

COOK TIME: 15 minutes

This quick salmon bowl is ready in less than 30 minutes. Chunks of fish are cooked in a sweet and spicy sauce with hints of ginger and garlic. It's served over cauliflower rice and topped with fresh avocado, cucumber, carrot, and green onion, but you can add your favorite veggies. This recipe is easy to double or triple for meal prep, making it a versatile option for the week ahead.

---

1 (8-ounce) skinless salmon fillet

⅓ cup soy sauce or tamari

3 tablespoons sugar-free or regular honey

4 cloves garlic, minced

½ teaspoon ginger powder

1 teaspoon sesame seeds, plus more for garnish if desired

½ teaspoon red pepper flakes

1 cup cooked cauliflower rice

½ avocado, thinly sliced

¼ medium cucumber, thinly sliced

2 tablespoons grated carrot

2 green onions, thinly sliced on the diagonal

FOR THE SRIRACHA MAYO (OPTIONAL)

1 tablespoon mayonnaise

2 teaspoons plain Greek or low-carb yogurt

2 teaspoons sriracha

1. Cut the salmon into bite-size cubes and place in a large bowl. Add the soy sauce, honey, garlic, ginger powder, sesame seeds, and red pepper flakes. Toss to coat.
2. Preheat a large skillet over medium-high heat. Put the salmon and sauce in the skillet. Cook for 2 minutes, flip each piece, and cook for another 2 minutes, or until the fish becomes slightly firm, tender, and flaky and its internal temperature reaches 125°F to 130°F.
3. Remove the salmon from the skillet, then lower the heat under the pan to medium and continue to cook the sauce until thickened and sticky, about 5 minutes.
4. To build the bowl, put the cooked cauliflower rice in a serving bowl. Add the cooked salmon along with the avocado, cucumber, carrot, and green onions. Pour the sauce over the bowl. Drizzle the sriracha mayo on top, if desired. Sprinkle with more sesame seeds, if desired.

notes

To make this egg free, omit the sriracha mayo. To make it gluten free, use coconut aminos or liquid aminos in place of soy sauce or tamari.

CALORIES: **519** | PROTEIN: **56.6g** | FAT: **17.5g** | TOTAL CARBS: **78.2g** | NET CARBS: **18.8g** | FIBER: **29.4g** | SUGAR ALCOHOLS: **30g**

TUNA SALAD

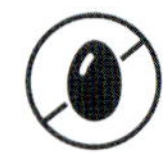

SERVES 1

PREP TIME: 5 minutes

This tuna salad is a flavorful high-protein meal filled with crunchy bits of celery, pickles, and red onions for added texture. It's perfect for a quick and easy lunch. You can enjoy it wrapped in lettuce or an egg wrap, or use it to make a tuna sandwich with your favorite low-carb bread. Double or triple the recipe to meal prep your lunches for the week.

---

1 (5-ounce) can tuna (packed in water), drained

2½ tablespoons plain Greek or low-carb yogurt

2 teaspoons Dijon mustard

2 teaspoons prepared yellow mustard

⅓ cup finely chopped celery

⅓ cup finely chopped dill pickles

2 tablespoons finely chopped red onions

1 tablespoon chopped fresh dill or parsley

Everything bagel seasoning, for garnish (optional)

Put all the ingredients in a medium bowl. Mix until combined. Sprinkle with everything bagel seasoning, if desired.

CALORIES: **229** | PROTEIN: **37g** | FAT: **6.3g** | TOTAL CARBS: **6g** | NET CARBS: **3.6g** | FIBER: **2.4g**

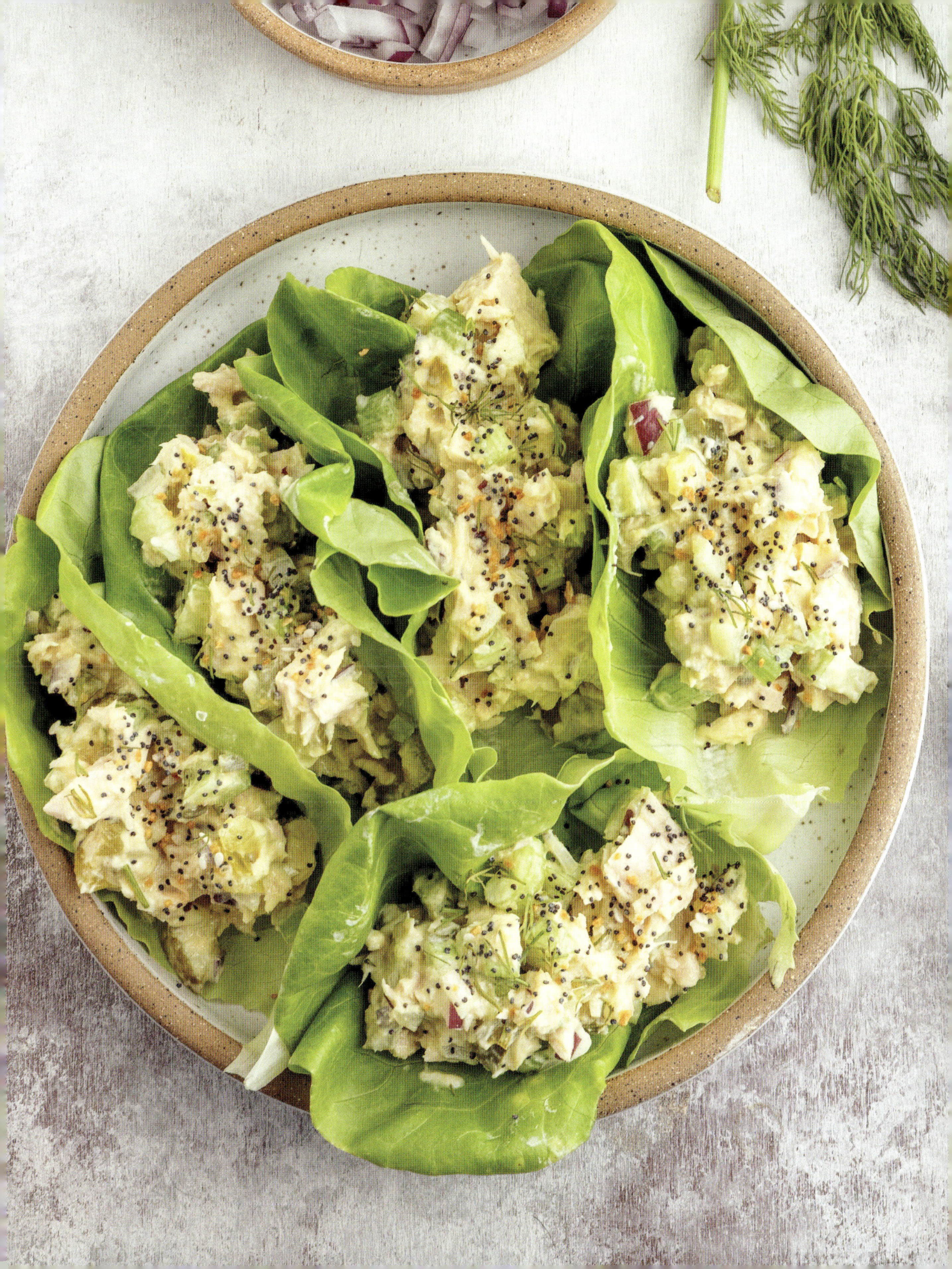

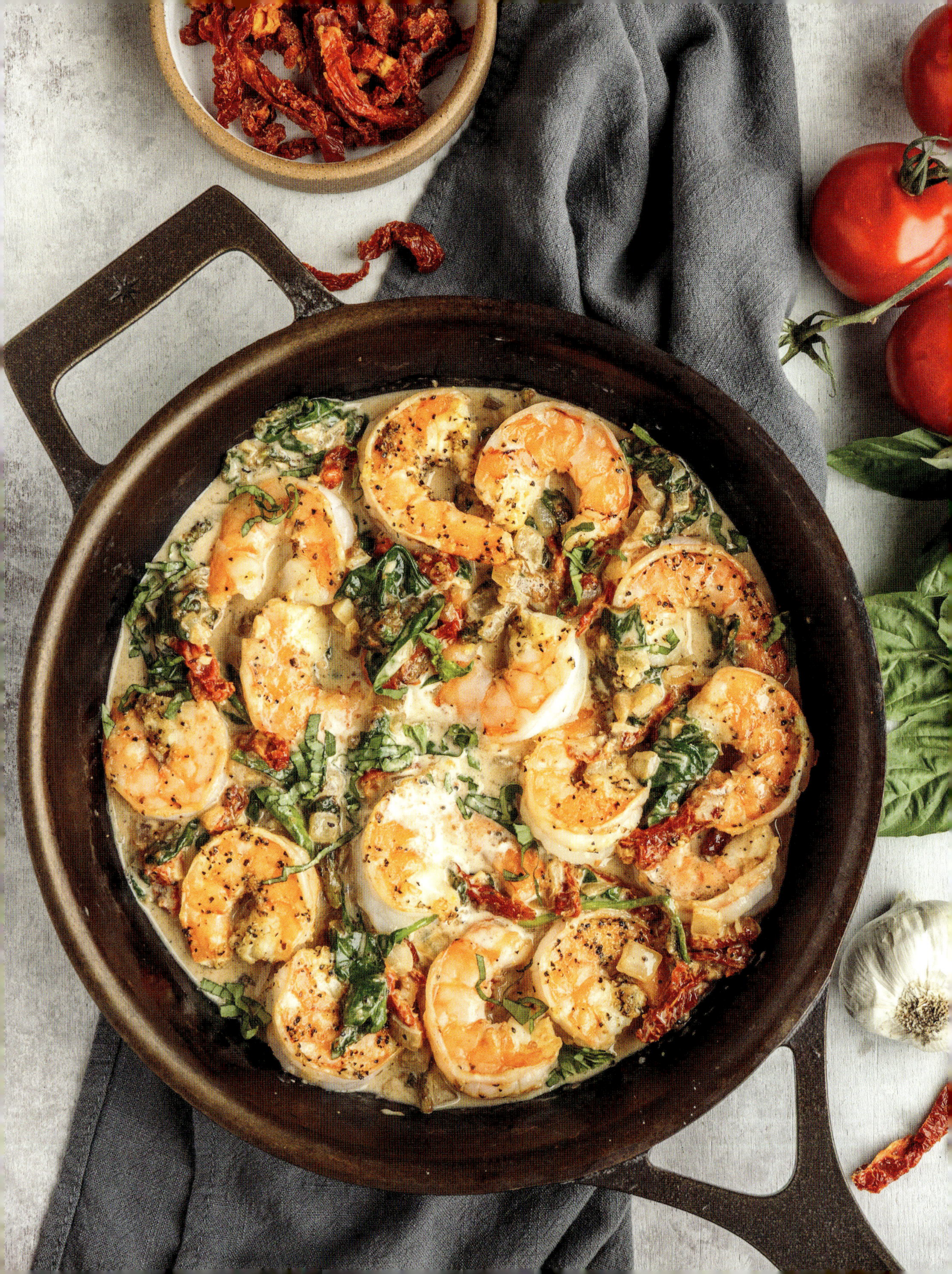

TUSCAN SHRIMP

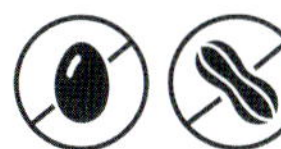

SERVES 6
PREP TIME: 5 minutes
COOK TIME: 35 minutes

This is one of my favorite shrimp dishes when I want a simple, elegant dinner or Mediterranean-inspired flavors. It features juicy shrimp in a creamy garlic sauce with sun-dried tomatoes, spinach, and fresh basil. Serve over cauliflower rice or your favorite low-carb noodles.

2 pounds large or jumbo shrimp, peeled and deveined (tails off)

2 tablespoons lemon pepper seasoning

1 teaspoon salt

2 tablespoons extra-virgin olive oil

½ medium onion, diced

4 cloves garlic, minced

1 cup chicken broth

1 cup heavy cream

2 tablespoons minced fresh basil

1 teaspoon arrowroot powder

½ cup julienned sun-dried tomatoes

2 cups baby spinach

½ cup grated Parmesan cheese

1. Pat the shrimp dry with a paper towel, then place in a large bowl. Season with the lemon pepper seasoning and salt. Toss to evenly coat.
2. Preheat a large skillet over medium heat, then pour in the olive oil. Once the oil ripples, add the shrimp in batches, cooking for 2 to 3 minutes on each side, until pink on the outside and white on the inside. Remove the shrimp from the skillet and set aside.
3. In the same skillet, sauté the onion until translucent, 3 to 5 minutes. Stir in the garlic and cook until fragrant, about 1 minute. Add the broth, cream, basil, arrowroot powder, and sun-dried tomatoes. Stir until the mixture is bubbly and thickened enough to coat the back of a spoon, about 15 minutes; it should hold its shape when you run a finger through the sauce coating the spoon.
4. Reduce the heat to low. Add the spinach. Continue to simmer until the spinach has wilted. Return the shrimp to the skillet and stir in the Parmesan cheese. Serve immediately.

(per serving)
CALORIES: **420** | PROTEIN: **40.4g** | FAT: **23.7g** | TOTAL CARBS: **7.5g** | NET CARBS: **5.6g** | FIBER: **1.9g**

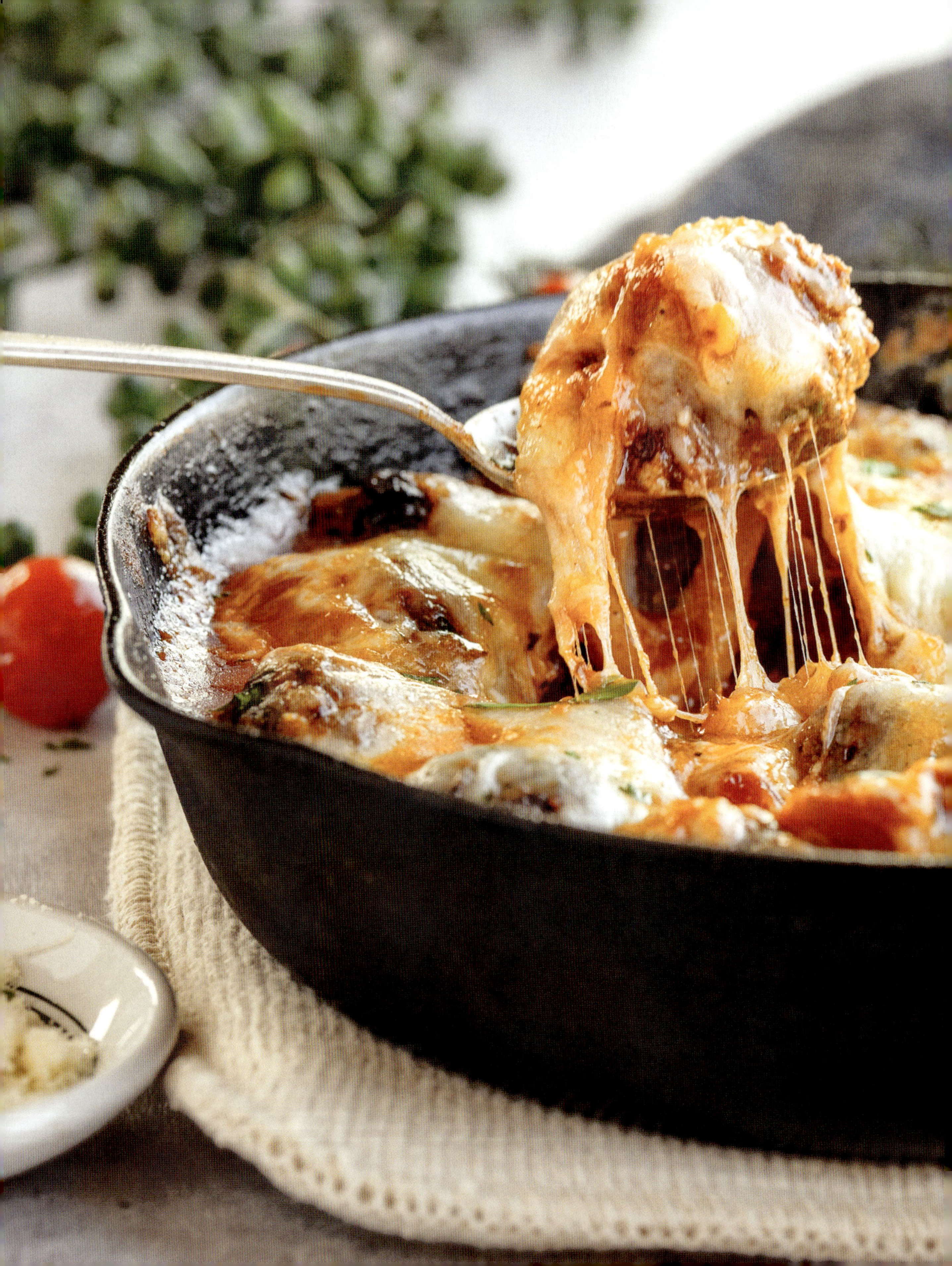

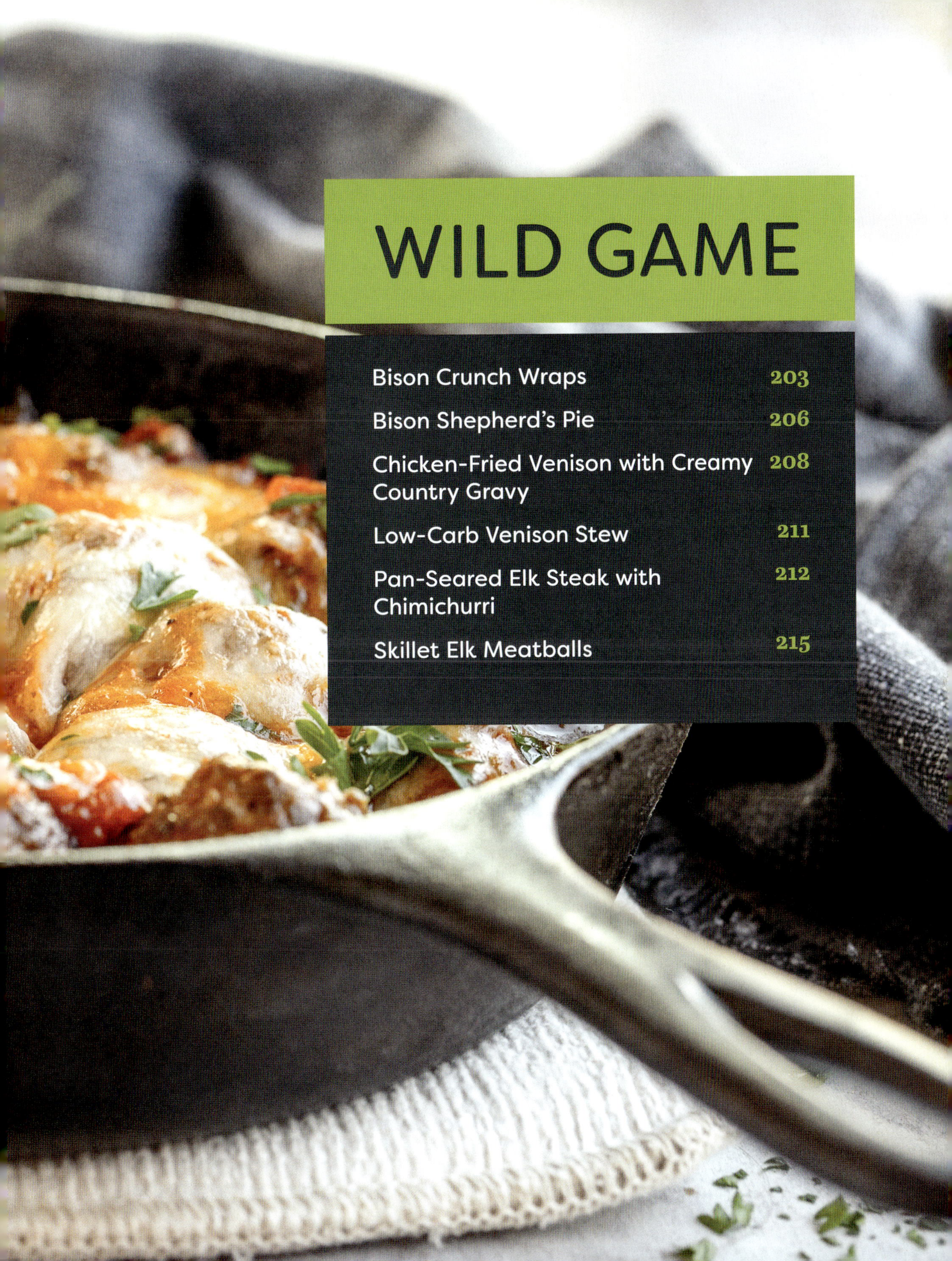

WILD GAME

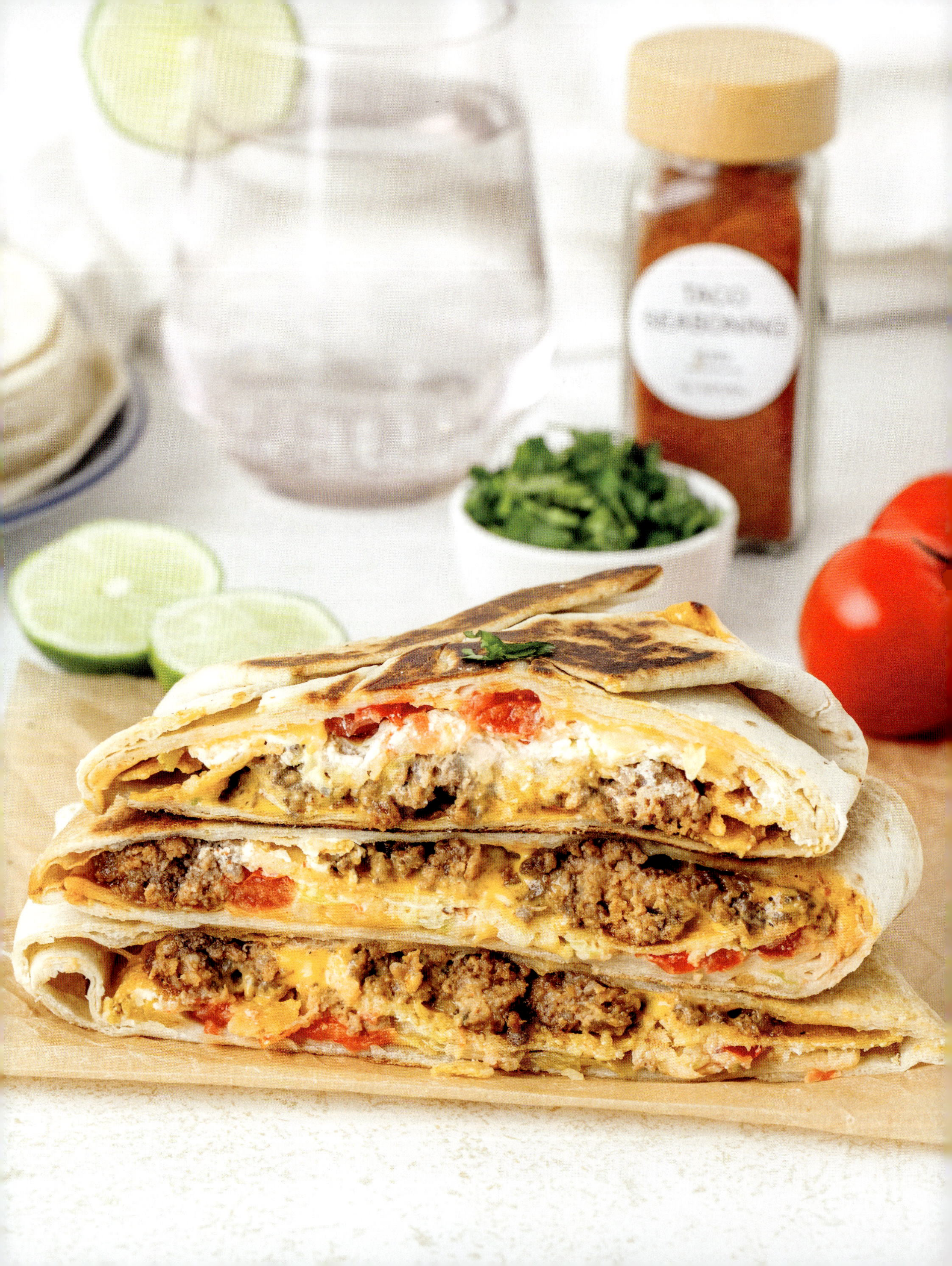
TACO
SEASONING

BISON CRUNCH WRAPS

SERVES 8

PREP TIME: 30 minutes

COOK TIME: 1 hour 10 minutes

This high-protein sandwich is a low-carb take on a Taco Bell favorite, the Crunchwrap Supreme. Ground bison provides a lean protein base, but you can easily swap it for any ground meat you prefer, such as beef or elk. A couple of soft low-carb tortillas on the outside and a homemade crispy low-carb tostada shell inside keep things low carb and ensure every bite delivers that signature crunch.

FOR THE BISON FILLING

1 tablespoon avocado oil

1 pound ground bison

2 tablespoons taco seasoning

¼ cup water

FOR THE TOSTADA SHELLS

1⅓ cups blanched, super-fine almond flour

2 tablespoons unflavored protein powder

1 tablespoon xanthan gum

½ teaspoon salt

6 tablespoons hot water

Avocado oil, for the pan

FOR ASSEMBLY

8 (10- to 12-inch) low-carb tortillas, store-bought or homemade (page 249)

1 cup low-carb nacho cheese sauce, store-bought or homemade (page 317), warmed and melty

½ cup sour cream

2 cups shredded lettuce

½ medium tomato, diced

1 cup shredded Mexican cheese blend

8 (4-inch) low-carb tortillas, store-bought or homemade (page 249)

Special equipment: Tortilla press (optional)

1. To make the filling, preheat a large skillet over medium-high heat. Pour in the avocado oil and add the ground bison. Cook, breaking the meat into crumbles with a spatula, until browned. Stir in the taco seasoning and pour in the water. Turn the heat to low, cover, and simmer for 5 minutes to develop the flavor.
2. Meanwhile, prepare the tostada shells. In a small bowl, whisk together the almond flour, protein powder, xanthan gum, and salt. Stir in the hot water and mix with a spoon or fork until a dough ball forms. Divide the dough into 8 equal-size portions by dividing the dough in half, then into quarters, and so on.
3. If using a tortilla press, cut two circles of parchment paper to match the size of your press. Line the bottom of the press with one of the parchment circles, set a dough ball in the center of the parchment, then lay the second parchment circle on top and press lightly with your fingers. Close the press and press down on the handle to flatten the tortilla. If you don't have a tortilla press, you can use a rolling pin to flatten the dough; simply roll out the balls between two sheets of parchment paper into 4-inch circles. Repeat with the remaining dough.
4. Set a medium nonstick skillet over medium heat. Pour in enough avocado oil to create a depth of about ⅜ inch (just enough that the tortilla will be submerged while frying). Once the oil is rippling, carefully peel off one side of the parchment paper to loosen it. Return the tortilla to the parchment paper, flip, and peel off the second side. The tortilla will now be loosened from each side without breaking. Place the tortilla in the hot oil. Press down the tortilla with a spatula and fry for 2 to 3 minutes, until golden brown. Flip over and fry the other side for 1 to 3 minutes, until golden brown and slightly hardened. Remove from the oil and place on a paper towel. Repeat with the remaining tortillas. The shells will continue to harden as they dry and cool.

(recipe continues)

5. To assemble a crunch wrap, scoop ⅓ to ½ cup of the bison filling into the center of a large tortilla, leaving a 3-inch border all the way around. Drizzle 2 tablespoons of the nacho cheese sauce over the meat and top with a hard tostada shell. Spread 1 tablespoon of the sour cream on top of the shell. Then top with ¼ cup of shredded lettuce, a sprinkle of diced tomato, and 2 tablespoons of shredded Mexican cheese blend.
6. Wipe out most of the oil from the skillet, leaving a little bit, or spray with cooking oil. Place over medium heat. While the pan is heating up, finish the assembly of the wrap. Place a small tortilla on top of the cheese and fold the edges of the large tortilla up and over the edge of the small tortilla. Place the crunch wrap in the hot skillet seam side down and cook for 2 to 3 minutes, until it starts to brown and the seam is set (so that your crunch wrap won't open). Flip and cook on the other side until golden brown. Repeat steps 5 and 6 to make the remaining crunch wraps.

STORAGE INSTRUCTIONS:

- To save time, make the keto tostada shells ahead. You can stop at the uncooked tortilla stage and refrigerate them for up to a week or freeze them for 1 to 2 months. Keep the tortillas sandwiched between parchment paper and store flat in a freezer-safe bag. Store fried tostada shells at room temperature for up to 3 days.
- The assembled crunch wraps can be stored in the refrigerator for up to 5 days. To reheat, air-fry at 375°F for 3 to 4 minutes or bake in the oven for 5 to 8 minutes. The lettuce and tomatoes will lose some crispness, but the crunch wrap will still taste delicious.
- Freezing the assembled crunch wraps is not recommended.

notes

Most store-bought nacho cheese sauce is low in carbohydrates; however, some brands have added sugars. Check the nutrition label to find one that has less than 5 grams of carbs per serving.

The low-carb tortillas I used in this recipe are store-bought and contain gluten. For the larger tortillas, I used the brand La Banderita, and for the smaller, I used Mission Zero Carb tortillas. For a gluten-free option, you can use my low-carb tortilla recipe on page 249 to make both sizes.

(per serving)
CALORIES: **462** | PROTEIN: **28.4g** | FAT: **27.8g** | TOTAL CARBS: **38.4g** | NET CARBS: **9.7g** | FIBER: **28.7g**

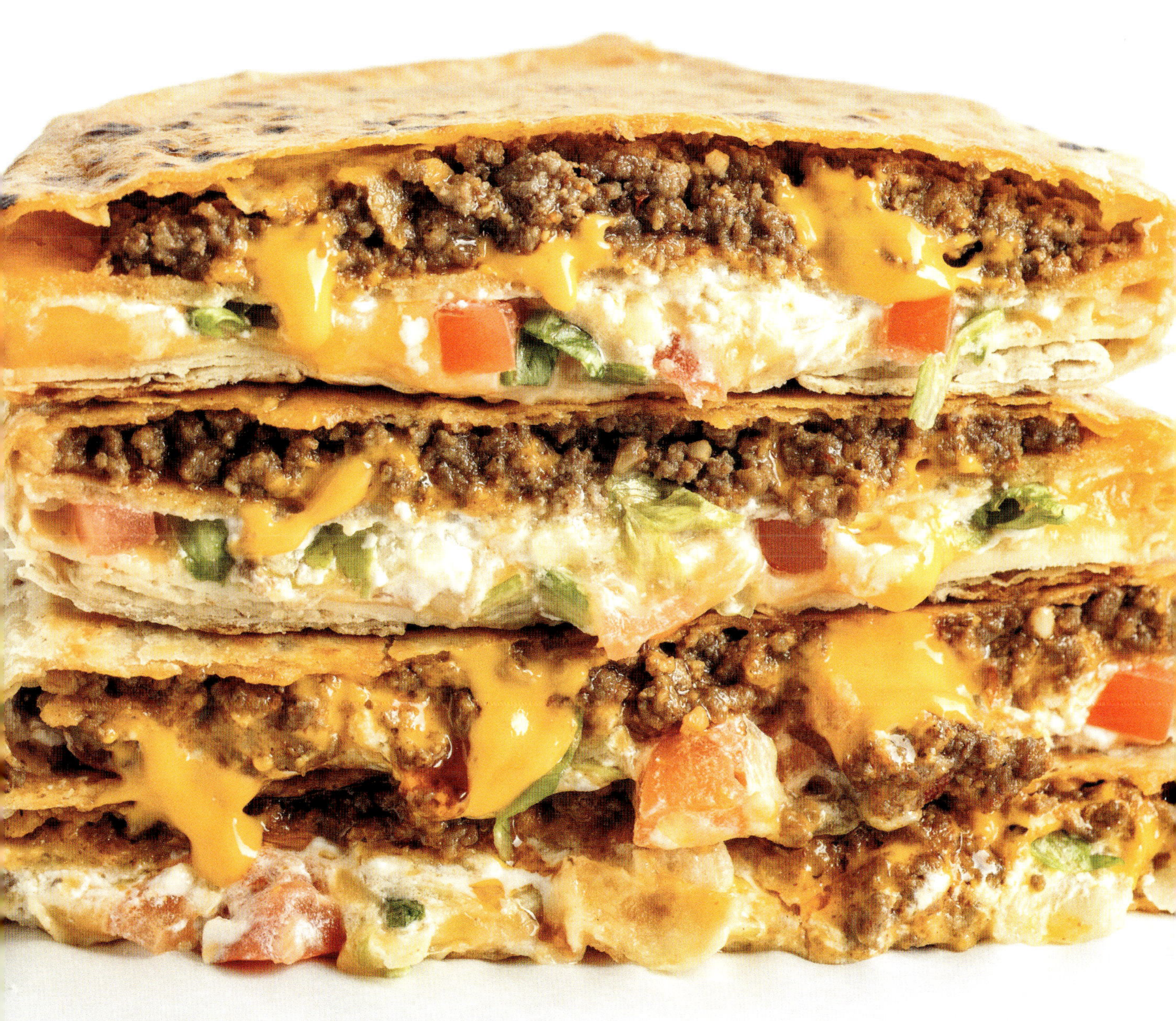

Pack It with Protein: Use Greek or low-carb yogurt instead of sour cream. Make my Protein Nacho Cheese Sauce (page 317) instead of using a store-bought option.

BISON SHEPHERD'S PIE

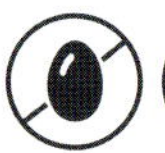

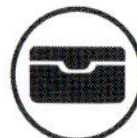

SERVES 6

PREP TIME: 25 minutes

COOK TIME: 1 hour 10 minutes

This low-carb shepherd's pie swaps traditional mashed potatoes for a creamy, cheesy layer of mashed turnips, creating a comforting dish with all the classic flavors. Turnips have a similar texture and flavor to potatoes when mashed. I use ground bison because it's lean and high in protein, but the recipe works well with other ground meats, too.

FOR THE MASHED TURNIP TOPPING

2 pounds small turnips

1 small russet potato, rinsed and cut in half (do not peel)

1 cup beef broth

Salt

3½ tablespoons salted butter

⅓ cup heavy cream

½ teaspoon ground black pepper

1 cup shredded cheddar cheese

FOR THE FILLING

2 tablespoons salted butter

3 celery stalks, chopped

¼ cup finely chopped onions

⅓ cup finely chopped carrots

4 cloves garlic, minced

⅔ cup frozen cut green beans

½ teaspoon dried thyme leaves

½ teaspoon dried rosemary needles

1½ pounds ground bison

½ teaspoon salt

½ teaspoon ground black pepper

⅓ cup tomato paste

2 tablespoons Worcestershire sauce

¾ cup beef broth

½ cup chopped fresh parsley, plus more for garnish

1. To make the topping, peel the turnips and cut them into ¾-inch cubes. Put the turnips in a large saucepan. Place the potato halves on top of the turnips.
2. Pour in the beef broth. Then add enough water to the pan to cover the turnips and potato. Season with a pinch of salt.
3. Bring to a boil and cook until the turnips have softened enough for a fork to easily pierce through, about 20 minutes.
4. Drain the water and discard the potato. Return the cooked turnips to the pan and place back on the stovetop over medium heat. Dry cook the turnips until most of the remaining moisture is gone.
5. Transfer the turnips to a food processor or blender. Add the butter, cream, and pepper. Pulse until pureed into a mashed "potato" texture. Stir in the cheese. Season with more salt if needed. Set aside.
6. Preheat the oven to 375°F.
7. To make the filling, melt the butter in a large skillet over medium heat. Add the celery, onions, and carrots and cook until almost softened.
8. Stir in the garlic, green beans, thyme, and rosemary. Cook for 1 minute, or until the garlic is fragrant.
9. Add the ground bison. Season with the salt and pepper. Cook, breaking up the meat with a spatula, until browned.
10. Stir in the tomato paste and Worcestershire sauce.
11. Pour in the broth and cook until the mixture has thickened. Stir in the parsley. Season with additional salt and pepper if needed.

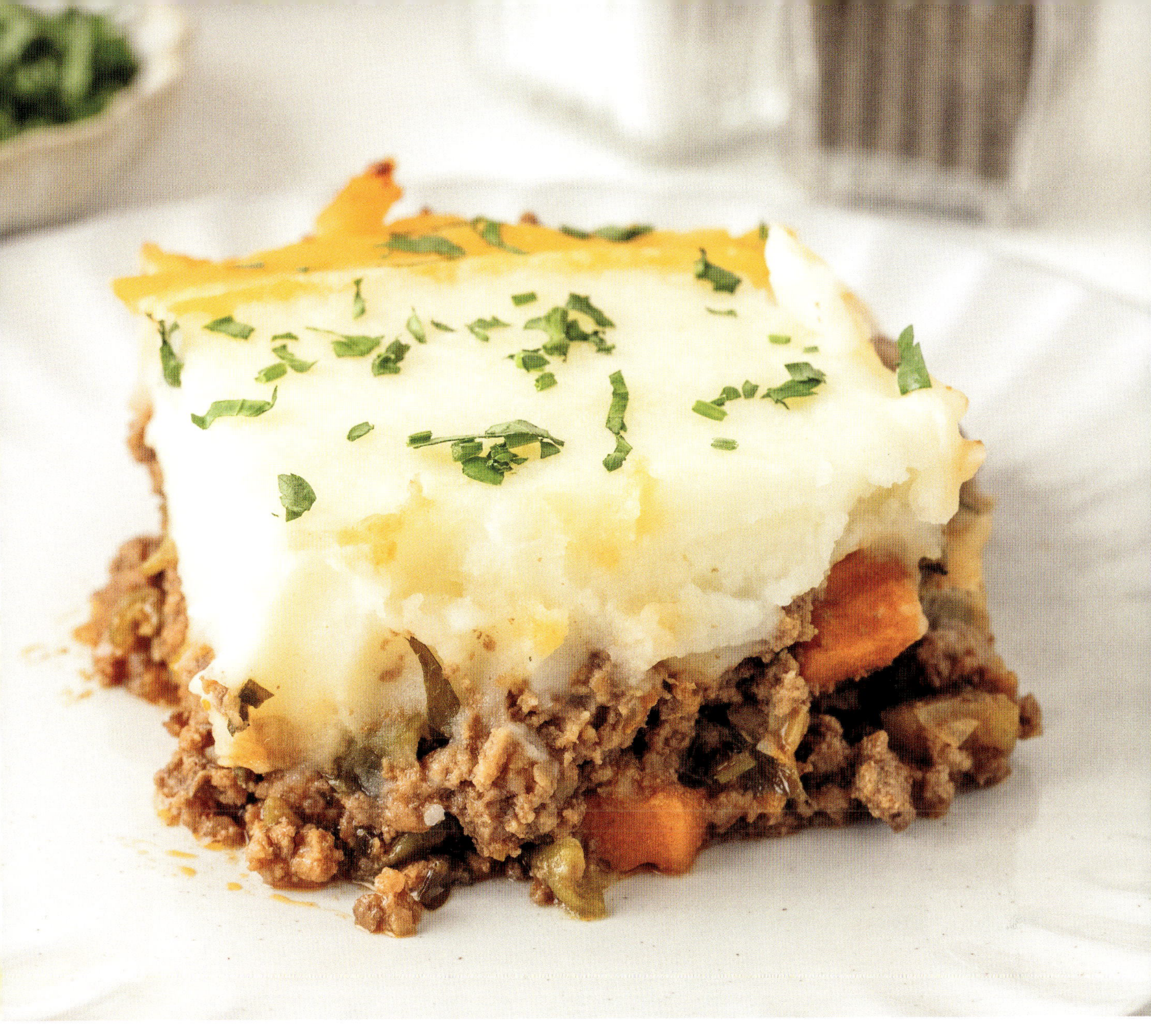

12. Transfer the filling to a 2.5-quart casserole dish. Dollop the mashed turnips on top of the filling, then spread out the mashed turnips to evenly cover the top. Place in the oven. If the topping is right up at the top of the casserole dish, put a rimmed baking sheet underneath the dish to catch any drips during baking. Bake for 30 to 45 minutes, until the top starts to brown. Sprinkle more parsley on top before serving.

note

Other low-carb options for replacing potatoes in this recipe are rutabaga and celery root.

(per serving)
CALORIES: **442** | PROTEIN: **31.1g** | FAT: **29.9g** | TOTAL CARBS: **14g** | NET CARBS: **6.7g** | FIBER: **7.3g**

CHICKEN-FRIED VENISON WITH CREAMY COUNTRY GRAVY

SERVES 5

PREP TIME: 15 minutes

COOK TIME: 20 minutes

When I was growing up, my dad and brother hunted, and my mom's chicken-fried venison was one of my favorite meals. She would dust the steaks with all-purpose flour and fry them to crispy perfection. I'm now married to an avid hunter, and my husband, Ty, has also fallen in love with my mom's simple recipe. To make it fit my low-carb and his gluten-free lifestyle, I adapted her version by swapping the flour for a combination of protein powder and pork panko, which creates a breading that's not only crispy and golden but packed with extra protein. After frying the steaks, I use the same skillet to make a creamy gravy with heavy cream, chicken broth, and arrowroot powder as a thickener. It's the best complement to the crunchy steaks. If venison isn't available, elk, antelope, or cubed beef steak are just as delicious in this recipe.

---

20 ounces venison backstrap (aka loin), cut into 5 (4-ounce) medallions

Salt and pepper

½ cup unflavored protein powder

2 large eggs, beaten

2 tablespoons water

1¾ cups pork panko

2 teaspoons garlic powder

2 to 4 tablespoons salted butter

Chopped fresh parsley, for garnish (optional)

FOR THE GRAVY

¼ cup heavy cream

½ to ¾ cup chicken broth

1 teaspoon arrowroot powder

Salt and pepper

1. Place the venison medallions in a zip-top bag or sandwich between two sheets of plastic wrap. Using a meat mallet, hammer the steaks to a ¼- to ½-inch thickness. Remove from the plastic and season both sides generously with salt and pepper.
2. Grab three shallow bowls. Put the protein powder in the first bowl. Whisk the beaten eggs with the water in the second bowl. In the third bowl, mix together the pork panko and garlic powder.
3. Coat one steak with protein powder on all sides. Then dip in the egg wash. Gently shake off the excess egg. Then place the steak in the bowl with the pork panko. Press the panko onto all sides of the steak. Set aside on a clean plate. Repeat with the remaining steaks and breading.
4. Preheat a large cast-iron or other heavy-bottomed skillet over medium heat. Drop 2 tablespoons of the butter into the skillet and let melt.
5. Once the butter is melted, add the breaded steaks to the skillet in batches. Be careful not to overcrowd the pan, or the steaks will steam and not get crispy around the edges. Add more butter between batches, if needed. Fry the steaks for 4 to 5 minutes on each side, until the breading is golden brown. Remove the steaks and transfer to a wire rack while you work on the gravy.
6. To make the gravy, pour the cream and ½ cup of the broth into the skillet. Whisk together while scraping up the brown bits stuck to the bottom of the pan to incorporate that flavor into the gravy. Add the arrowroot powder and continue to simmer until the sauce reduces and the gravy thickens to your liking. You may need to add more chicken broth if you like your gravy thinner. Season with salt and pepper to taste.

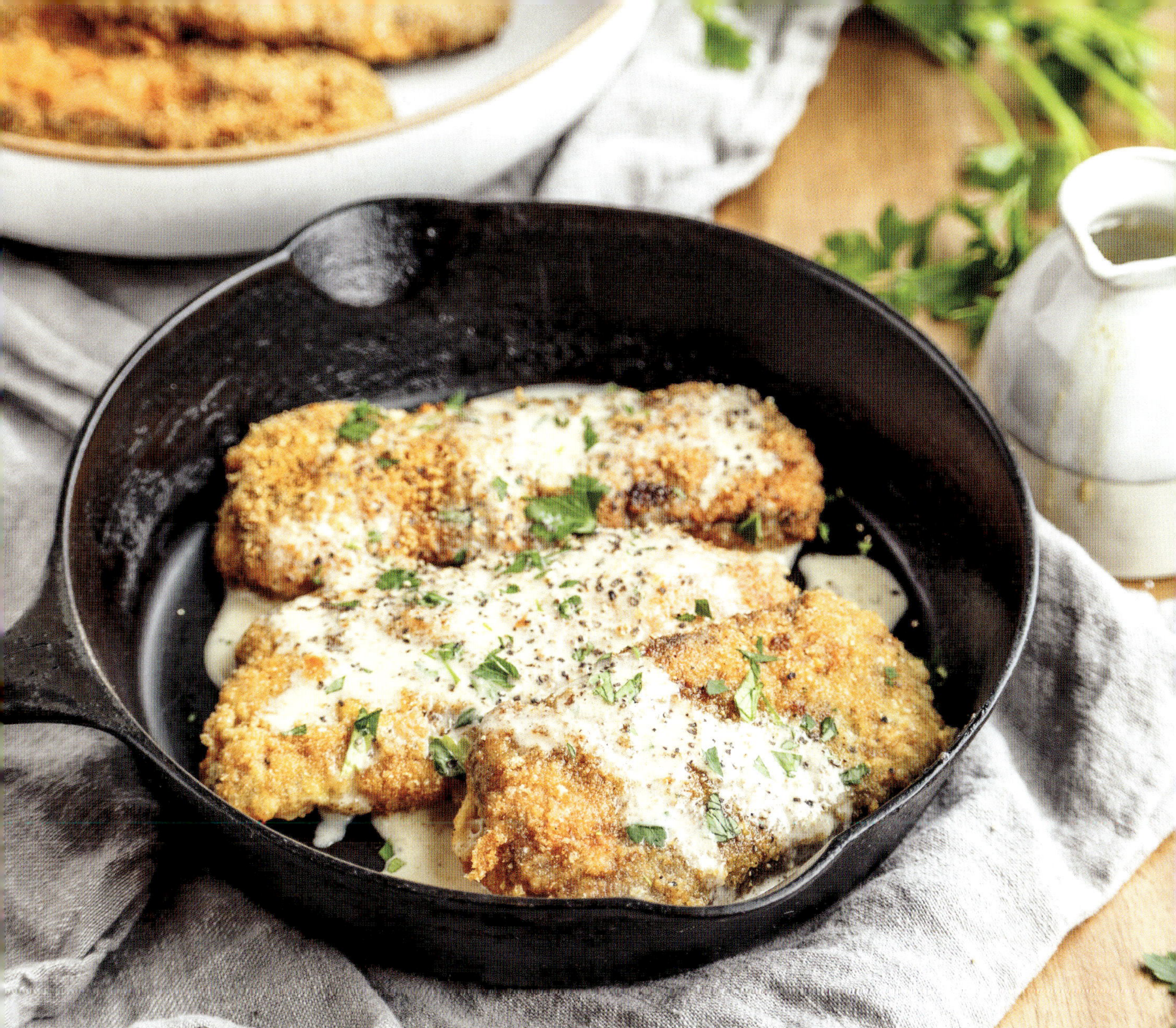

7. Pour the country gravy over the fried steaks and sprinkle chopped parsley on top, if desired.

STORAGE INSTRUCTIONS: Leftovers can be stored in the refrigerator for 3 to 4 days. The breading will become soft; however, you can get it crispy again by reheating it in the air fryer at 350°F for 3 to 5 minutes.

note

You can use almond flour in place of protein powder for the initial breading.

(per serving)
CALORIES: **451** | PROTEIN: **58.8g** | FAT: **22.6g** | TOTAL CARBS: **1.8g** | NET CARBS: **1.7g** | FIBER: **0.1g**

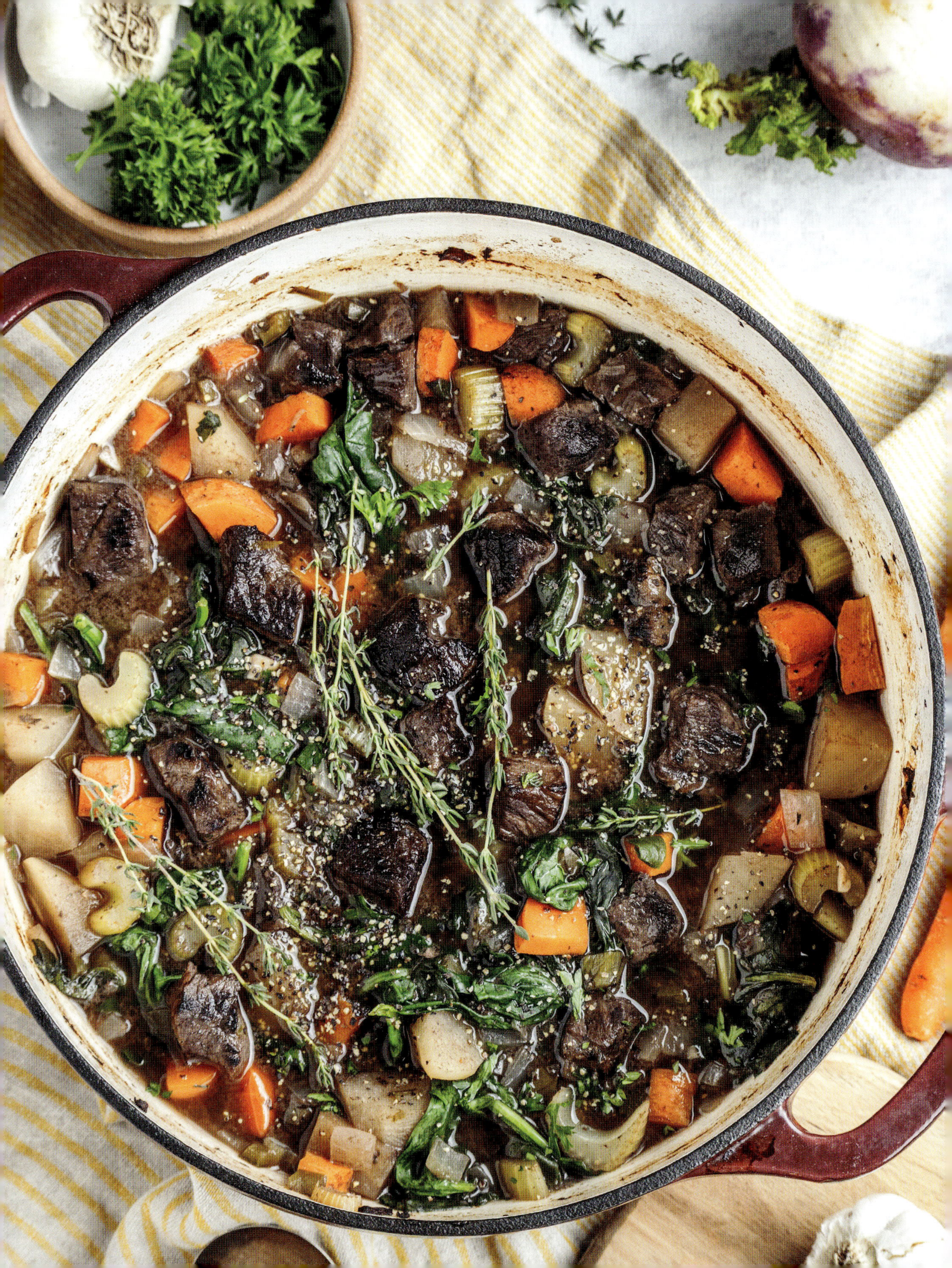

LOW-CARB VENISON STEW

 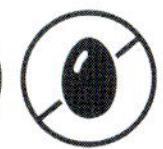  
OPTION
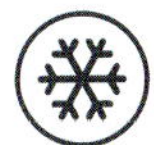 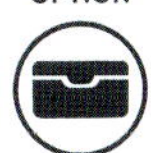

SERVES 6

PREP TIME: 15 minutes

COOK TIME: 40 minutes or 3 hours 10 minutes, depending on method

This hearty stew is a lean, low-calorie dish packed with vibrant vegetables and bold flavors. Onion, celery, carrot, turnips, jalapeño, and spinach come together for a nutrient-rich, low-carb meal. Turnips replace traditional potatoes, offering the same satisfying texture and flavor without the carbs. The gamey notes of venison are mellowed by plenty of garlic and the spicy kick of jalapeño—flavors inspired by my neighbor Ryan, who shared his hunting-trip stew secrets with my husband. My aunt Gail, famous for her amazing beef stew, influenced this recipe with her Italian heritage and flavorful approach to cooking. You can make this in the oven or in an Instant Pot.

---

2 pounds venison backstrap (aka loin), cut into ¾-inch chunks

1 medium onion, diced

3 celery stalks, sliced

2 carrots, chopped

2 small turnips, peeled and diced

4 cloves garlic, minced

2 jalapeño peppers, finely diced

2 teaspoons arrowroot powder

1 teaspoon ground black pepper

½ teaspoon salt

2 cups beef broth

1 cup red wine

2 tablespoons tomato paste

1 teaspoon dried thyme leaves, or 4 sprigs fresh thyme

2 bay leaves

2 cups baby spinach

Sprigs of fresh herbs, such as parsley or thyme, for garnish

OVEN INSTRUCTIONS:

1. Preheat the oven to 325°F.
2. Put the venison, onion, celery, carrots, turnips, garlic, jalapeños, arrowroot powder, black pepper, and salt in a Dutch oven or other large oven-safe pot with a lid.
3. Stir in the broth, wine, tomato paste, thyme, and bay leaves.
4. Put the lid on the pot and put in the oven to cook for 2½ to 3 hours, until the meat is fork-tender and easily falls apart. Remove from the oven.
5. Set the oven to broil on high. Move the oven rack closer to the broiler so the pot can sit right below the broiler. Stir in the spinach. Leaving the lid off, return the pot to sit under the broiler for 5 to 10 minutes, stirring occasionally, until most of the meat is browned and the sauce has thickened.
6. Remove from the oven and remove the bay leaves. Season with more salt and pepper to taste. Garnish with fresh herbs before serving.

INSTANT POT INSTRUCTIONS:

Put all the ingredients except the spinach leaves in the Instant Pot. Secure the lid and pressure-cook on high for 35 minutes, then allow the pressure to vent naturally for 10 minutes before turning or pressing the vent to release the remaining pressure. Carefully open the lid and remove and discard the bay leaves. Stir in the spinach and let wilt. Garnish with fresh herbs before serving.

(per serving)
CALORIES: **307** | PROTEIN: **47.4g** | FAT: **4.2g** | TOTAL CARBS: **11g** | NET CARBS: **8.1g** | FIBER: **2.9g**

PAN-SEARED ELK STEAK WITH CHIMICHURRI

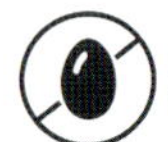

SERVES 4

PREP TIME: 15 minutes

COOK TIME: 5 minutes

A simple way to enjoy lean game meat is to pan-sear it and pour chimichurri over the top. Cooked in butter on the stovetop, these elk steaks are perfectly seared and tender, reaching medium-rare to medium doneness. They're paired with a simple chimichurri sauce made from fresh parsley, cilantro, and oregano blended with garlic, red wine vinegar for a tangy bite, and red pepper flakes for a touch of heat. You can use lemon juice in place of the vinegar if you're out of vinegar or prefer a brighter, citrusy flavor; just keep in mind that it's slightly less tangy but still works great to balance the herbs and garlic.

FOR THE CHIMICHURRI

⅓ cup roughly chopped fresh parsley

⅓ cup roughly chopped fresh cilantro

1 teaspoon fresh oregano leaves

2 cloves garlic, peeled

½ teaspoon red pepper flakes

¼ teaspoon salt

½ cup avocado oil or extra-virgin olive oil

¼ cup red wine vinegar or lemon juice

4 (6-ounce) boneless elk steaks (about 1 inch thick)

Salt and pepper

2 tablespoons salted butter

1. To make the chimichurri, put the parsley, cilantro, oregano, garlic, red pepper flakes, salt, oil, and vinegar in a food processor or blender. Blend until smooth and combined. The longer the chimichurri sauce sits, the more flavor will develop. Ideally, let the sauce sit for 30 minutes at room temperature to let the flavors meld.
2. Pat the elk steaks dry with a paper towel and season both sides generously with salt and pepper.
3. Preheat a large cast-iron or other heavy-bottomed skillet over medium-high heat. Put the butter in the skillet and swirl it around the bottom. Once melted, place the steaks in the skillet and cook for 2 minutes on the first side. Reduce the heat to medium, then flip the steaks. Cook for another 2 to 3 minutes. You may need to work in batches if the skillet is not big enough to hold all four steaks without overcrowding. Remove the steaks from the skillet and place on a cutting board to rest for 5 to 10 minutes.
4. Serve the steaks with the chimichurri sauce poured on top.

note

The chimichurri can be made ahead and stored in the refrigerator for up to 5 days.

(per serving)

CALORIES: **498** | PROTEIN: **33.3g** | FAT: **40.3g** | TOTAL CARBS: **1.1g** | NET CARBS: **0.8g** | FIBER: **0.3g**

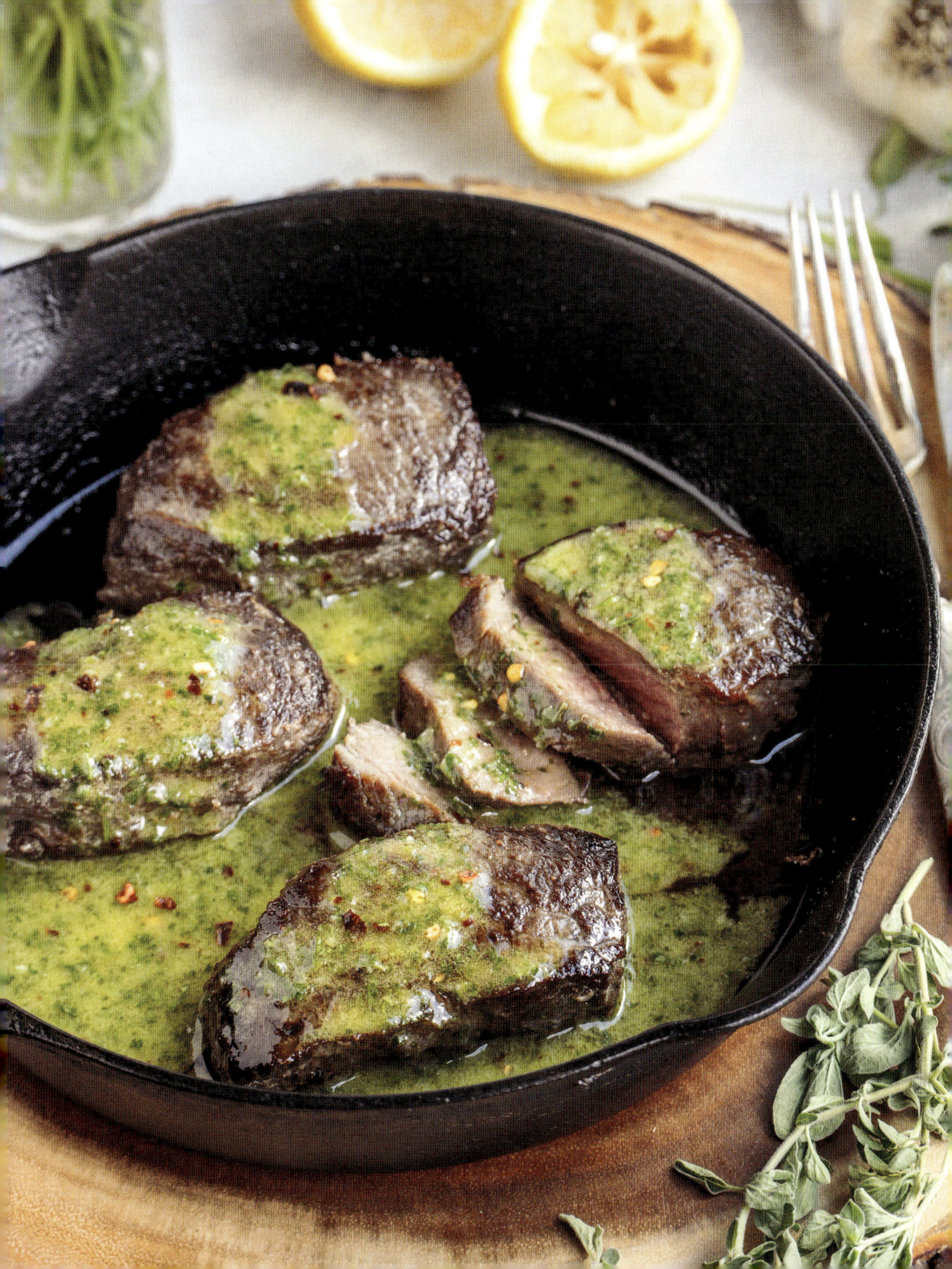

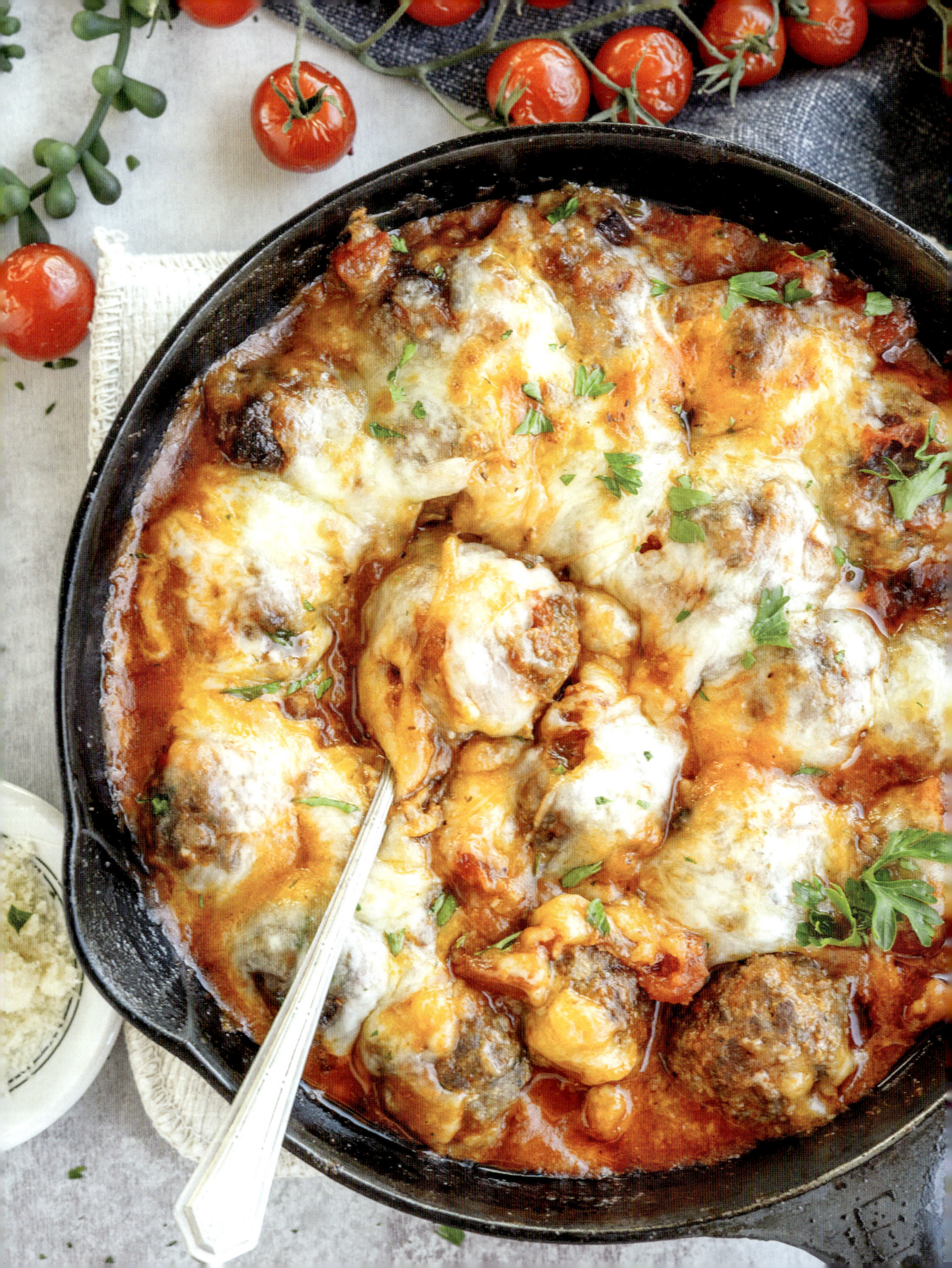

SKILLET ELK MEATBALLS

 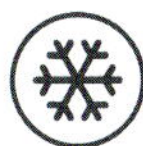 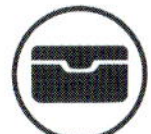

SERVES 8
PREP TIME: 15 minutes
COOK TIME: 25 minutes

This skillet dish is ideal for weeknight dinners or meal prep. I like to make a big batch for my husband and his brothers when they go hunting. The meatballs freeze well and are simple to reheat—thaw overnight, then just pour them into a skillet to warm them up.

I make these meatballs with ground elk, but you can use any ground meat you like—beef, chicken, turkey, pork, bison, or venison. The secret to their deliciousness (and for mellowing the gamey taste of wild meats) is to add lots of garlic and use a seasoning salt like Lawry's. Enjoy them on their own or serve over your favorite low-carb noodles.

- 2 pounds ground elk
- 2 large eggs
- 1 cup grated Parmesan cheese
- ⅔ cup pork panko
- 2 tablespoons minced garlic
- 1 teaspoon salt
- 1 teaspoon seasoning salt
- 1 teaspoon ground black pepper
- 1 teaspoon dried oregano leaves
- ½ cup chopped fresh parsley, plus more for garnish if desired
- 3 tablespoons avocado oil or extra-virgin olive oil, for the pan
- 1 (25-ounce) jar low-carb marinara sauce
- 1½ cups shredded mozzarella cheese

1. Put the ground elk, eggs, Parmesan cheese, pork panko, garlic, salt, seasoning salt, pepper, oregano, and parsley in a large mixing bowl. Mix with your hands or a large spoon until combined.
2. Pinch off some of the elk mixture and roll it between your palms to form a 1-inch ball. Repeat with the remaining mixture to make a total of about 42 meatballs.
3. Preheat a large skillet over medium heat. Pour 1 tablespoon of the oil into the skillet and allow it to heat up. Working in several batches, add the meatballs to the skillet and cook for 3 to 4 minutes on all sides, until cooked through. Don't add too many meatballs to the skillet at once or they will steam instead of fry. Continue with the remaining oil and meatballs.
4. Return all the meatballs to the skillet. Pour in the marinara sauce and top with the mozzarella. Cover, turn the heat to low, and let simmer for 5 minutes, or until the cheese is melted. Garnish with more chopped parsley, if desired.

(per serving)
CALORIES: **471** | PROTEIN: **45.3g** | FAT: **28.7g** | TOTAL CARBS: **5.8g** | NET CARBS: **4.4g** | FIBER: **1.4g**

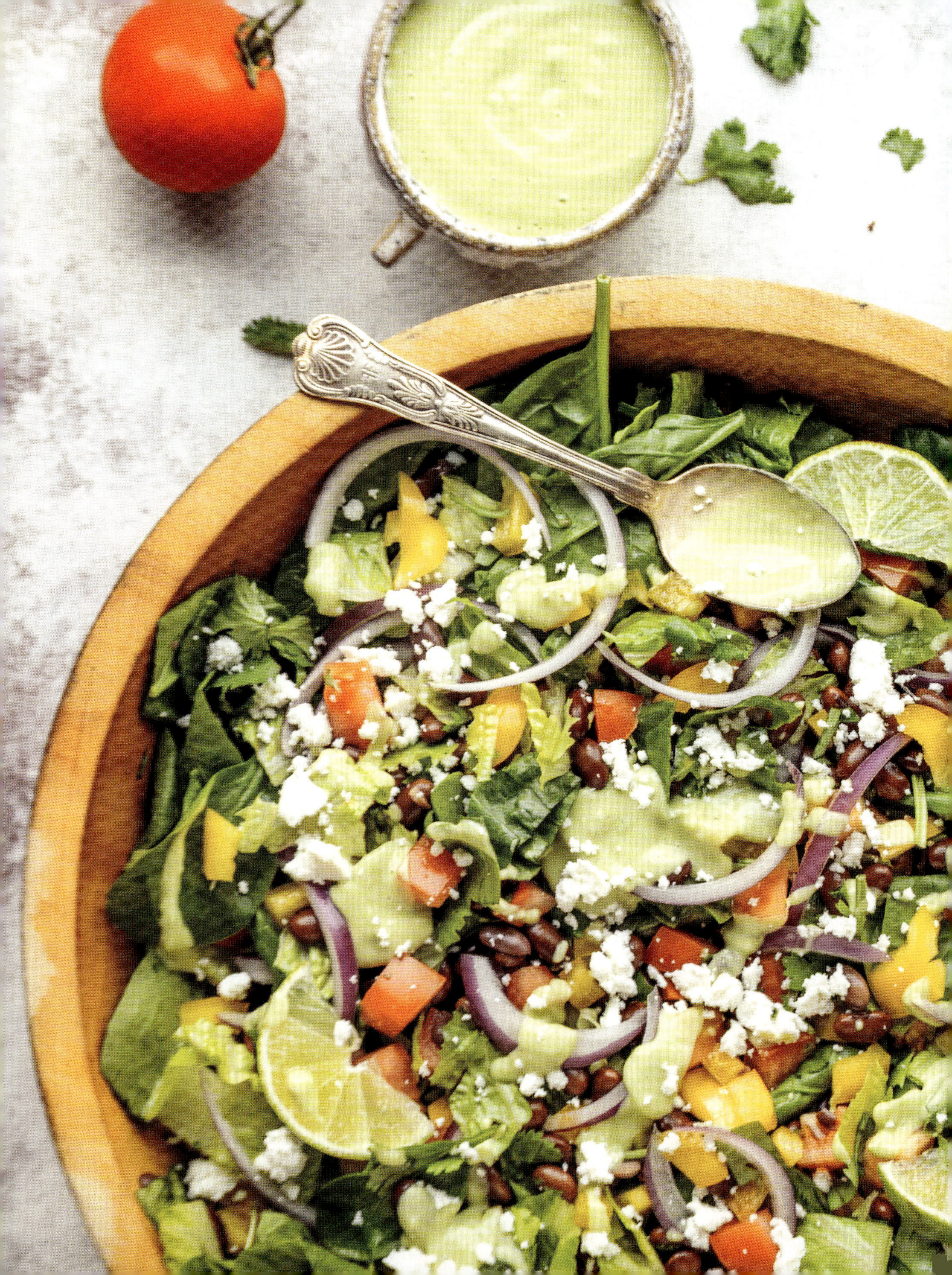

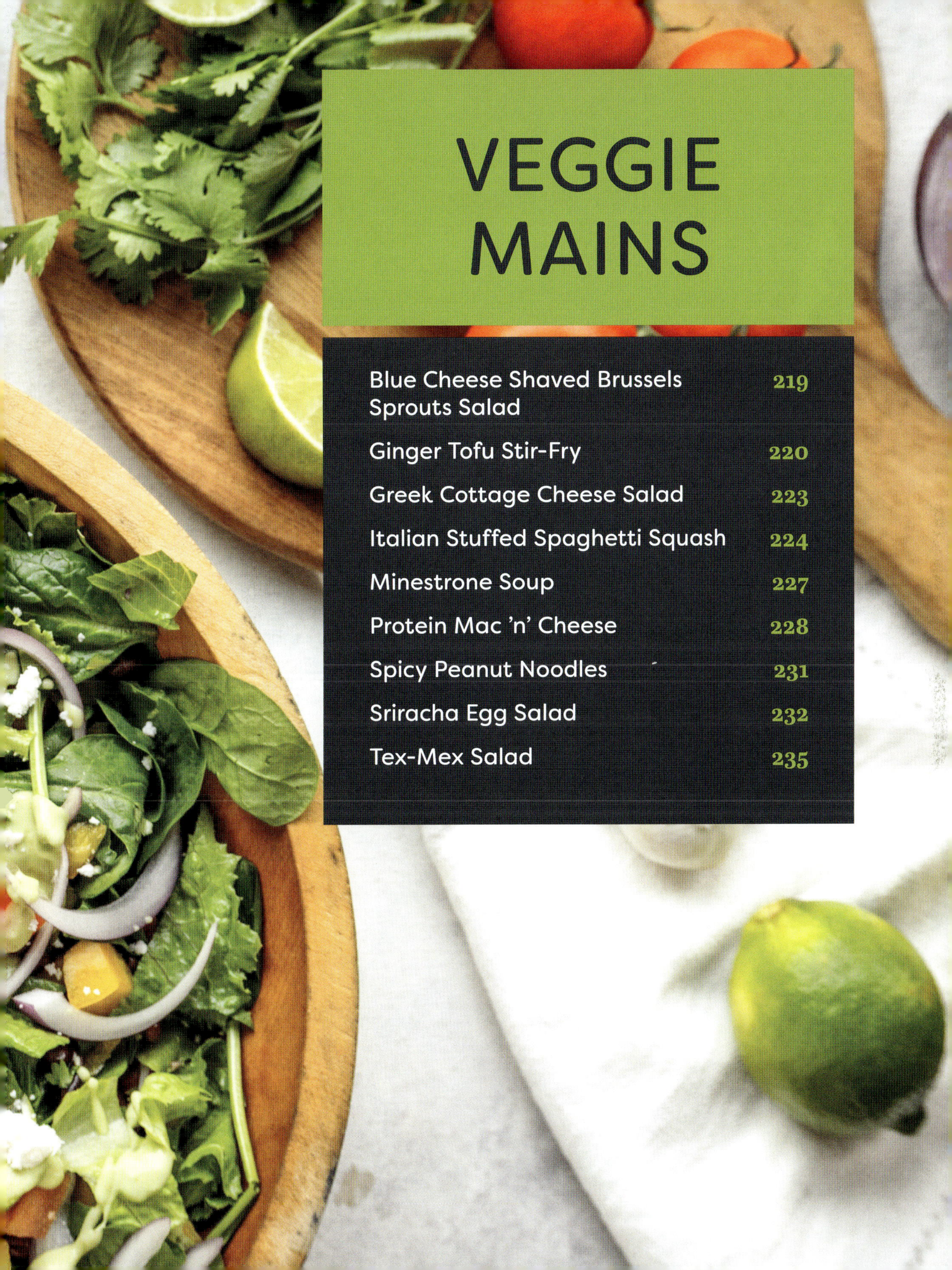

VEGGIE MAINS

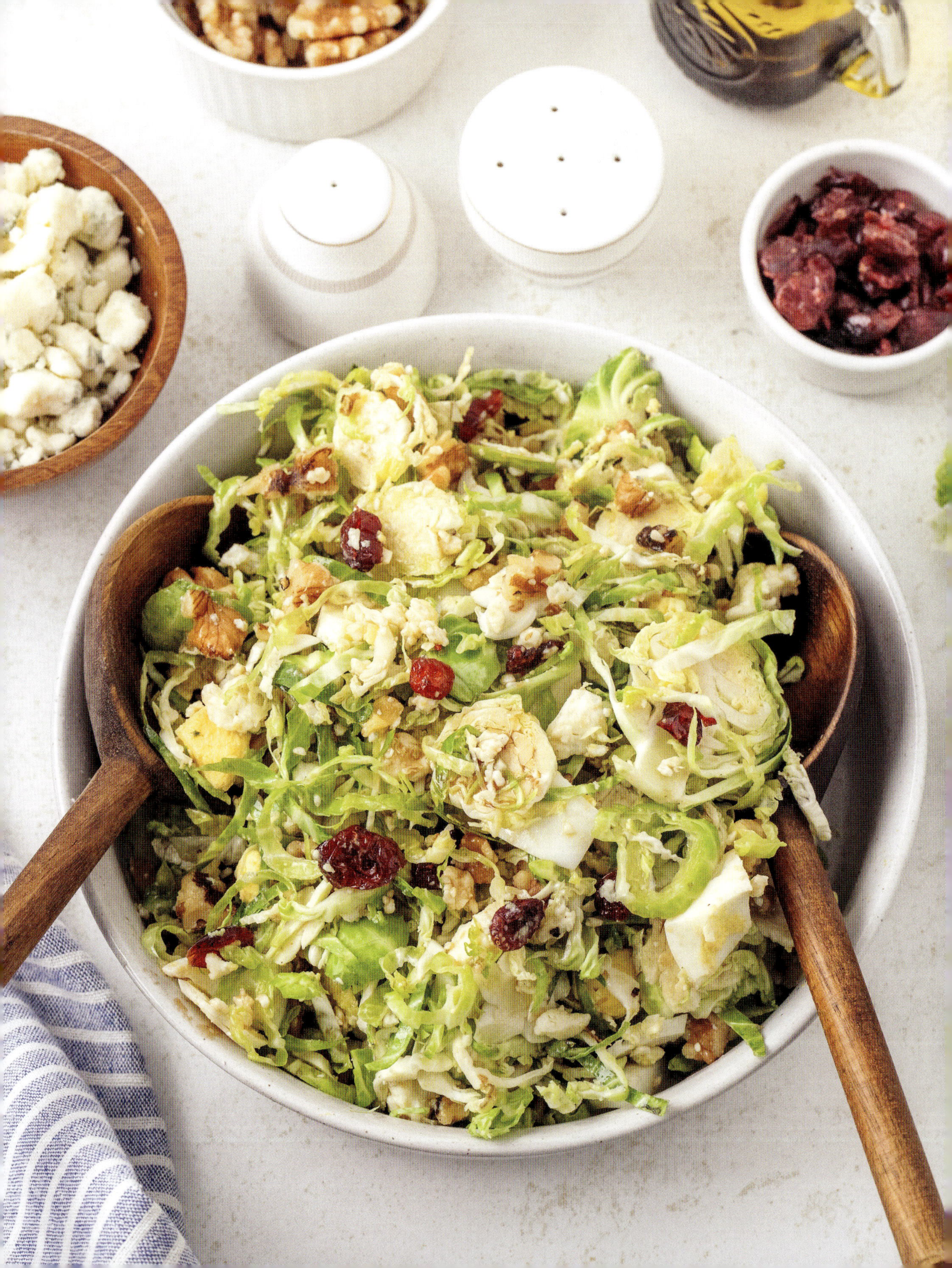

BLUE CHEESE SHAVED BRUSSELS SPROUTS SALAD

SERVES 2

PREP TIME: 15 minutes (not including time to hard-boil eggs)

This shaved Brussels sprouts salad is a protein-packed blend of exciting flavors, featuring blue cheese, walnuts, dried cranberries, and chopped hard-boiled eggs. Tossed in a tangy balsamic vinaigrette, it combines the crunch of raw Brussels sprouts with the creaminess of blue cheese. With protein coming from the Brussels sprouts (3 grams per cup), blue cheese (5 to 6 grams per ¼ cup), walnuts (4 grams per ounce), and eggs, this salad has plenty of protein for anyone eating a plant-based diet.

---

4 cups thinly sliced (shaved) Brussels sprouts

½ cup crumbled blue cheese

½ cup chopped walnuts

2 large hard-boiled eggs, chopped

2 tablespoons dried unsweetened cranberries

FOR THE DRESSING

2 tablespoons balsamic vinegar

2 tablespoons extra-virgin olive oil

½ teaspoon ground black pepper

¼ teaspoon salt

1. Put the sliced Brussels sprouts in a large bowl. Add the blue cheese, walnuts, chopped eggs, and dried cranberries.
2. In a small bowl, whisk together the balsamic vinegar, olive oil, pepper, and salt.
3. Drizzle the dressing over the salad. Toss to coat. Enjoy right away or let it sit for up to 15 minutes to absorb the flavor of the dressing.

notes

I used a mandoline slicer to carefully shave 10 ounces of whole Brussels sprouts to get the 4 cups needed for this recipe. If you don't have a mandoline, you can use the slicing side of a box grater or a very sharp knife. (Watch your fingers!)

To lower the calories, decrease the amount of walnuts and add 1 or 2 more hard-boiled eggs.

To lower the carbs, use a bottled low-carb balsamic dressing, like the one from Yo Mama's Foods or G. Hughes, instead of the homemade dressing.

(per serving)
CALORIES: **613** | PROTEIN: **21.3g** | FAT: **47g** | TOTAL CARBS: **31.2g** | NET CARBS: **21.1g** | FIBER: **10.1g**

GINGER TOFU STIR-FRY

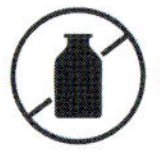
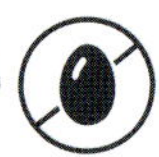
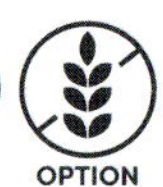

SERVES 2

PREP TIME: 15 minutes, plus 30 minutes to marinate tofu

COOK TIME: 20 minutes

When I was growing up, my mom made a lot of stir-fries, becoming a pro at combining whatever vegetables and proteins she had on hand with pantry seasonings and sauces. During her vegetarian phase, she created a dish like this vegetable and tofu stir-fry, which I loved just as much as she did. This recipe features broccoli, edamame, zucchini, and carrots cooked with cubed tofu in a flavorful mix of ginger, garlic, lime, and soy sauce. It's easy to make, perfect for meal prep, and packed with plant-based protein from the tofu and edamame.

3 tablespoons soy sauce or tamari

1 tablespoon grated fresh ginger

3 cloves garlic, minced

1½ tablespoons unseasoned rice vinegar

1 (14-ounce) package extra-firm tofu, cubed

2 tablespoons avocado oil

6 ounces broccoli florets

1 cup shelled edamame

½ medium zucchini, diced

¼ cup grated carrots

2 tablespoons lime juice

1 teaspoon sugar-free or regular honey

1 teaspoon arrowroot powder

1. In a small bowl, whisk together the soy sauce, ginger, garlic, and rice vinegar. Put the cubed tofu in an 8- or 9-inch square baking dish. Pour the sauce over and toss to coat. Let marinate for 30 minutes, periodically turning the pieces to marinate evenly.
2. Preheat a large wok or skillet over medium heat and pour in the avocado oil. Once rippling, add the broccoli florets, edamame, and zucchini. Cook, stirring often, until softened, about 8 minutes.
3. Using a slotted spoon, transfer the marinated tofu to the pan, reserving the marinade. Cook, stirring often, until the tofu is browned on all sides.
4. Add the grated carrots. Pour in the reserved marinade, lime juice, honey, and arrowroot powder. Stir to combine and cook until thickened.

note

To make this gluten free, use coconut aminos or liquid aminos in place of soy sauce or tamari.

(per serving)

CALORIES: **486** | PROTEIN: **33.7g** | FAT: **26.6g** | TOTAL CARBS: **27.9g** | NET CARBS: **17.8g** | FIBER: **8.4g**
SUGAR ALCOHOLS: **1.7g**

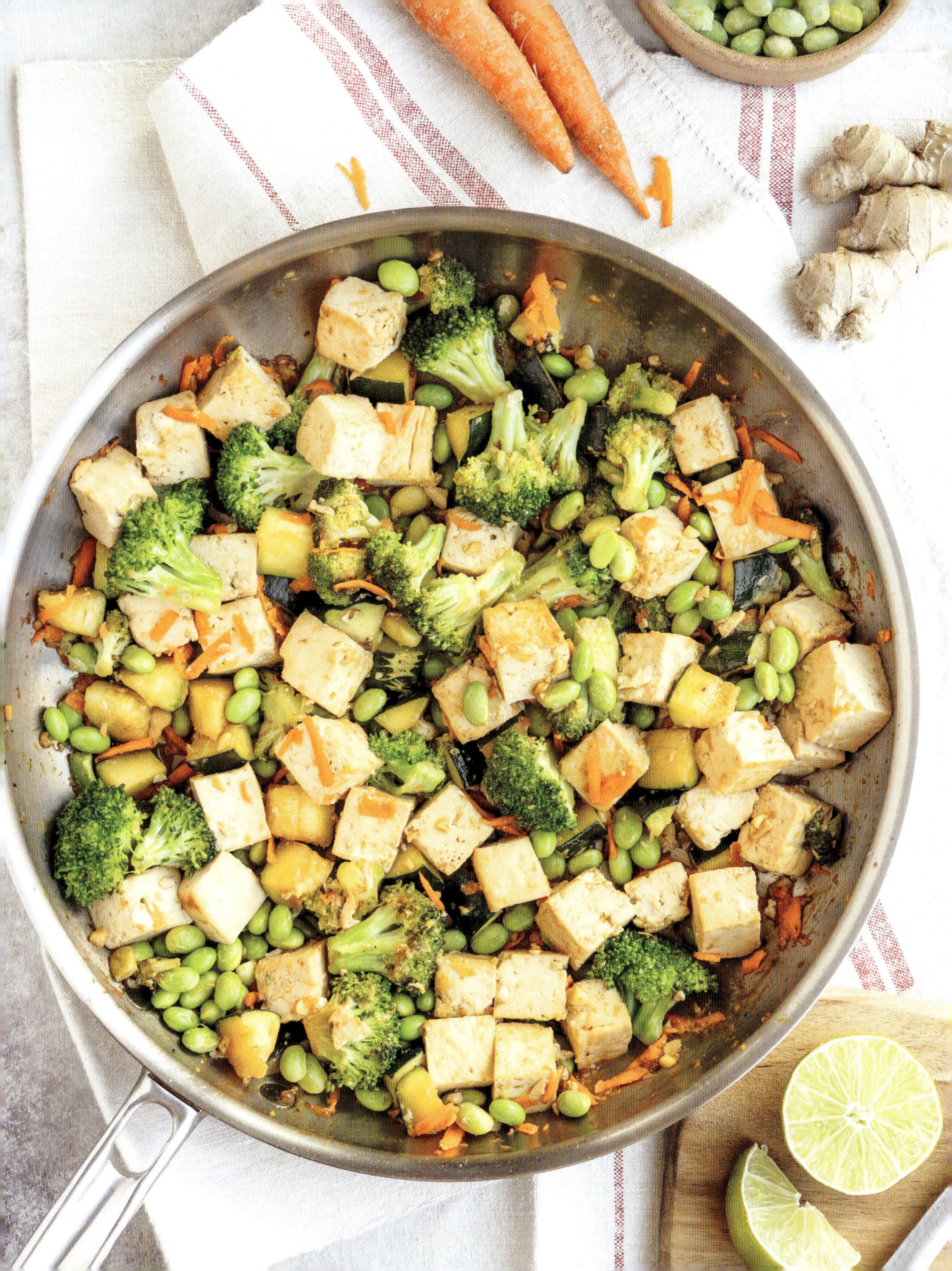

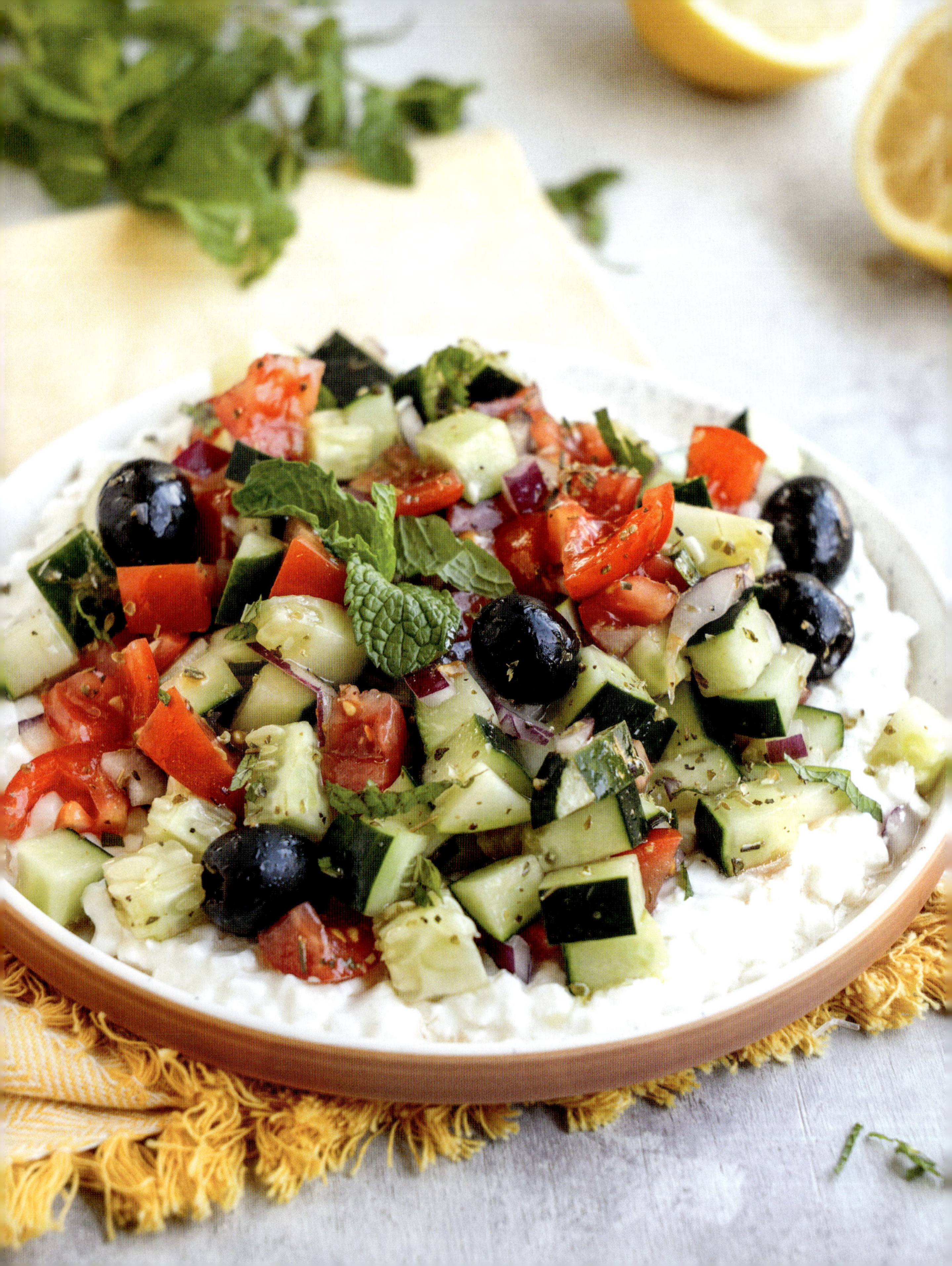

GREEK COTTAGE CHEESE SALAD

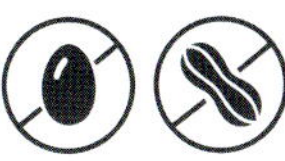

SERVES 1

PREP TIME: 5 minutes

I know the idea of a cottage cheese salad might sound strange, but stay with me—this Greek-inspired version will win you over. It's a refreshing, protein-packed dish featuring creamy cottage cheese combined with crispy cucumber, tomatoes, red onion, olives, and fresh mint. A drizzle of olive oil and lemon juice ties it all together. Ready in just 5 minutes, it's a quick, flavorful option for lunch or a light dinner.

1 cup cottage cheese (4% milkfat)

1 Roma tomato, diced

½ medium cucumber, diced

2 tablespoons finely diced red onions

6 pitted black olives

2 fresh mint leaves, finely chopped

2 tablespoons extra-virgin olive oil

Juice of ½ lemon

½ teaspoon dried oregano leaves

Pinch of salt

1. Spread the cottage cheese across a shallow bowl or plate.
2. Top with the remaining ingredients, distributing them evenly on top of the cottage cheese.

CALORIES: **527** | PROTEIN: **29.5g** | FAT: **39.5g** | TOTAL CARBS: **16.2g** | NET CARBS: **13.5g** | FIBER: **2.7g**

ITALIAN STUFFED SPAGHETTI SQUASH

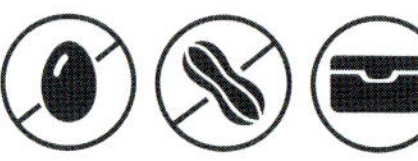

SERVES 4
PREP TIME: 15 minutes
COOK TIME: 1 hour

When cooked, spaghetti squash transforms into noodle-like strands that are a perfect low-carb base for flavorful fillings or toppings. Here, I've mixed a blend of veggies—onion, mushrooms, and spinach—with a creamy, protein-rich marinara sauce made with tofu. The dish is topped with cheese and baked until bubbly, delivering a hearty, protein-filled meal. It's a delicious way to enjoy comforting Italian flavors while keeping it light and wholesome.

---

1 spaghetti squash (about 3 pounds)

1 tablespoon extra-virgin olive oil

Salt and pepper

FOR THE FILLING

1 tablespoon extra-virgin olive oil

½ medium onion, diced

8 ounces sliced cremini mushrooms

1 cup low-carb marinara sauce

1 (14-ounce) package extra-firm tofu

4 cloves garlic, minced

1 tablespoon Italian seasoning

1 teaspoon salt

½ teaspoon ground black pepper

4 cups baby spinach

1 cup shredded mozzarella cheese

¼ cup grated Parmesan cheese

Chopped fresh parsley, for garnish

1. Preheat the oven to 400°F. Line a rimmed baking sheet with parchment paper.
2. Cut the spaghetti squash in half lengthwise and scoop out and discard the seeds. Rub 1 tablespoon of olive oil on the cut sides and season lightly with salt and pepper. Place each half cut side down on the prepared pan, pierce a few holes in the skin with a fork to allow for venting, and roast for 40 to 50 minutes, until softened.
3. During the last 10 minutes of roasting, make the filling. Preheat a large skillet over medium heat, then pour in the olive oil. Add the onion and mushrooms and sauté until almost softened.
4. While the onion and mushrooms are cooking, pour the marinara sauce into a blender or food processor. Add the tofu and blend until smooth. Set aside.
5. Stir the garlic into the onion mixture and cook until fragrant. Pour in the tofu marinara sauce, Italian seasoning, salt, and pepper and bring to a simmer. Stir in the spinach and cook until wilted.
6. Remove the squash from the oven and turn the halves cut side up. Shred into spaghetti strands with two forks. Scoop about a cup of the shredded squash from each half and stir into the marinara sauce.
7. Fill each halved squash with the marinara mixture and top with the cheeses. Place back in the oven for another 5 to 10 minutes, until the cheese is melted.
8. Garnish with chopped parsley and serve.

(per serving)
CALORIES: **425** | PROTEIN: **26.3g** | FAT: **22g** | TOTAL CARBS: **34.7g** | NET CARBS: **25.6g** | FIBER: **9.1g**

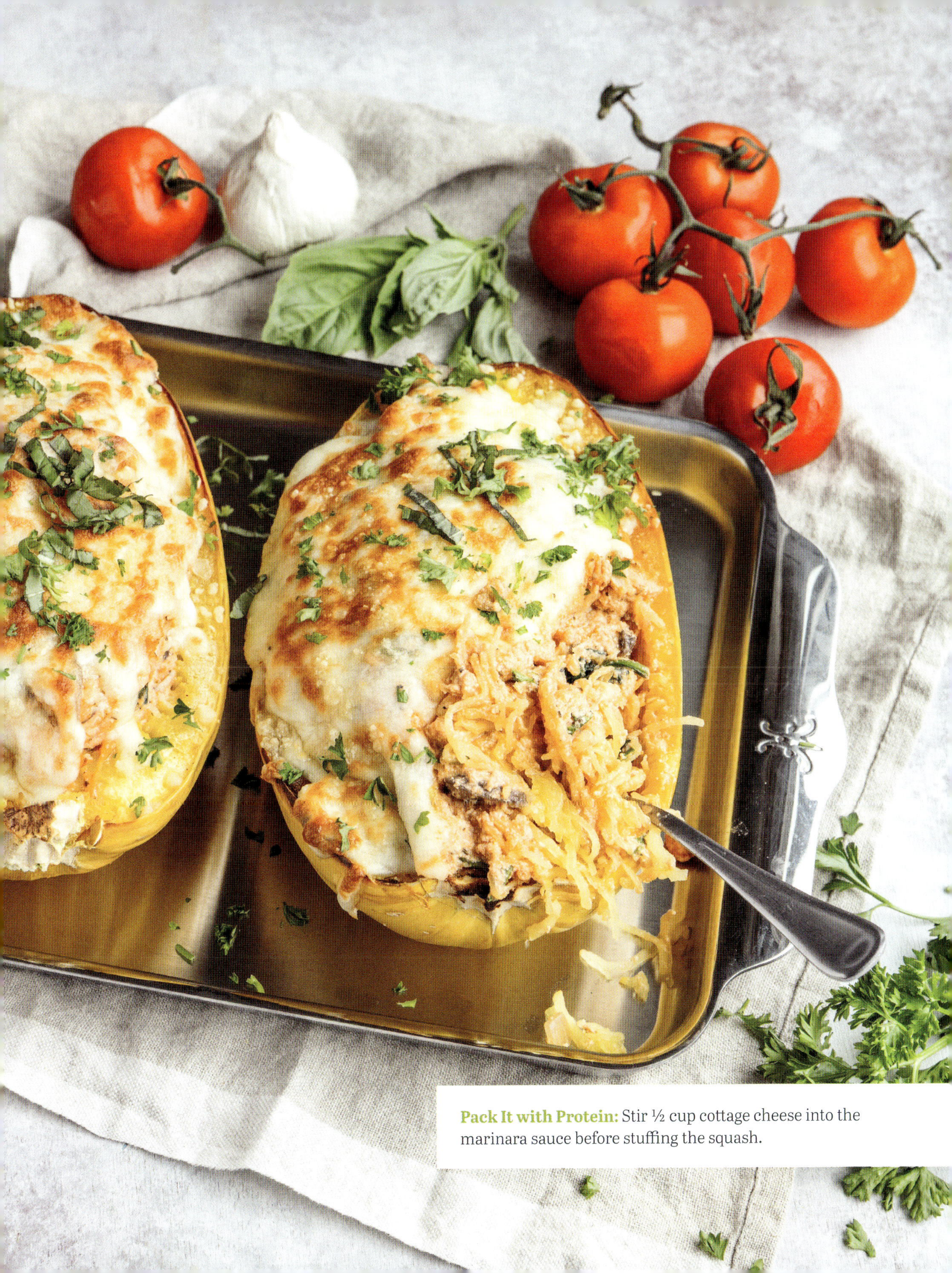

Pack It with Protein: Stir ½ cup cottage cheese into the marinara sauce before stuffing the squash.

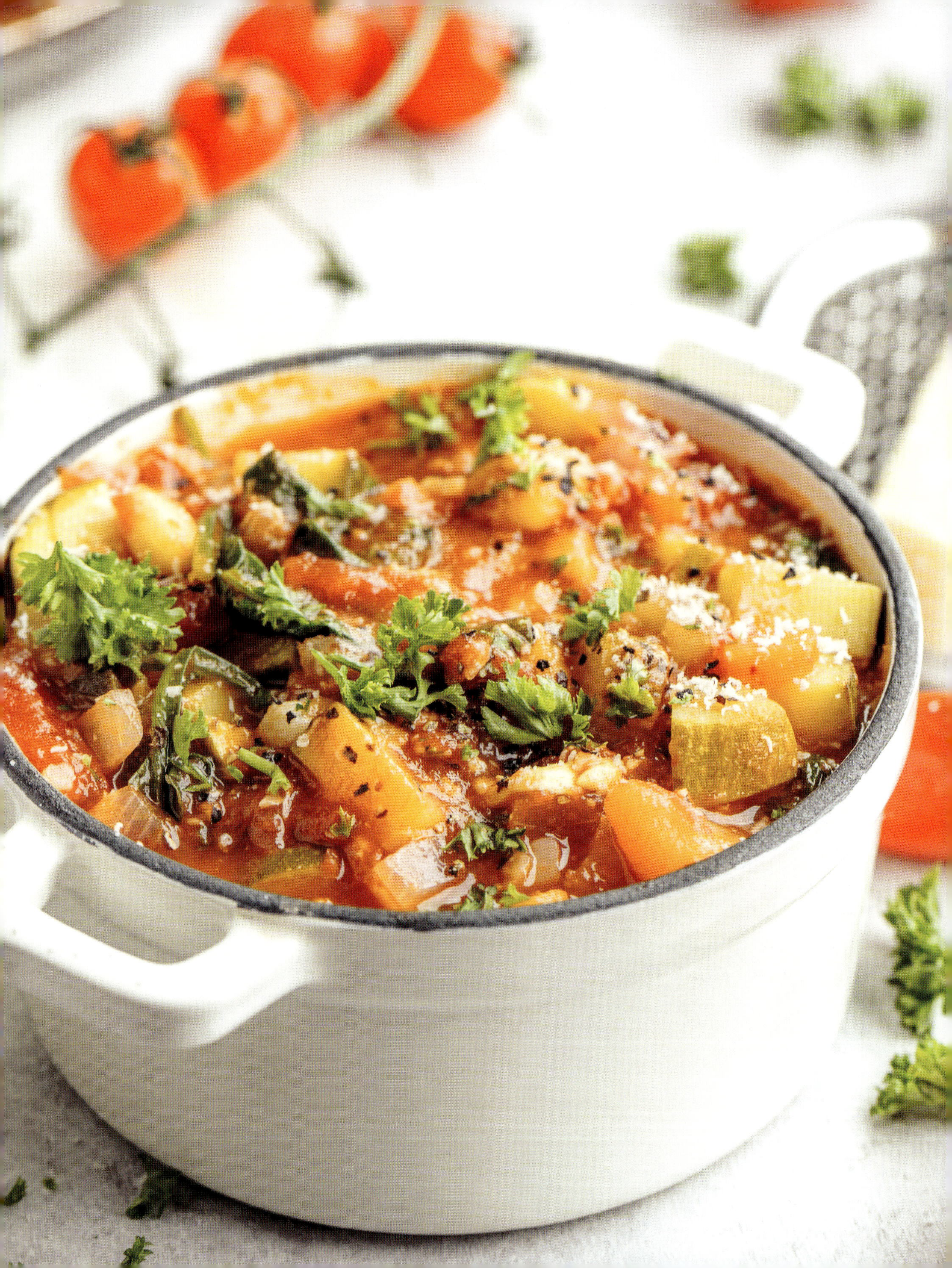

MINESTRONE SOUP

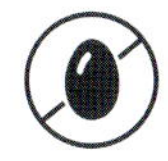 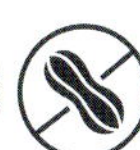 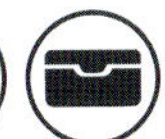

SERVES 2

PREP TIME: 10 minutes

COOK TIME: 40 minutes

This protein-packed minestrone is the ultimate low-carb comfort food for a chilly day. Instead of traditional high-carb beans like kidney or great northern beans, this recipe uses lupini beans, a keto-friendly option rich in fiber and protein. The soup features a medley of vegetables like zucchini, celery, onions, and a bit of carrot, which are simmered in a flavorful broth made from canned tomatoes. A Parmesan cheese rind adds a rich umami depth. This recipe yields a hearty portion with over 23 grams of protein per serving. You can double the recipe to feed more people.

---

2 tablespoons extra-virgin olive oil

½ cup diced onions

½ cup diced carrots

3 celery stalks, diced

2 medium zucchini, cut into quarter-moons

1 (28-ounce) can whole tomatoes

4 cups vegetable broth

1 teaspoon salt

1 Parmesan cheese rind (about 1 by 4 inches)

1 cup cauliflower rice

2 cups jarred lupini beans, rinsed and drained (see note)

3 cups spinach leaves

Ground black pepper

FOR GARNISH (OPTIONAL)

Chopped fresh parsley

Freshly cracked black pepper

Grated Parmesan cheese

1. Preheat a Dutch oven or other large heavy-bottomed pot over medium-high heat. Pour in the olive oil.
2. Add the onions, carrots, and celery to the pot and cook, stirring occasionally, until almost tender.
3. Add the zucchini, tomatoes with their juices, broth, salt, and Parmesan rind. Stir to combine. Bring to a boil, then reduce the heat to low. Simmer, uncovered, until the vegetables are tender, at least 20 minutes. The longer you simmer the soup, the more flavor the Parmesan rind will release.
4. Stir in the cauliflower rice and lupini beans. Cook for 5 more minutes to heat the cauliflower rice and beans and continue deepening the flavor of the soup.
5. Stir in the spinach and continue stirring until it has wilted into the soup. Remove the cheese rind and discard, then season the soup with salt and pepper to taste. Garnish with parsley, cracked pepper, and/or grated Parmesan cheese, if desired.

Pack It with Protein: Add more lupini beans or top your soup with grated Parmesan cheese.

note

Lupini beans are packed with protein and fiber and can be enjoyed as a snack, tossed into salads, or added to recipes like other legumes. For this recipe, use jarred or pickled lupini beans. I use the Cento brand of unpeeled lupini beans, but the peeled beans are also fine. You can order canned lupini beans from Amazon.

(per serving)
CALORIES: **457** | PROTEIN: **23.7g** | FAT: **14.7g** | TOTAL CARBS: **54.9g** | NET CARBS: **27.9g** | FIBER: **27g**

PROTEIN MAC 'N' CHEESE

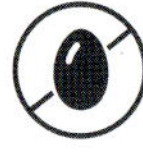
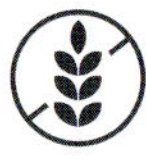
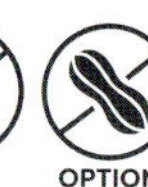

SERVES 1

PREP TIME: 5 minutes (not including time to cook pasta)

COOK TIME: 2 minutes

This five-ingredient mac and cheese is a quick, high-protein version of the classic comfort food. The creamy base is made with cottage cheese, which adds a boost of protein, while real cheddar cheese and a touch of cheddar cheese powder provide a rich, cheesy flavor. You can experiment with different cheeses—try Colby Jack or smoked Gouda. High-protein pasta ties it all together with more than 40 grams of protein.

½ cup cottage cheese (4% milkfat)

½ cup shredded medium cheddar cheese

1½ tablespoons cheddar cheese powder

2 tablespoons nut or seed milk of choice (unflavored and unsweetened)

2 ounces medium lupini pasta, such as ziti, cooked and drained

Paprika, for garnish (optional)

1. In a mini food processor, blend the cottage cheese, shredded cheddar, cheddar cheese powder, and milk until smooth and creamy.
2. Put the cooked pasta in a small bowl and allow to cool slightly if just made. (If hot, the cottage cheese in the sauce could curdle.) Pour the cheese sauce over the pasta and toss to coat.
3. Pour the mixture into a skillet and heat over medium-low heat until the cheese sauce is warmed, about 2 minutes. Or microwave at 40 percent power in 30-second intervals until warmed.
4. Dust with paprika, if desired.

notes

You can omit the cheddar cheese powder; however, it makes the cheddar flavor more pronounced. The powder I use is from Hoosier Hill Farm. It and other brands can be purchased on Amazon.

The low-carb, high-protein ziti noodles I used for this recipe are from the brand Kaizen. I chose the version that has 6 grams of net carbs.

CALORIES: **520** | PROTEIN: **44.2g** | FAT: **30.6g** | TOTAL CARBS: **26.5g** | NET CARBS: **14.4g** | FIBER: **12.1g**

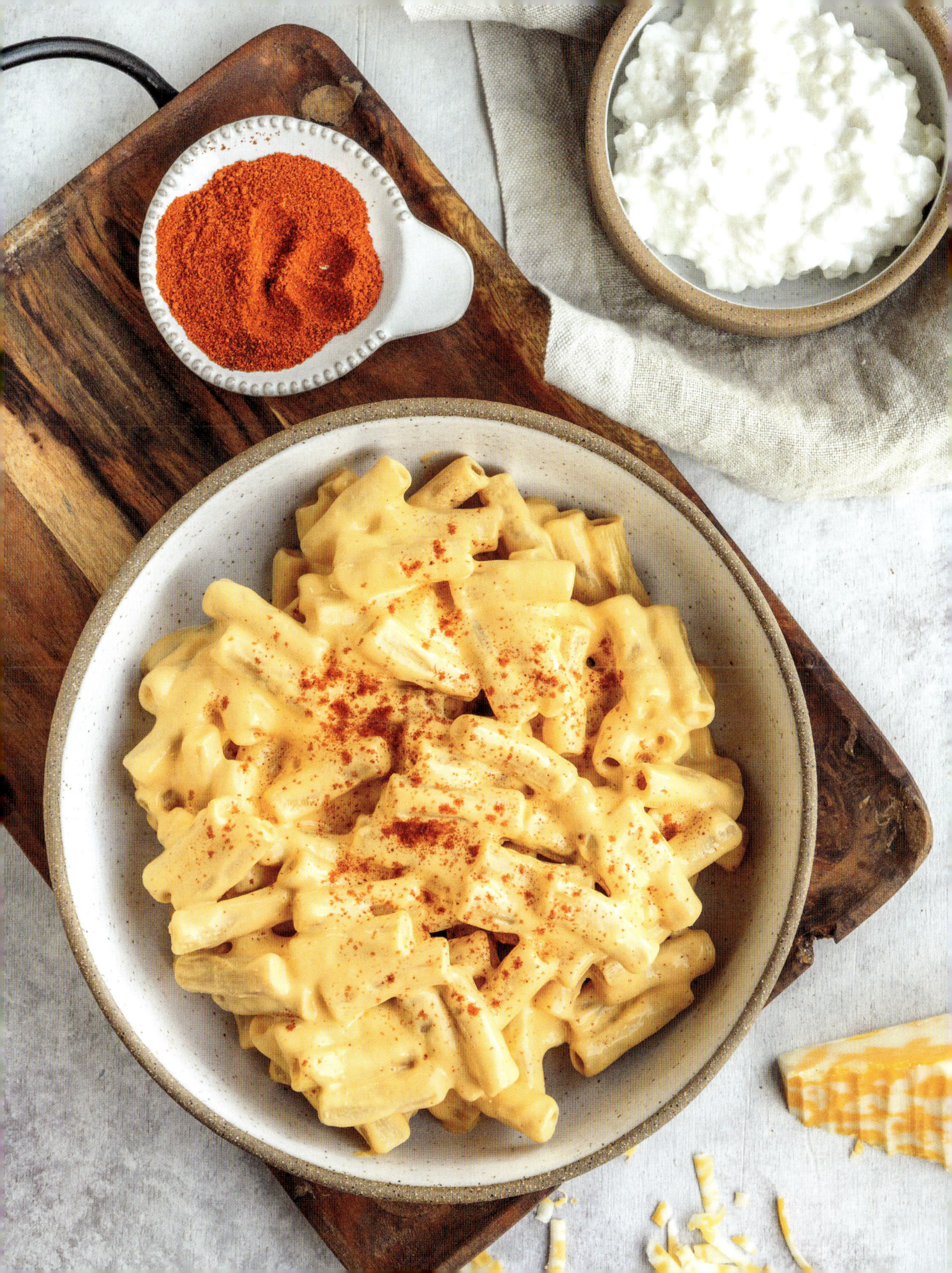

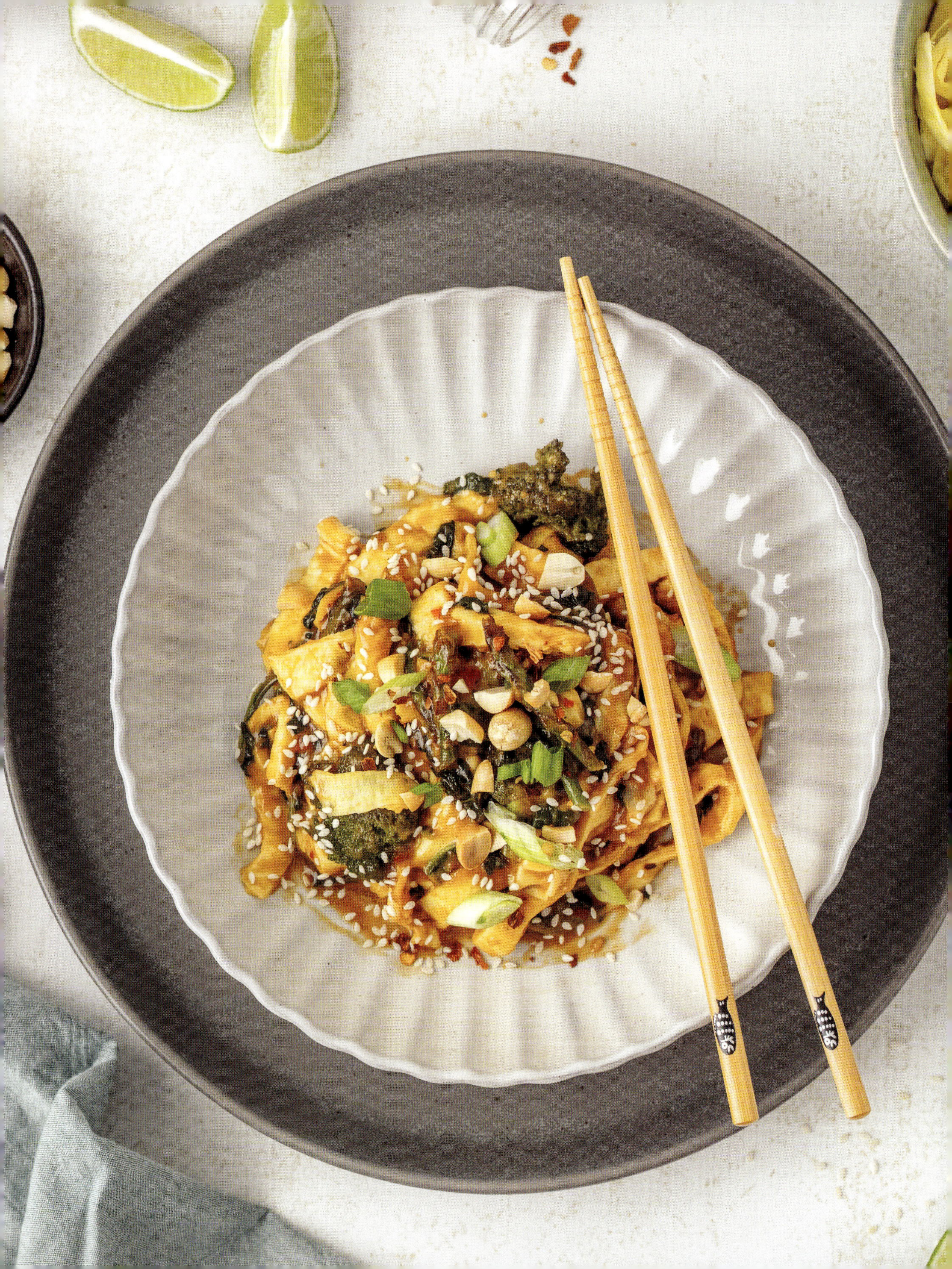

SPICY PEANUT NOODLES

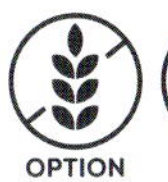

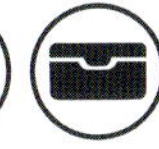

SERVES 6

PREP TIME: 10 minutes (not including time to make noodles)

COOK TIME: 10 minutes

This high-protein, plant-based pasta dish is loaded with asparagus, broccoli, and spinach—all coated in a sweet and spicy peanut sauce. Because this recipe comes together in about 20 minutes once the protein noodles are prepared, it's perfect for weeknight dinners. It's as convenient as it is tasty. You can use your favorite store-bought low-carb noodles in place of my protein noodles to save even more time.

½ cup no-sugar-added peanut butter

⅓ cup soy sauce or tamari

3 tablespoons unseasoned rice vinegar

2 tablespoons chili garlic sauce or chili paste

2 tablespoons toasted sesame oil

2 tablespoons brown sugar substitute

4 cloves garlic, peeled, divided

1¼ teaspoons ginger powder

2 tablespoons avocado oil

1 bundle thin asparagus, cut into 1½-inch pieces

18 ounces broccoli florets

4 cups baby spinach

6 servings Protein Noodles (page 253)

FOR SERVING (OPTIONAL)

Roughly chopped roasted salted peanuts

Sesame seeds

Red pepper flakes

Sliced green onions

Lime wedges

1. Put the peanut butter, soy sauce, rice vinegar, chili garlic sauce, sesame oil, brown sugar substitute, 2 of the garlic cloves, and the ginger powder in a blender or food processor. Blend until smooth. Set aside.
2. Heat the avocado oil in a large wok or skillet over medium-high heat. Mince the remaining 2 cloves of garlic. Add the asparagus, broccoli, and minced garlic. Sauté until tender, 3 to 5 minutes.
3. Lower the heat to medium. Add the peanut butter sauce and spinach. Continue to cook, stirring occasionally, until the spinach has wilted and the sauce is heated through. Stir in the noodles.
4. Sprinkle with peanuts, sesame seeds, red pepper flakes, and/or sliced green onions and serve with lime wedges, if desired. Serve immediately.

Pack It with Protein: Add hard-boiled eggs or scramble in an egg at the end of cooking.

notes

For a non-vegetarian option, add chicken or beef.

If you're allergic to peanuts (which are technically legumes) but can have tree nuts, you can substitute almond or cashew butter for the peanut butter.

Other low-carb noodle options include store-bought shirataki noodles and heart of palm noodles.

To make this gluten free, use coconut aminos or liquid aminos in place of soy sauce or tamari.

(per serving)
CALORIES: **544** | PROTEIN: **25.9g** | FAT: **40.6g** | TOTAL CARBS: **25.9g** | NET CARBS: **9.4g** | FIBER: **12.5g**
SUGAR ALCOHOLS: **4g**

SRIRACHA EGG SALAD

SERVES 2

PREP TIME: 5 minutes (not including time to hard-boil eggs)

This protein-packed dish combines classic egg salad with spicy, flavorful inspiration from my friend Deney's secret sriracha mayo recipe. Made with hard-boiled eggs and Greek yogurt, it's creamy and nutritious with a punch of heat from the sriracha. Deney's mayo blend—featuring Greek yogurt, sriracha, and a hint of honey—adds the perfect balance of sweetness and spice, elevating this timeless favorite. This egg salad is perfect for sandwiches, wraps, or enjoying on its own.

---

8 large hard-boiled eggs

3 tablespoons mayonnaise

1½ tablespoons plain Greek or low-carb yogurt

1 to 2 teaspoons sriracha, according to taste

½ teaspoon sugar-free or regular honey

Salt and pepper to taste

SANDWICH FIXINGS (OPTIONAL)

Keto bread or wraps

Green leaf lettuce

1. Using the largest holes on a cheese grater, grate the hard-boiled eggs into a large bowl.
2. Add the remaining ingredients. Stir to combine.
3. Enjoy by the spoonful or assemble as a sandwich or wrap using keto bread or wraps and green leaf lettuce.

note

Make a wrap using Cottage Cheese Flatbread (page 241) or Egg Wraps (page 245).

(per serving)

CALORIES: **438** | PROTEIN: **26g** | FAT: **35.1g** | TOTAL CARBS: **3.7g** | NET CARBS: **2.7g** | FIBER: **0.4g**
SUGAR ALCOHOLS: **0.6g**

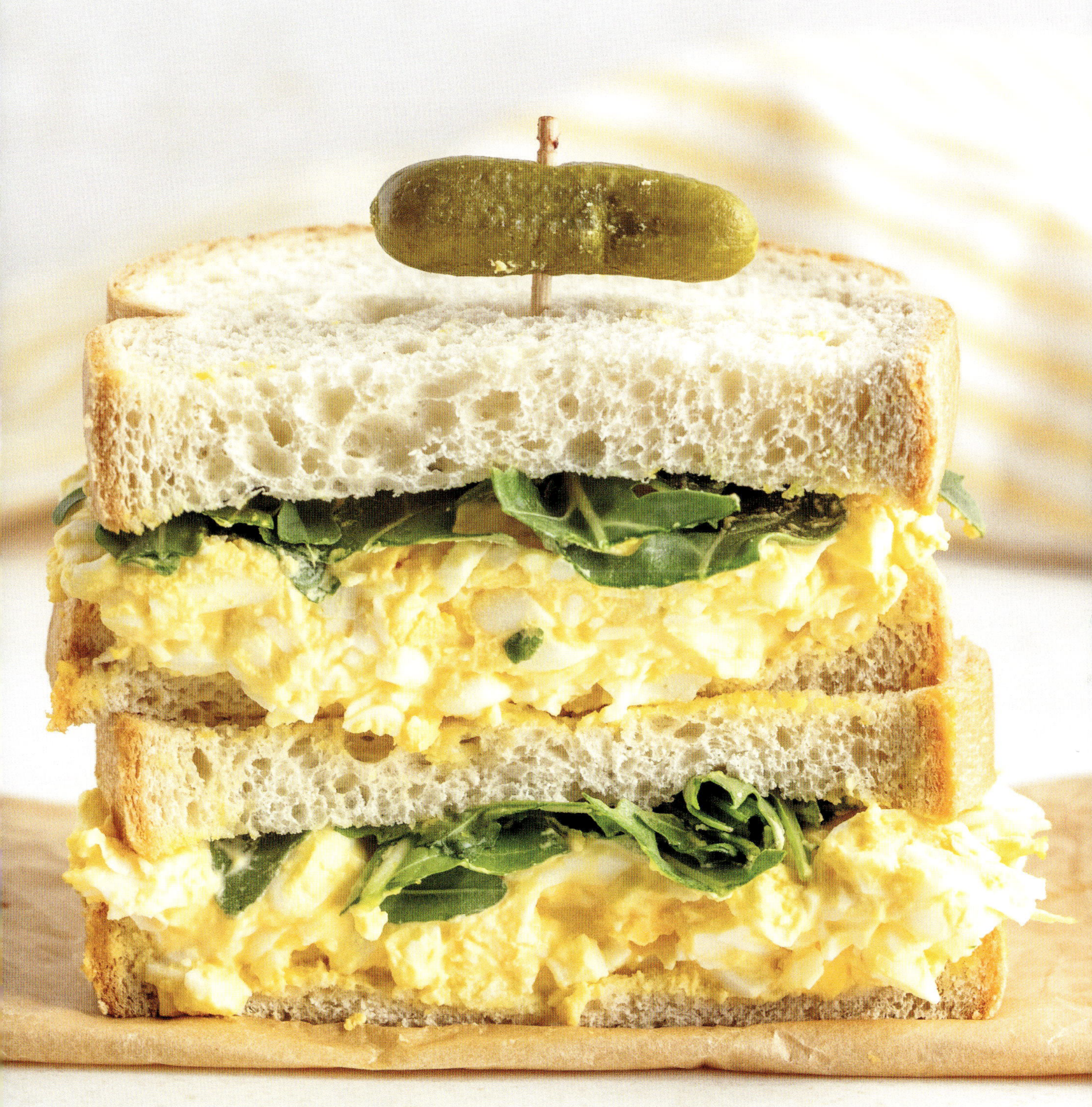

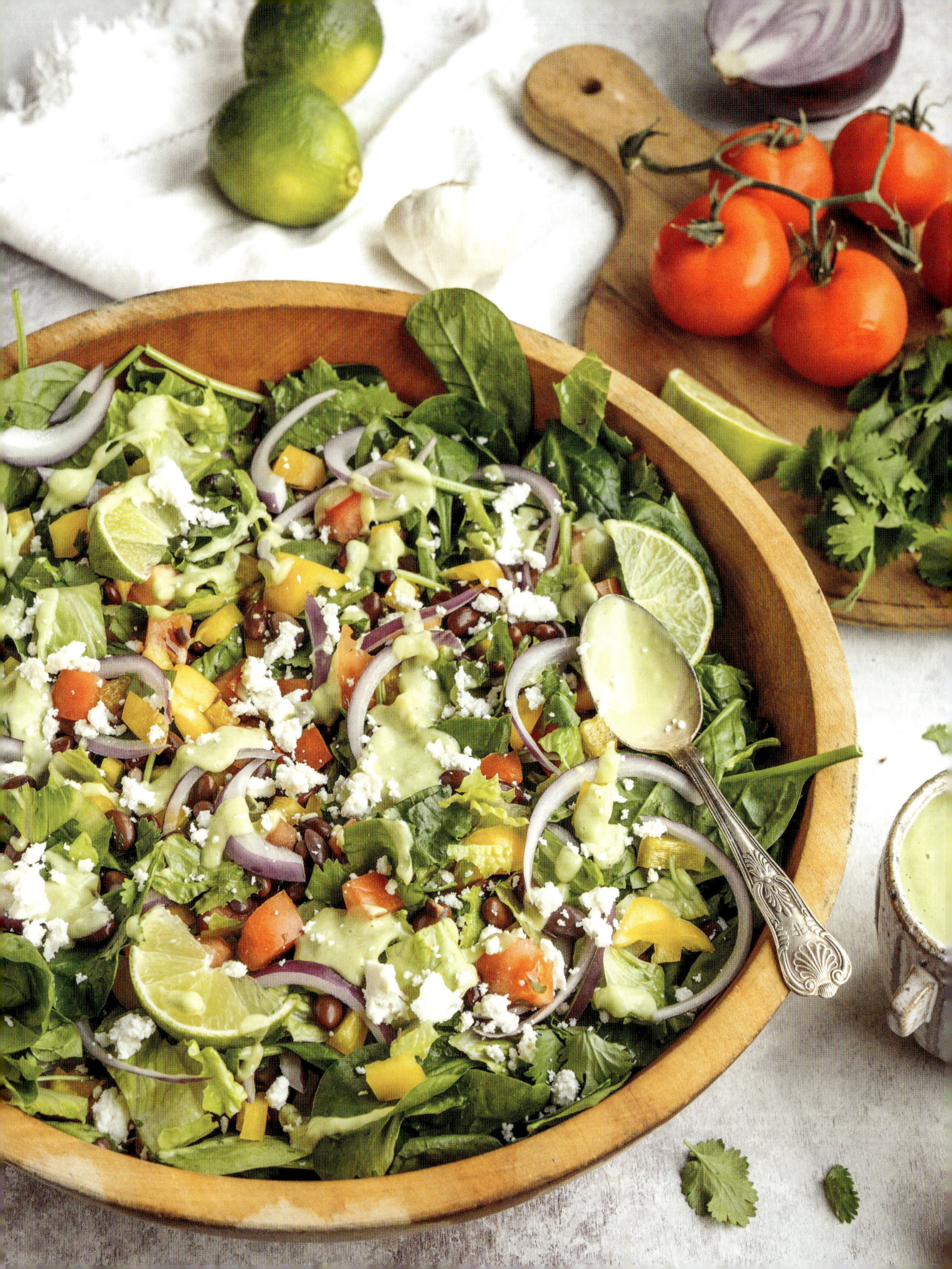

TEX-MEX SALAD

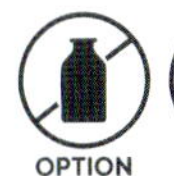

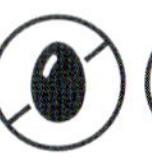

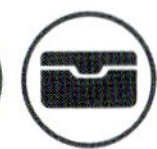

SERVES 2

PREP TIME: 15 minutes

This Tex-Mex–inspired salad combines bold flavors with a focus on protein, making it a great option for a quick and nutritious plant-based meal. Black soybeans are a handy low-carb alternative to black beans. They serve as the protein-packed base, complemented by Cotija cheese and spinach. The salad is finished with a creamy avocado cilantro lime dressing, bringing together freshness and zesty flavor in each bite.

FOR THE DRESSING

2 tablespoons avocado oil

¼ cup water

1 medium avocado, pitted and peeled

5 tablespoons lime juice (from 2 medium limes)

2 cloves garlic, peeled

1 tablespoon chopped jalapeño pepper

½ teaspoon salt

½ teaspoon ground cumin

FOR THE SALAD

3 cups baby spinach

3 cups chopped romaine lettuce hearts

1 medium yellow bell pepper, diced

1 medium tomato, diced

½ cup chopped fresh cilantro

¼ medium red onion, sliced

1 (15-ounce) can black soybeans, rinsed and drained

⅓ cup crumbled Cotija cheese

1. To make the dressing, pour the avocado oil and water into a mini food processor or blender. Add the avocado, lime juice, garlic cloves, jalapeño, salt, and cumin. Blend until smooth and creamy. Set aside.
2. Put the spinach and chopped lettuce in a large bowl. Toss with the bell pepper, tomato, cilantro, red onion, soybeans, and cheese.
3. Drizzle the dressing over the salad before serving.

notes

For meal prep, store the salad components separately from the dressing. To prevent the salad from getting soggy, pour on the dressing right before serving.

Can't find black soybeans? I order them from Amazon, but you could use black beans if you don't mind the extra carbs.

To make this dairy free, omit the cheese.

(per serving)

CALORIES: **617** | PROTEIN: **28.9g** | FAT: **35.9g** | TOTAL CARBS: **47.1g** | NET CARBS: **24.4g** | FIBER: **22.7g**

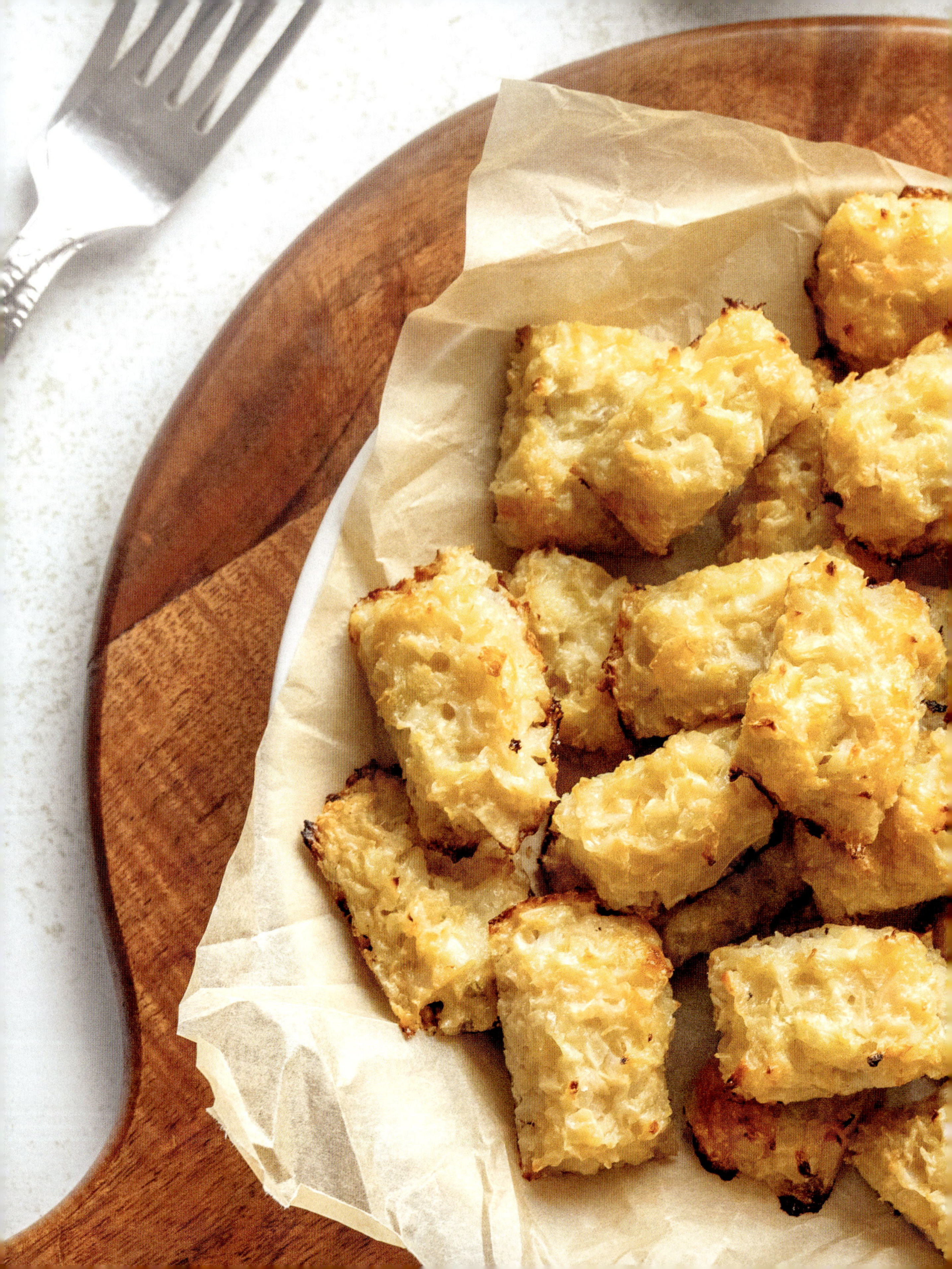

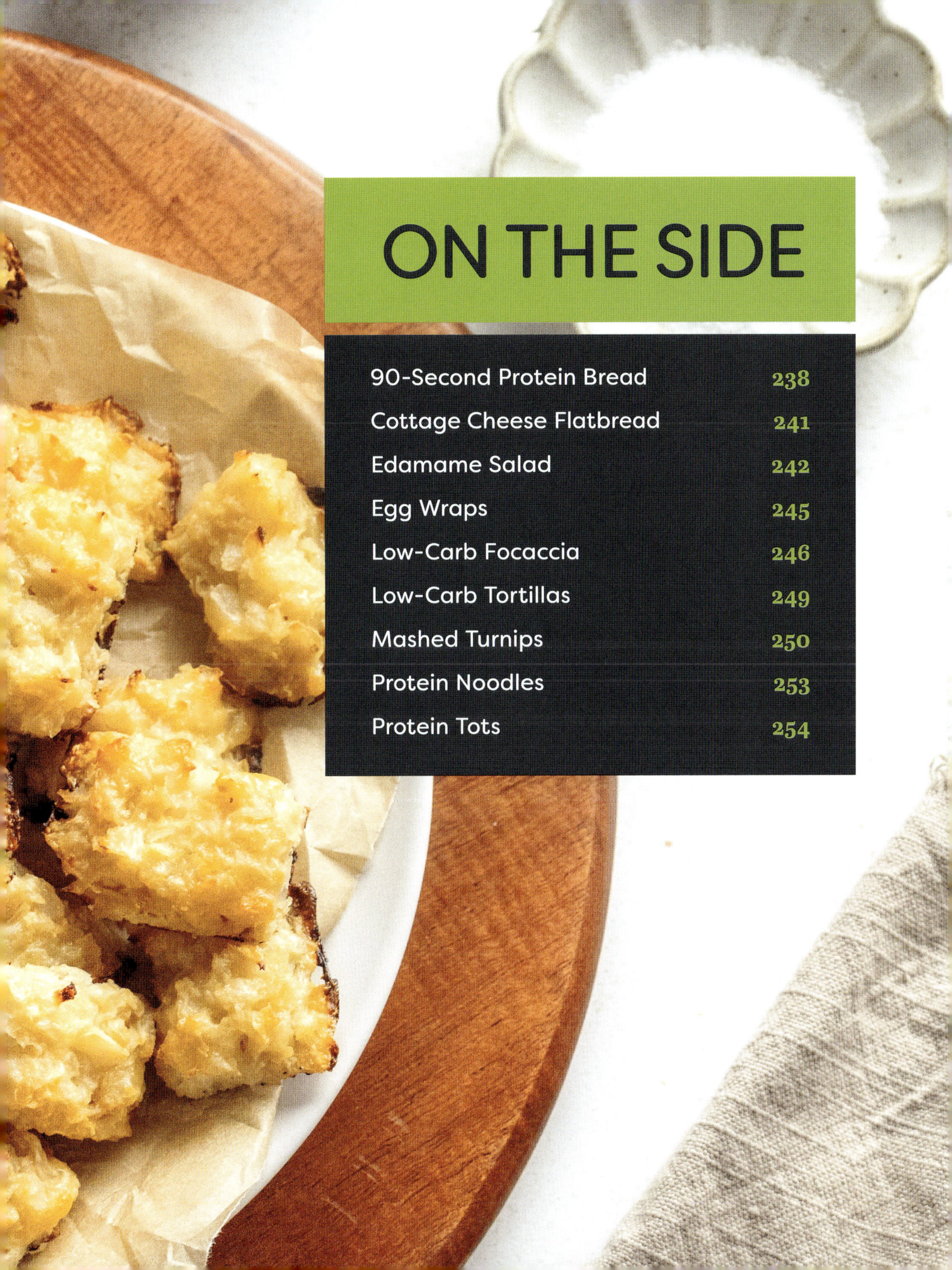

ON THE SIDE

90-SECOND PROTEIN BREAD

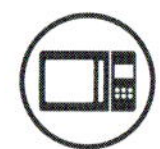

SERVES 1 (2 slices)
PREP TIME: 2 minutes
COOK TIME: 90 seconds

A quick and delicious option for a single serving of low-carb bread. Each slice packs more than 9 grams of protein and bakes in just 90 seconds in the microwave, creating two airy, fluffy slices perfect for sandwiches or toast. Unlike many other gluten-free keto bread recipes, this bread has no eggy flavor and closely resembles the taste and texture of traditional bread. If you dislike using a microwave, I've included the oven method below.

¼ cup blanched, super-fine almond flour

1 tablespoon unflavored protein powder

1 teaspoon baking powder

¼ teaspoon granulated allulose or other granulated sugar-free sweetener (optional)

⅛ teaspoon salt

2 tablespoons unsalted butter, softened

1 large egg white

1 tablespoon heavy cream

2 teaspoons plain Greek or low-carb yogurt or sour cream

Special equipment: 4-inch square microwave-safe dish

1. Mix together the almond flour, protein powder, baking powder, sweetener (if using), and salt in a small bowl.
2. Add the butter, egg white, cream, and yogurt. Mix with a fork until combined.
3. Spray a 4-inch square microwave-safe dish with cooking oil and lay down two 4-inch-wide strips of parchment paper, one crossing over the other, to line all sides of the dish, allowing the parchment to extend over the sides. Using a rubber spatula, scoop the dough into the lined dish and spread evenly edge to edge.
4. Put the dish in the microwave and cook for 90 seconds, or until the bread is set in the center and springs back when you touch the top.
5. Let the bread cool for about a minute, then use the ends of the parchment paper to lift it out of the dish. Let cool completely on a wire rack before slicing.
6. Using a serrated knife, cut the bread in half horizontally to make two thin, square slices. If not using immediately, wrap in a paper towel and store in a zip-top bag in the refrigerator for up to 3 days.

Variation: 9-Minute Protein Bread

Preheat the oven to 350°F. Complete Steps 1 through 3 but use an oven-safe dish in Step 3. Put the dish in the oven and bake for 9 to 11 minutes, until the bread is set in the center and springs back when you touch the top. Complete Steps 5 and 6 as written.

(per slice)
CALIORIES: **240** | PROTEIN: **9.1g** | FAT: **21g** | TOTAL CARBS: **4.1g** | NET CARBS: **2.1g** | FIBER: **2g**

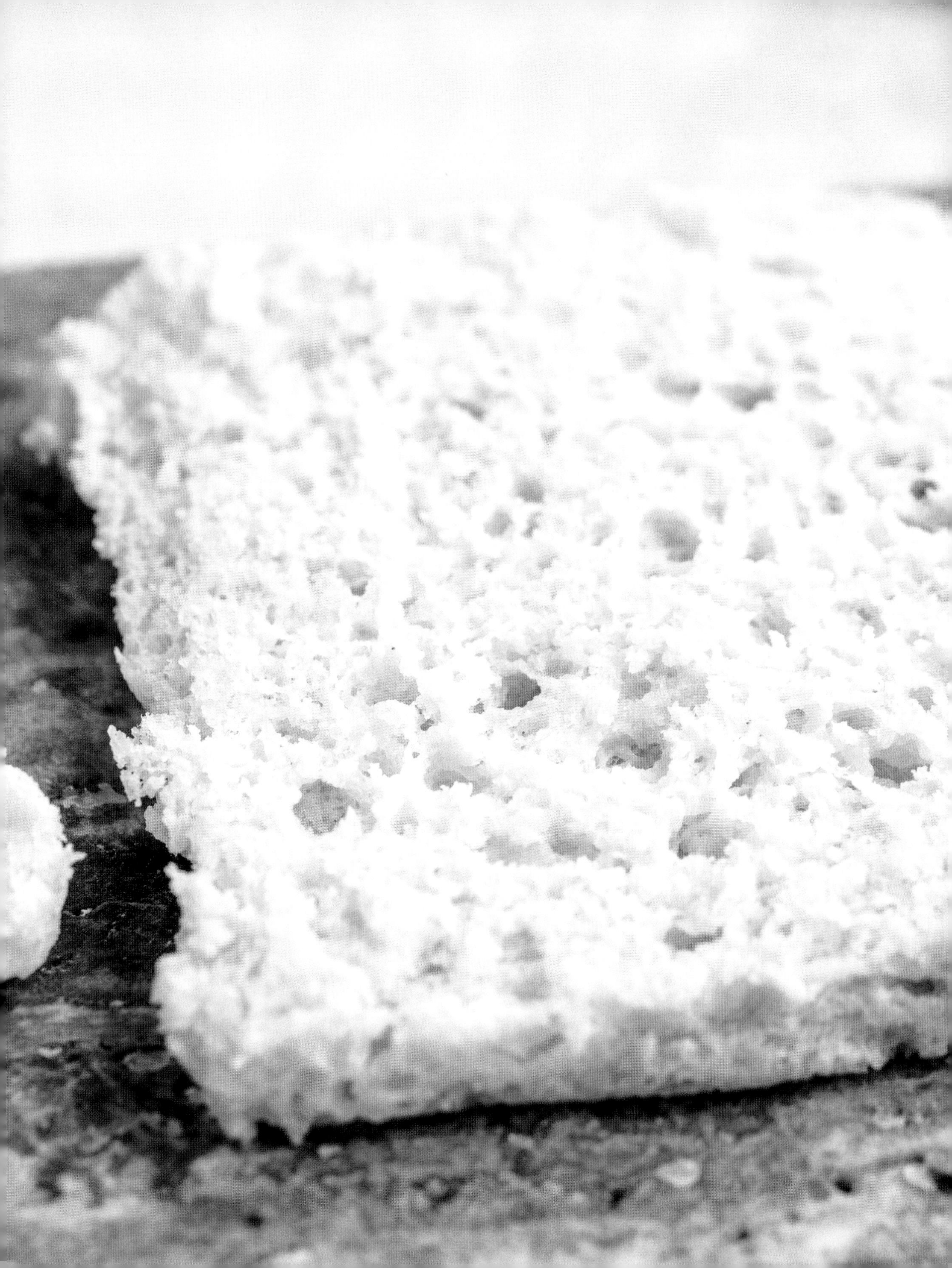

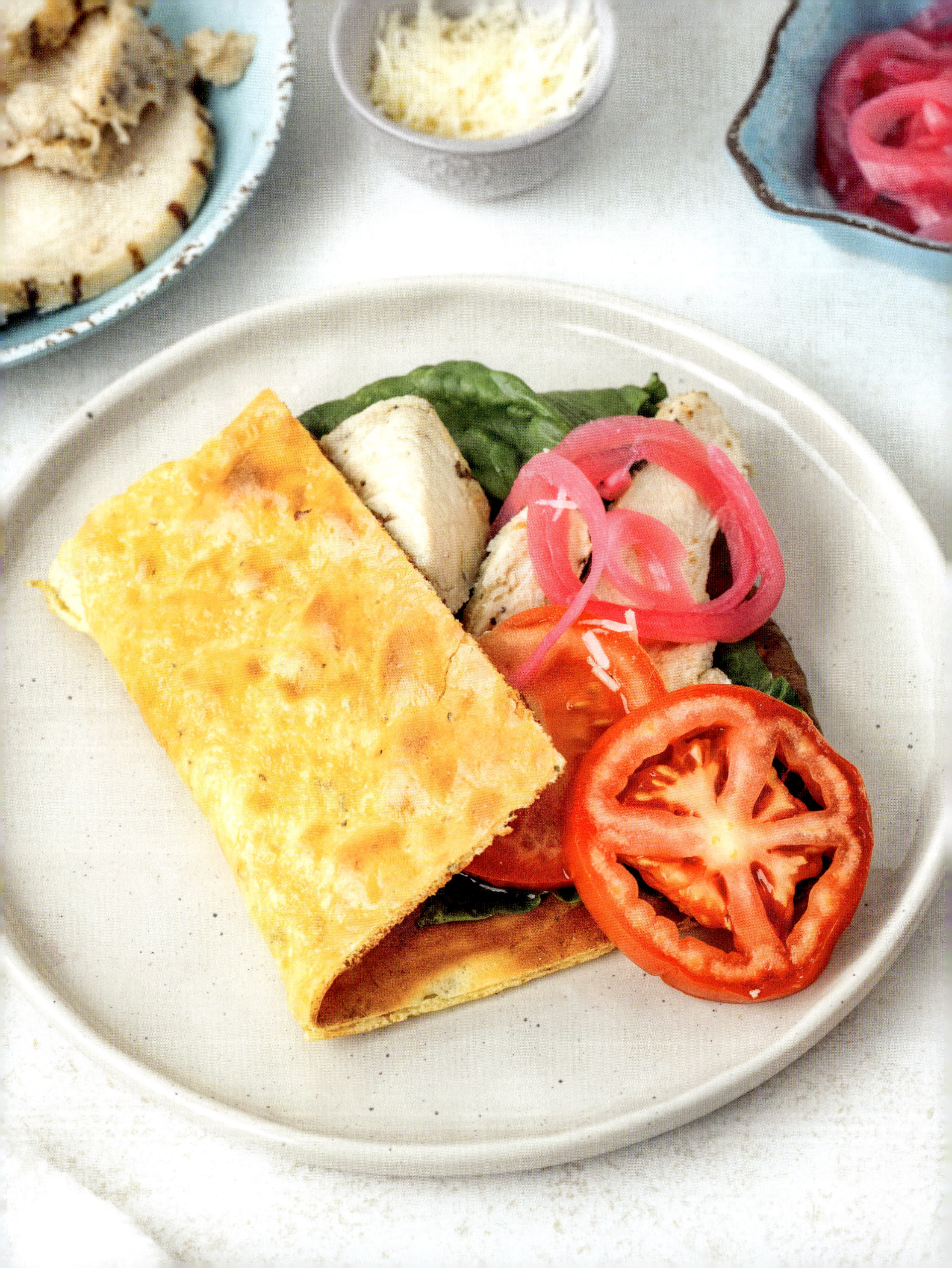

COTTAGE CHEESE FLATBREAD

SERVES 2
PREP TIME: 5 minutes
COOK TIME: 40 minutes

This five-ingredient high-protein flatbread is made from cottage cheese, eggs, grated Parmesan cheese, and a touch of seasoning. Blending the ingredients into a smooth batter and then baking it produces a soft, flexible flatbread. It's perfect for rolling into sandwich wraps, like the one shown here with chicken, lettuce, tomato, and pickled red onion, or using as a base for a flatbread pizza.

8 ounces cottage cheese (4% milkfat)

2 large eggs

¼ cup grated Parmesan cheese

½ teaspoon garlic powder

½ teaspoon Italian seasoning

1. Preheat the oven to 350°F. Line a rimmed baking sheet with parchment paper or a silicone mat.
2. In a food processor or blender, blend all the ingredients until smooth.
3. Pour the batter onto the prepared pan and spread into a thin layer from edge to edge.
4. Bake for 35 to 40 minutes, until the top is set. Remove from the oven and let cool completely in the pan.
5. Since this recipe makes two servings, you can cut the flatbread in half lengthwise now, or you can assemble your wrap (or add your toppings if using as a pizza crust) and then portion out a serving. Store leftover flatbread wrapped in plastic wrap or in a zip-top bag in the refrigerator for up to 3 days.

(per serving)
CALORIES: **245** | PROTEIN: **26.4g** | FAT: **14g** | TOTAL CARBS: **4.3g** | NET CARBS: **4.1g** | FIBER: **0.2g**

EDAMAME SALAD

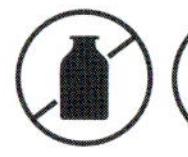
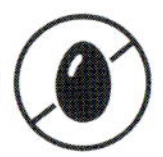
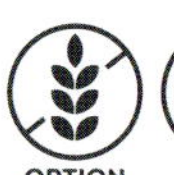

SERVES 4

PREP TIME: 15 minutes

This quick and easy salad is a high-protein, low-carb side dish with a perfect balance of sweet and spicy flavors. Edamame are a great way to get a little extra protein in your day. They are tossed in a delicious sauce along with crunchy red bell pepper, cucumber, and sliced almonds. This salad is ideal for meal prep or busy nights when you need a side dish!

FOR THE DRESSING

2 tablespoons rice wine vinegar

1½ tablespoons soy sauce or tamari

1½ tablespoons sugar-free or regular honey

1 tablespoon toasted sesame oil

½ teaspoon sriracha

½ teaspoon garlic powder

¼ teaspoon ginger powder

FOR THE SALAD

1 (12-ounce) package frozen shelled edamame, thawed

1 cup diced cucumbers

½ medium red bell pepper, diced

¼ cup sliced almonds

1 teaspoon black sesame seeds

1. In a small bowl, whisk together all the ingredients for the dressing. Set aside.
2. Put the thawed edamame, cucumbers, bell pepper, almonds, and sesame seeds in a large bowl. Pour on the dressing and toss to coat evenly. Store in an airtight container in the refrigerator for up to 5 days.

note

To make this gluten free, use coconut aminos or liquid aminos in place of soy sauce or tamari.

(per serving)

CALORIES: **179** | PROTEIN: **12.5g** | FAT: **10.8g** | TOTAL CARBS: **16.3g** | NET CARBS: **5g** | FIBER: **7.5g**
SUGAR ALCOHOLS: **3.8g**

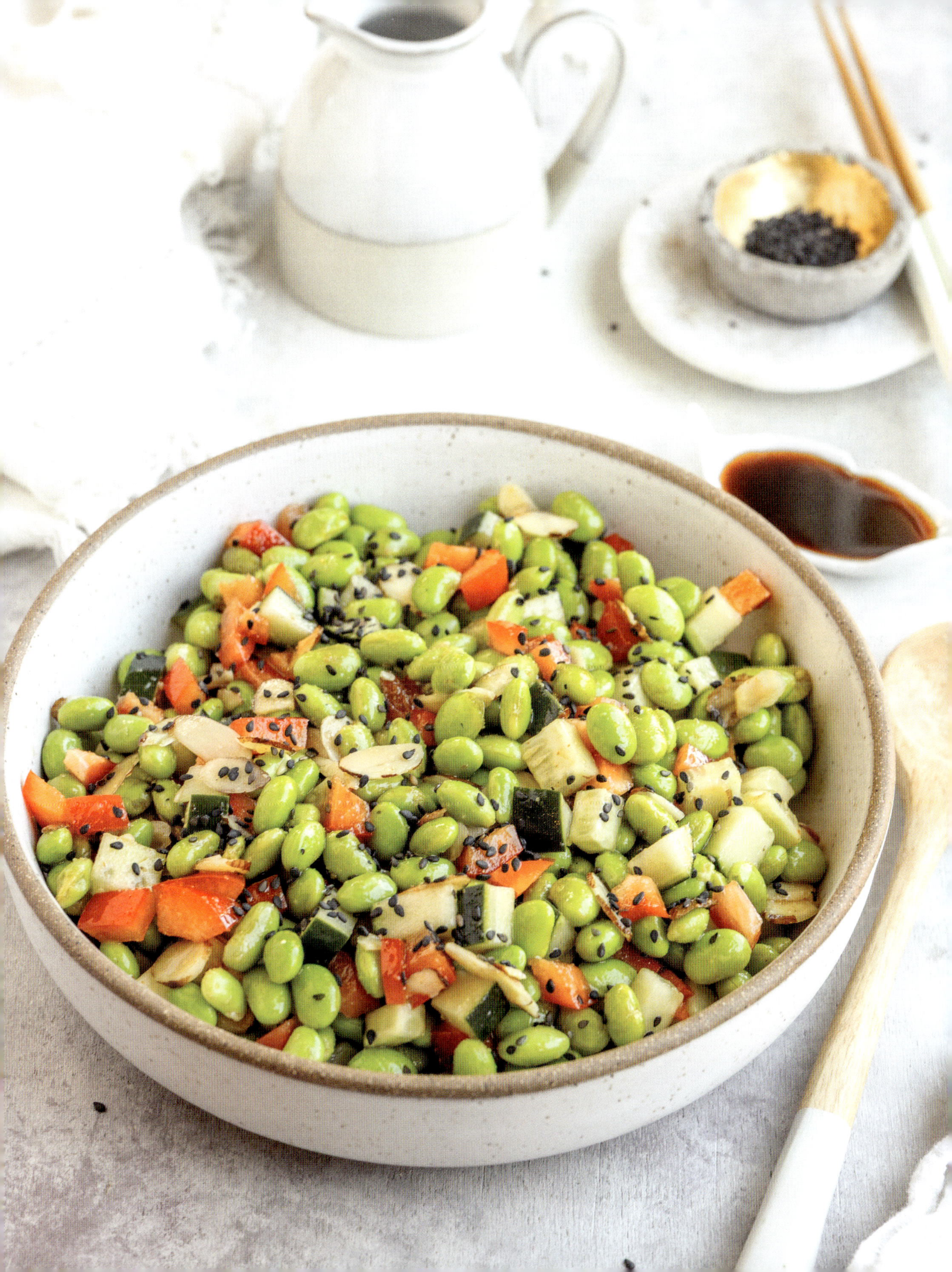

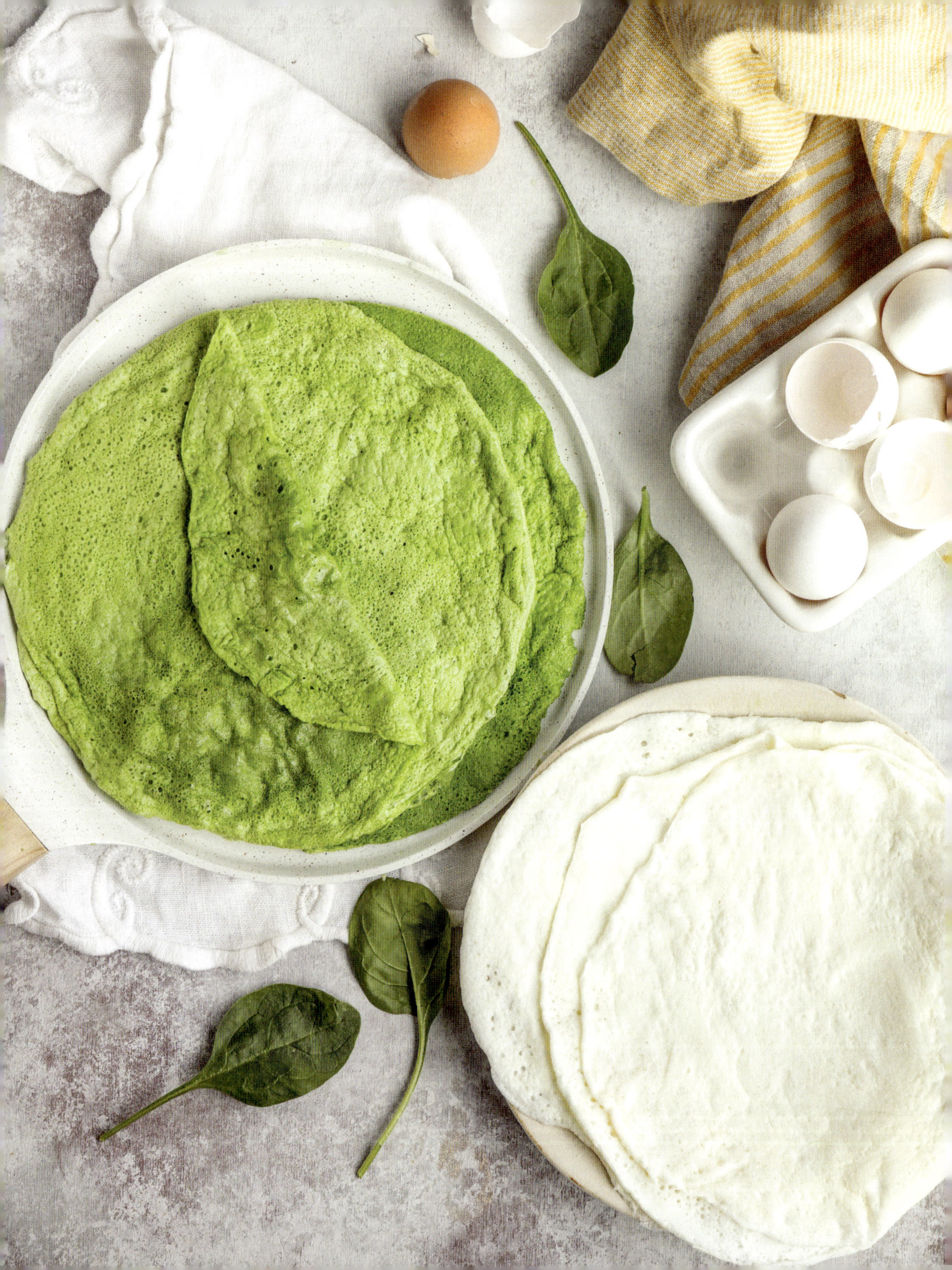

EGG WRAPS

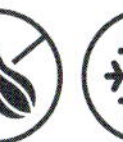
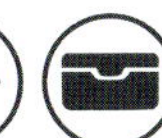

MAKES 3 wraps
PREP TIME: 5 minutes
COOK TIME: 6 minutes

Made with just two ingredients, these homemade egg wraps deliver about 10 grams of protein per wrap. They're not only simple to prepare and freezer-friendly for easy meal prep but also perfect as sandwich wraps or using as a base for other meals. You can also add spinach for a vibrant, nutrient-packed version (see below).

---

6 large egg whites

2 tablespoons unflavored protein powder

Special equipment: Crepe pan and crepe spreader (optional)

1. Put the egg whites and protein powder in a food processor or blender. Blend until smooth.
2. Preheat a crepe pan or 10-inch nonstick skillet over medium-low heat.
3. Spray the pan with cooking oil, then pour ⅓ cup of the batter into the center of the pan. Take a crepe spreader and, using a spinning action and a light touch, spread the batter to the edges of the pan in a very thin, even layer. If you don't have a crepe spreader, use a rubber spatula to spread the batter evenly, moving it from the center outward in a circular fashion. Cook until the egg is set on top, about 1 minute; lift one edge with a fork and carefully use your fingers to flip the wrap and cook the other side for a minute more. Remove and place on a paper towel–lined plate.
4. Repeat with the remaining batter to make a total of three wraps.
5. Store leftover wraps sandwiched between sheets of parchment paper.

Variation: Spinach Egg Wraps

Complete the recipe as written, except in Step 1, add 1 cup baby spinach, and in Steps 3 and 4, pour ½ cup of batter into the skillet instead of ⅓ cup.

(per plain wrap)
CALORIES: **45** | PROTEIN: **9.8g** | FAT: **0.1g** | TOTAL CARBS: **0.5g** | NET CARBS: **0.5g** | FIBER: **0g**

(per spinach wrap)
CALORIES: **48** | PROTEIN: **10.1g** | FAT: **0.1g** | TOTAL CARBS: **1g** | NET CARBS: **0.7g** | FIBER: **0.3g**

LOW-CARB FOCACCIA

SERVES 6

PREP TIME: 10 minutes

COOK TIME: 12 minutes

There's nothing authentic about this focaccia. Unlike the traditional Italian bread, this version doesn't use gluten-based flour or yeast. Yet the texture and flavor are reminiscent of focaccia because it employs some simple substitutions that bake similarly into a savory Italian-inspired bread. It's perfect for dipping into marinara sauce or olive oil.

FOR THE DOUGH

1½ cups blanched, super-fine almond flour

¼ cup lupin flour

3 tablespoons unflavored protein powder

1 teaspoon baking powder

½ teaspoon xanthan gum

½ teaspoon salt

1 tablespoon unsalted butter, melted

2 large eggs

1 large egg white

2 teaspoons Italian seasoning

1 to 2 tablespoons extra-virgin olive oil

1. Preheat the oven to 350°F.
2. In a medium bowl, whisk together the almond flour, lupin flour, protein powder, baking powder, xanthan gum, and salt.
3. Stir in the melted butter and whole eggs. When the dough becomes tough to stir, knead with your hands until all the ingredients are evenly incorporated.
4. Mold the dough into a round or square shape and place between two sheets of parchment paper. Roll into a flat oval or rectangle using a rolling pin until the dough is ¼ to ½ inch thick. Remove the top sheet of parchment and slide the bottom sheet with the rolled-out dough onto a baking sheet.
5. Brush the dough with the egg white. Using your fingers or the handle of a wooden spoon, make dimples in the dough. Sprinkle with the Italian seasoning.
6. Bake for 10 minutes, or until the bread is set in the center. Then move the focaccia under the broiler and broil on high for 1 to 2 minutes, until the top is golden brown. Remove from the oven and brush with the olive oil. Cut into 6 medium or 12 small strips.

(per serving)
CALORIES: **298** | PROTEIN: **12.8g** | FAT: **24.6g** | TOTAL CARBS: **8.2g** | NET CARBS: **3.6g** | FIBER: **4.6g**

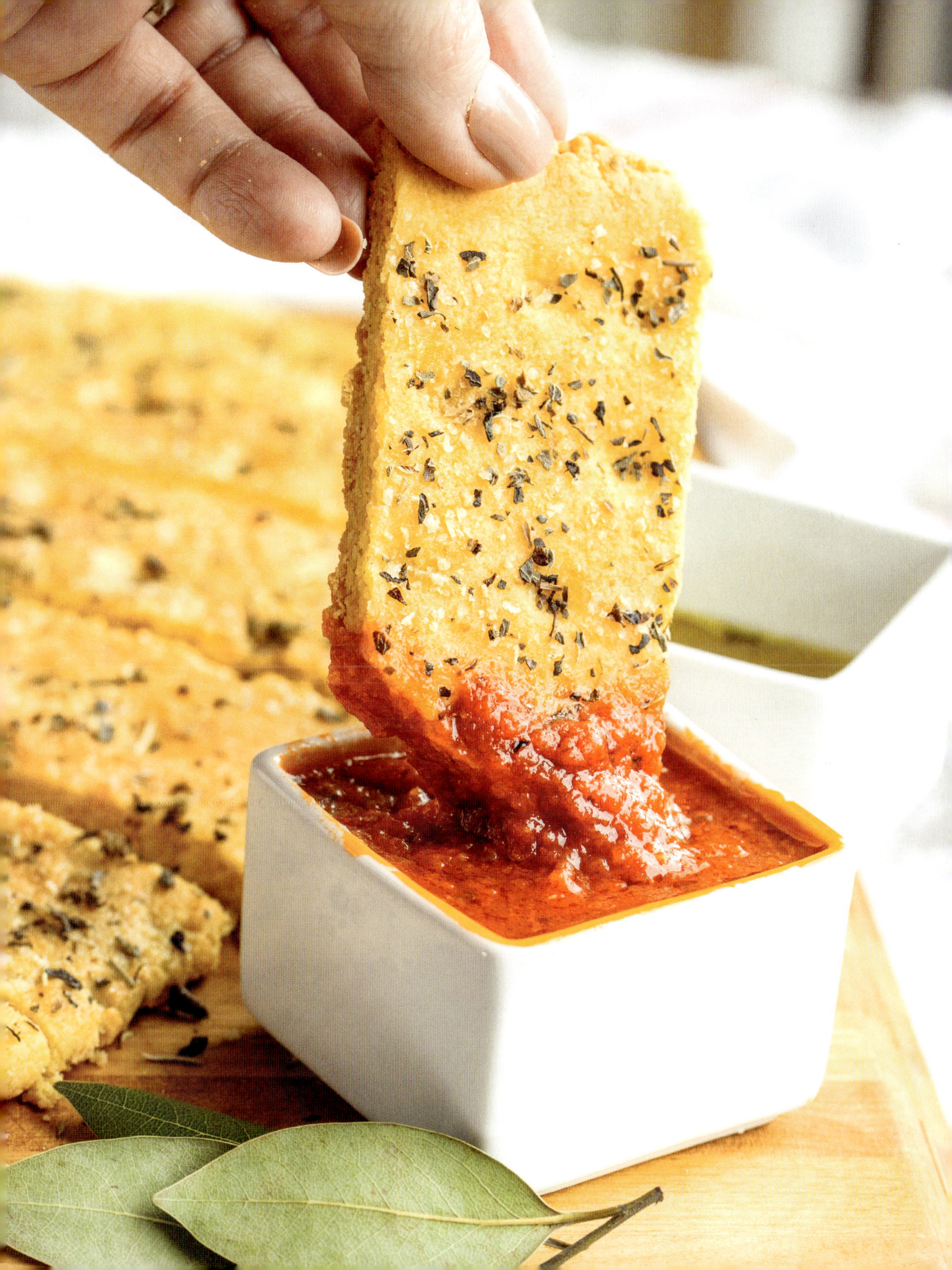

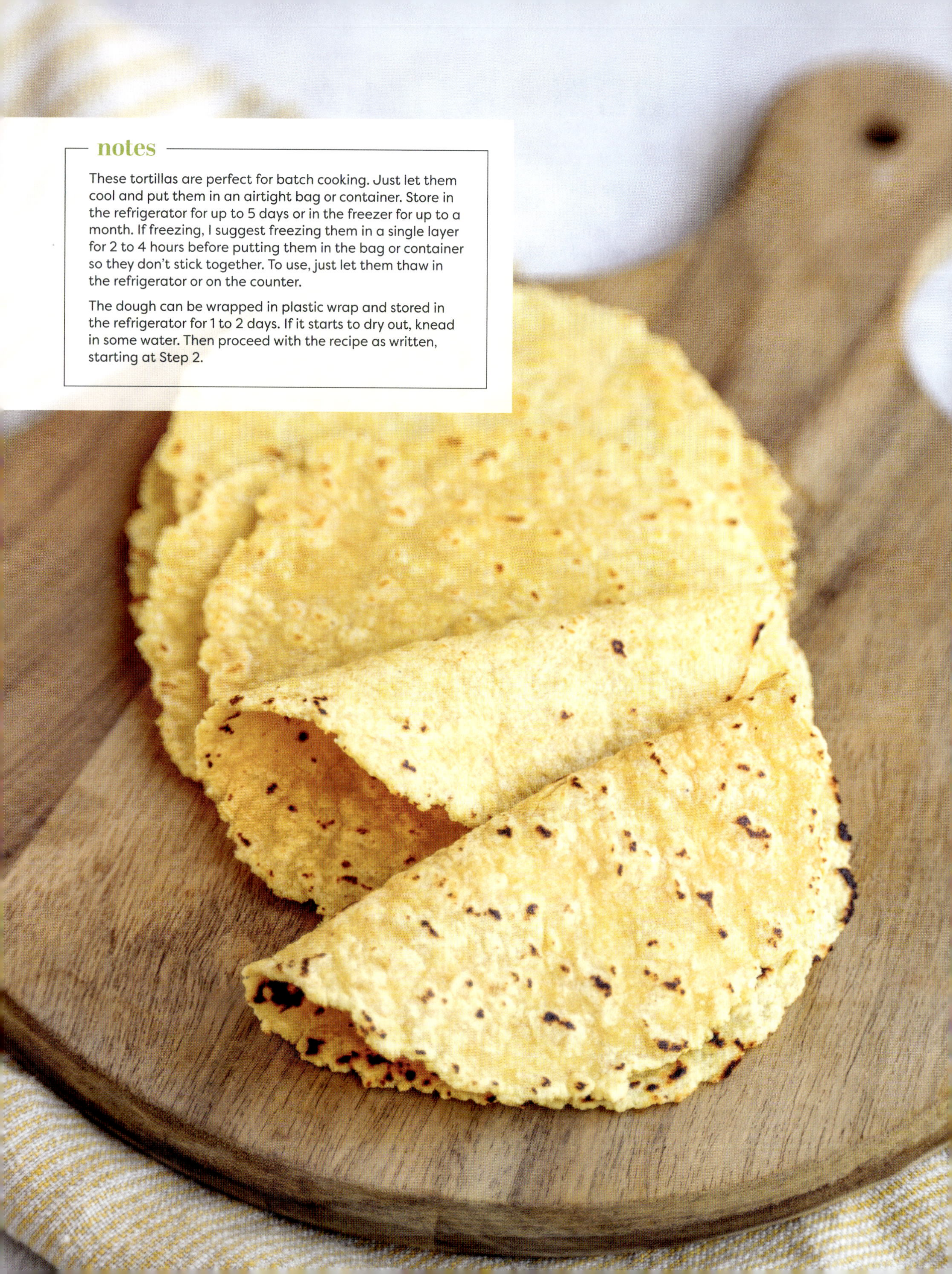

notes

These tortillas are perfect for batch cooking. Just let them cool and put them in an airtight bag or container. Store in the refrigerator for up to 5 days or in the freezer for up to a month. If freezing, I suggest freezing them in a single layer for 2 to 4 hours before putting them in the bag or container so they don't stick together. To use, just let them thaw in the refrigerator or on the counter.

The dough can be wrapped in plastic wrap and stored in the refrigerator for 1 to 2 days. If it starts to dry out, knead in some water. Then proceed with the recipe as written, starting at Step 2.

LOW-CARB TORTILLAS

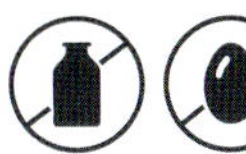
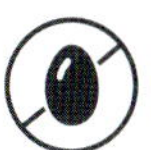
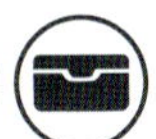

MAKES eight 4-inch tortillas

PREP TIME: 10 minutes

COOK TIME: 12 minutes

These gluten-free tortillas are quick to prepare and taste just like traditional corn tortillas. With only five ingredients and 0.6 gram of net carbs per tortilla, they're high in fiber and easy to make in bulk and freeze for convenient use anytime. The key ingredient is lupin flour, made from the lupini bean, a high-protein legume that perfectly replicates the texture and flavor of corn flour. Xanthan gum makes the tortillas pliable so you can roll and fold them without breaking. I recommend using a tortilla press for this recipe because it ensures even thickness and uniform shape, plus it's faster and easier than rolling them by hand.

½ cup blanched, super-fine almond flour

⅓ cup lupin flour

1 tablespoon xanthan gum

½ teaspoon salt

6 tablespoons water

Special equipment: Tortilla press (optional)

1. In a small bowl, whisk together the almond flour, lupin flour, xanthan gum, and salt. Pour in the water and mix with a fork or your hands until a dough forms. It should feel similar to Play-Doh. If it's too tacky and moist, sprinkle in more almond flour. If it's too dry, add a splash of water.
2. Divide the dough into eight equal portions to make 4-inch tortillas. For larger (6-inch) tortillas, divide the dough into four portions. Form each portion into a ball.
3. If using a tortilla press, cut two circles of parchment paper to match the size of your press, or use 8-inch parchment paper baking circles. Line the bottom of the press with one of the parchment circles, set a dough ball in the center of the parchment, and then lay the second parchment circle on top and press lightly with your fingers. Close the press and press down on the handle to flatten the dough. If you don't have a tortilla press, use a rolling pin to flatten the dough; simply roll it out between two sheets of parchment paper into a 4-inch (or 6-inch) circle.
4. Preheat a small nonstick skillet over high heat. (Do not use oil or cooking spray. The tortillas need to be dry seared.) To remove the tortilla from the parchment paper, carefully peel off one side of the paper, put the piece of parchment back on the tortilla, and flip the whole thing over. Now carefully peel off the top piece of parchment. Remove the tortilla from the bottom piece of parchment and place in the dry skillet. Cook for 30 to 60 seconds, until the underside starts to brown in some spots. Flip and cook the other side for 30 seconds. Remove from the skillet and place back on the parchment paper to cool.
5. Repeat with the remaining dough balls.

(per tortilla)
CALORIES: **57** | PROTEIN: **3.5g** | FAT: **4.1g** | TOTAL CARBS: **3.2g** | NET CARBS: **0.6g** | FIBER: **2.6g**

MASHED TURNIPS

SERVES 4
PREP TIME: 15 minutes
COOK TIME: 25 minutes

Mashed turnips are a creamy, fluffy, and lower-carb alternative to mashed potatoes, perfect for pairing with Pan-Seared Sirloin Steak (page 111), Crispy "Double Protein" Fried Chicken (page 140), or Chicken-Fried Venison (page 208). This recipe uses a few unique methods to neutralize the bitterness of the turnips (all explained below), which renders them so tasty that you'll be making this potato replacement over any other every time.

1½ pounds small turnips

1 small russet potato, rinsed and cut in half

1 cup chicken broth

Salt

3 tablespoons unsalted butter, plus more for garnish if desired

¼ cup plain Greek or low-carb yogurt or heavy cream

¼ teaspoon ground black pepper

Chopped fresh parsley, for garnish

Freshly cracked black pepper, for garnish

1. Peel the turnips, then cut them into ¾-inch cubes.
2. Put the cubed turnips in a large saucepan. Place the potato halves on top of the turnips.
3. Pour in the chicken broth, then add enough water to cover the turnips and potato. Season with a pinch of salt.
4. Bring to a boil and cook until the turnips have softened enough for a fork to easily pierce them, about 20 minutes.
5. Drain the water and discard the potato. Return the cooked turnips to the pan and place back on the stovetop over medium heat. Dry cook the turnips until most of the remaining moisture is gone.
6. Transfer the turnips to a food processor or blender. Add the butter, yogurt, and ground pepper. Pulse until pureed into a mashed "potato" texture. Season with more salt if needed. Top with chopped parsley, cracked pepper, and/or more butter, if desired.

Pack It with Protein: Add more Greek yogurt or even blended cottage cheese to the mashed turnips. Or try toasted beef gelatin to enhance the flavor and add protein. Put 1 to 2 tablespoons beef gelatin powder in a dry nonstick skillet over medium heat. Cook, stirring constantly with a spatula to keep it from burning, until golden, about 3 minutes.

(per serving, using Greek yogurt)
CALORIES: **130** | PROTEIN: **2.8g** | FAT: **8.5g** | TOTAL CARBS: **11.1g** | NET CARBS: **8.1g** | FIBER: **3.1g**

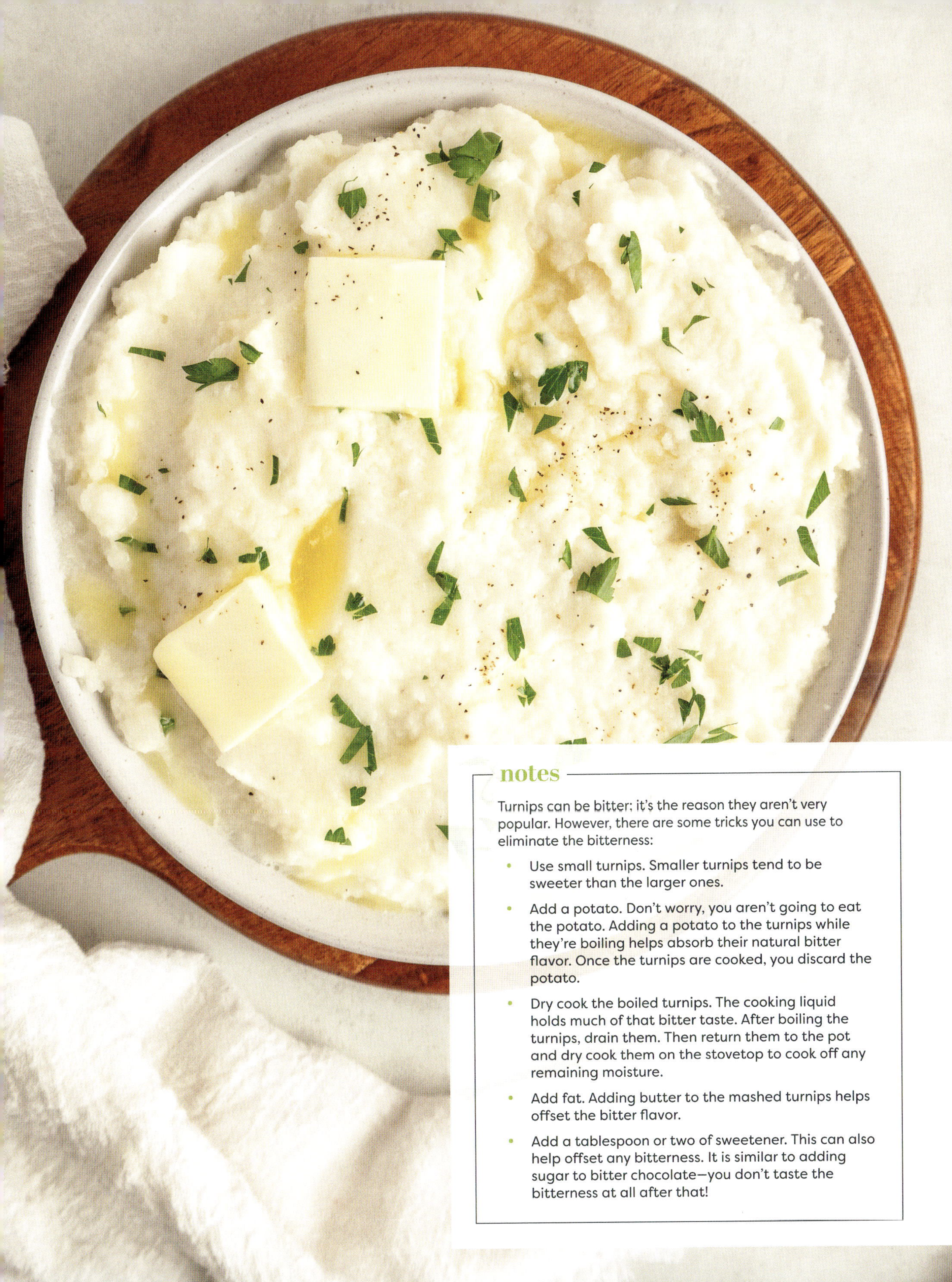

notes

Turnips can be bitter; it's the reason they aren't very popular. However, there are some tricks you can use to eliminate the bitterness:

- Use small turnips. Smaller turnips tend to be sweeter than the larger ones.
- Add a potato. Don't worry, you aren't going to eat the potato. Adding a potato to the turnips while they're boiling helps absorb their natural bitter flavor. Once the turnips are cooked, you discard the potato.
- Dry cook the boiled turnips. The cooking liquid holds much of that bitter taste. After boiling the turnips, drain them. Then return them to the pot and dry cook them on the stovetop to cook off any remaining moisture.
- Add fat. Adding butter to the mashed turnips helps offset the bitter flavor.
- Add a tablespoon or two of sweetener. This can also help offset any bitterness. It is similar to adding sugar to bitter chocolate—you don't taste the bitterness at all after that!

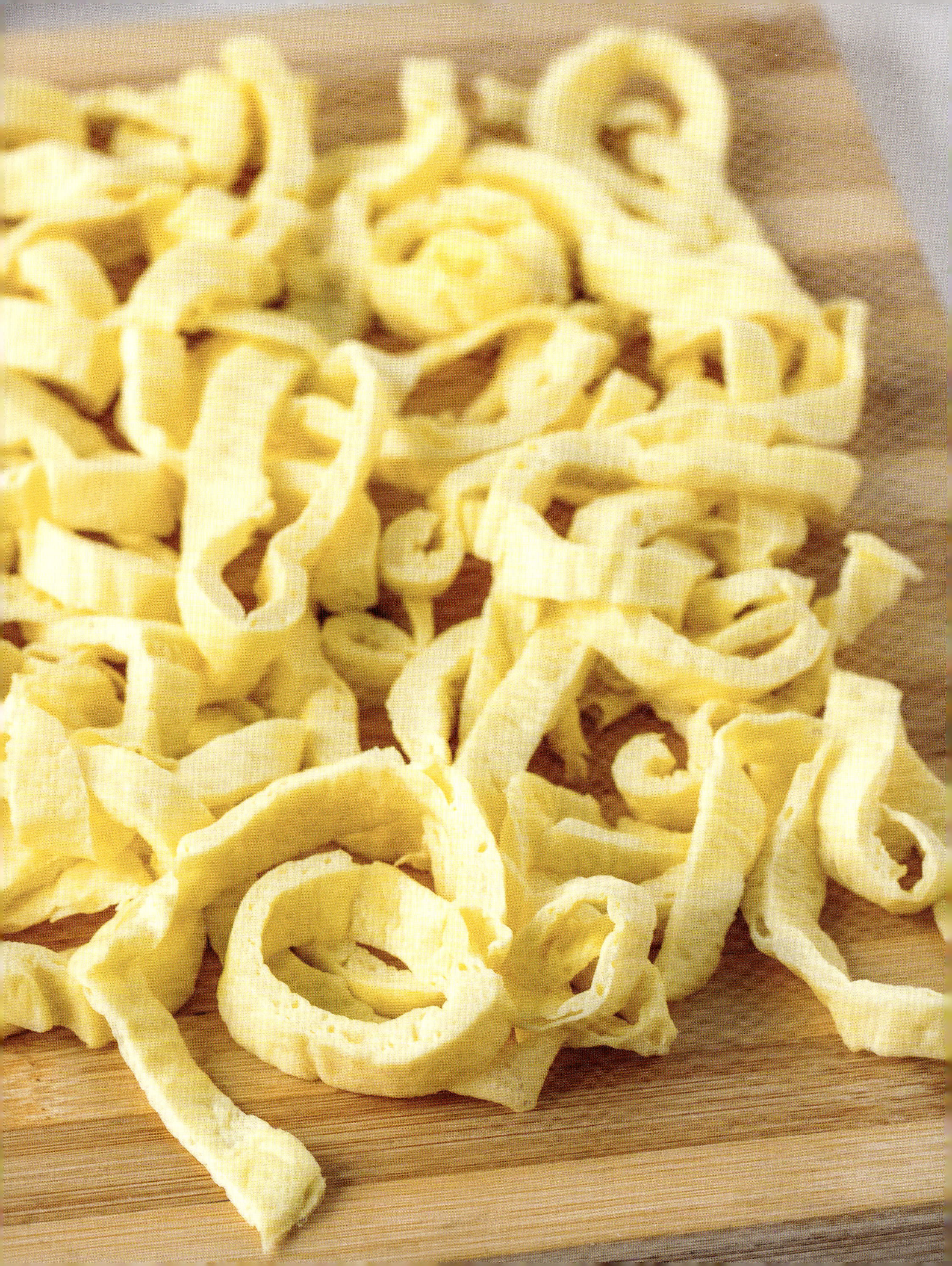

PROTEIN NOODLES

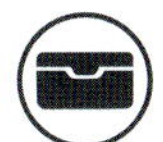

SERVES 2
PREP TIME: 15 minutes
COOK TIME: 10 minutes

These high-protein noodles are a simple, versatile option made primarily from eggs. With just five ingredients, they're easy to prepare and are both nut free and gluten free. They can be made in bulk and stored for later, and they're freezer friendly. They make meal prep a breeze! Use these noodles for your favorite pasta dishes or add them to soups.

---

4 large eggs, room temperature

2 ounces (¼ cup) cream cheese, softened

1 tablespoon xanthan gum

2 teaspoons apple cider vinegar

½ teaspoon salt

1. Preheat the oven to 325°F.
2. Put all the ingredients in a food processor or blender and blend until smooth. The dough will be rubbery and sticky. Let sit for 5 minutes to set up.
3. Scoop the dough onto the center of an 11 by 15-inch sheet of parchment paper. Cover with another sheet of parchment. Using a rolling pin, roll into an even rectangle that covers most of the paper. Place on a rimmed baking sheet.
4. Leave the dough sandwiched between the sheets of parchment paper and bake for 8 to 10 minutes, until the top sheet of parchment releases easily and the dough is cooked all the way through. (To test doneness, pull back the paper halfway and push down with your finger; if it doesn't leave an indent, the noodle is ready.)
5. Let cool for 1 to 2 minutes, then roll up, starting at one of the shorter edges. Using a sharp knife, slice the roll crosswise into fettuccine-style noodles.

(per serving)
CALORIES: **273** | PROTEIN: **14.4g** | FAT: **20g** | TOTAL CARBS: **8g** | NET CARBS: **2g** | FIBER: **6g**

PROTEIN TOTS

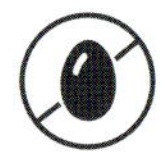

SERVES 5
PREP TIME: 10 minutes
COOK TIME: 40 minutes

These protein-packed tots are a low-carb alternative to traditional tater tots because they're made with cauliflower instead of potatoes. The protein boost comes from the cottage cheese, which provides nearly 10 grams of protein per serving. The tots are full of flavor and easy to prepare, and when you serve them with mustard, ketchup, or your favorite dipping sauce, they're a perfect side dish for any meal. They're also an excellent option for meal prep. Enjoy their crispy, cheesy goodness without the carbs!

- 1 (10-ounce) bag frozen cauliflower rice
- 1 cup cottage cheese (4% milkfat)
- ¼ cup shredded mozzarella cheese
- 1 tablespoon grated Parmesan cheese
- ½ teaspoon garlic powder
- ¼ teaspoon salt
- Chopped fresh parsley, for garnish (optional)

1. Preheat the oven to 375°F. Line a rimmed baking sheet with parchment paper.
2. Preheat a medium nonstick skillet over medium heat. Put the cauliflower rice in the dry skillet. Cook, stirring occasionally, until the majority of the moisture has evaporated and the cauliflower is fluffy. Set aside.
3. While the rice is cooking, put the cottage cheese in a blender or food processor and blend until smooth.
4. In a large bowl, combine the cooked cauliflower rice, blended cottage cheese, mozzarella, Parmesan, garlic powder, and salt.
5. Scoop 1 tablespoon of the cauliflower mixture, mold into a tater tot shape, and place on the prepared pan. Repeat with the remaining cauliflower mixture, leaving about ½ inch of space between tots.
6. Bake for 27 to 30 minutes, until golden brown. Remove and let cool for a few minutes before serving. Garnish with chopped parsley, if desired.

(per serving)
CALIORIES: **81** | PROTEIN: **9.1g** | FAT: **3.5g** | TOTAL CARBS: **4g** | NET CARBS: **2.8g** | FIBER: **1.2g**

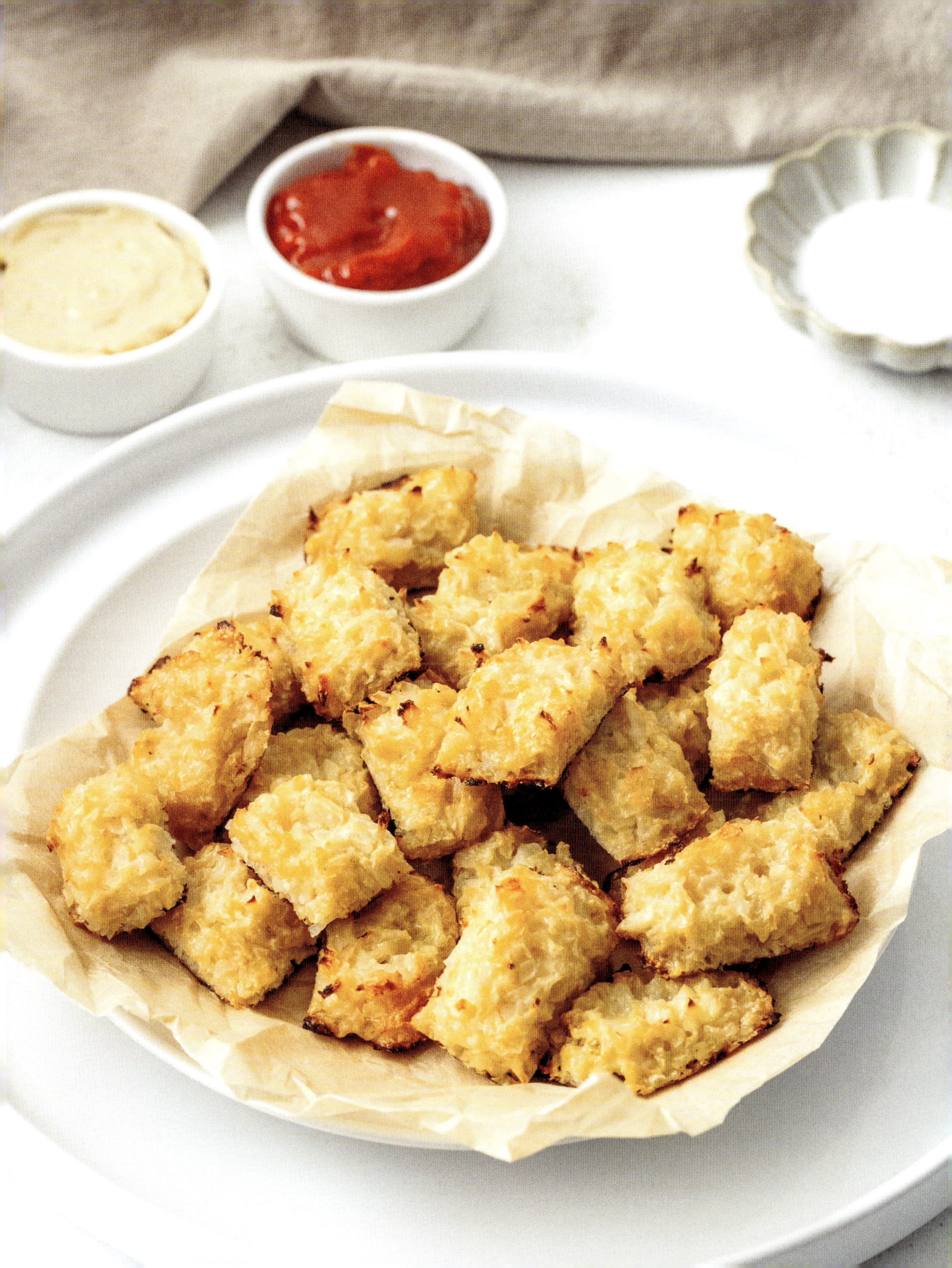

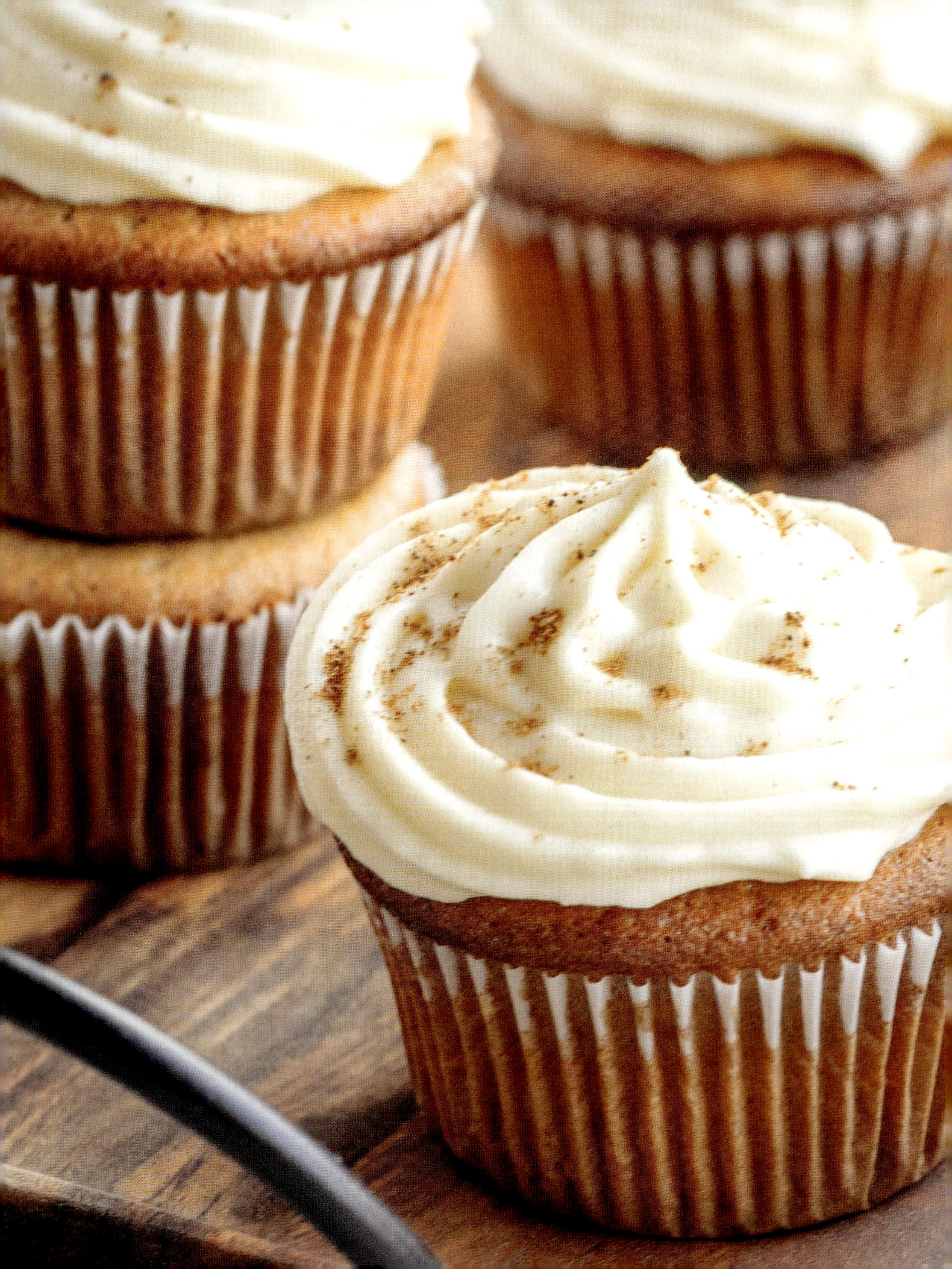

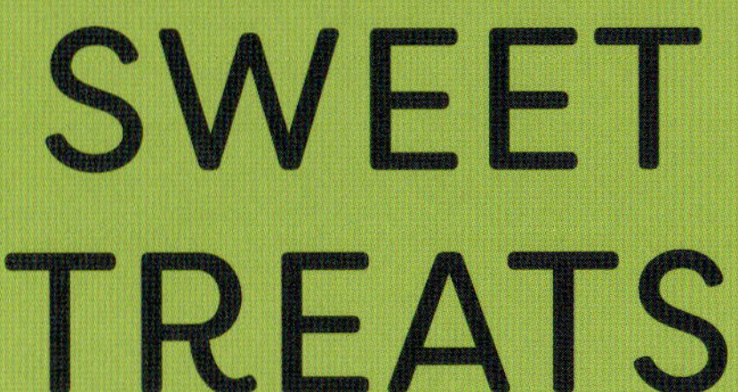

SWEET TREATS

ANGEL FOOD MUG CAKE

SERVES 1

PREP TIME: 10 minutes

COOK TIME: 15 minutes

This single-serve cake is a light, fluffy, and portion-controlled dessert with more than 25 grams of protein and just 1.5 grams of net carbs. Made with egg white protein powder, it mimics the taste and texture of classic angel food cake. For an even closer match, add pound cake or cake batter flavor extract if you have it. Top with whipped cream and berries.

¼ cup egg white protein powder

¼ cup powdered allulose

¼ teaspoon cream of tartar

⅛ teaspoon salt

¼ cup water

1 dropperful or ½ teaspoon pound cake flavor extract (optional)

SUGGESTED TOPPINGS

Whipped cream

Fresh strawberries

1. Preheat the oven to 325°F. Spray an 8-ounce ramekin or oven-safe dish with cooking oil. Then line the bottom and sides with parchment paper. Set aside.
2. In a medium bowl, whisk together the protein powder, allulose, cream of tartar, and salt.
3. Pour in the water and the flavor extract, if using. Using an electric mixer, start mixing on low speed until the mixture begins to foam. Then increase the speed to high and continue mixing until stiff peaks form.
4. Immediately scoop the mixture into the prepared ramekin. Bake for 15 minutes, or until the cake is golden brown on top and a knife inserted in the center comes out clean.
5. Let cool in the ramekin for 1 to 2 minutes before removing, then allow to cool for a few minutes more until ready to eat. Top with whipped cream and strawberries, if desired. This cake is best consumed right away because it doesn't store well.

notes

Egg whites don't work as a substitute for egg white powder for two reasons: 1) For the same volume, you would only use one egg white in this recipe, so the protein per serving would be less. 2) Egg white doesn't yield the same texture and deflates tremendously after baking.

To make this dairy free, skip the whipped cream topping.

CALORIES: **142** | PROTEIN: **26g** | FAT: **0g** | TOTAL CARBS: **37.5g** | NET CARBS: **1.5g** | FIBER: **0g**
SUGAR ALCOHOLS: **36g**

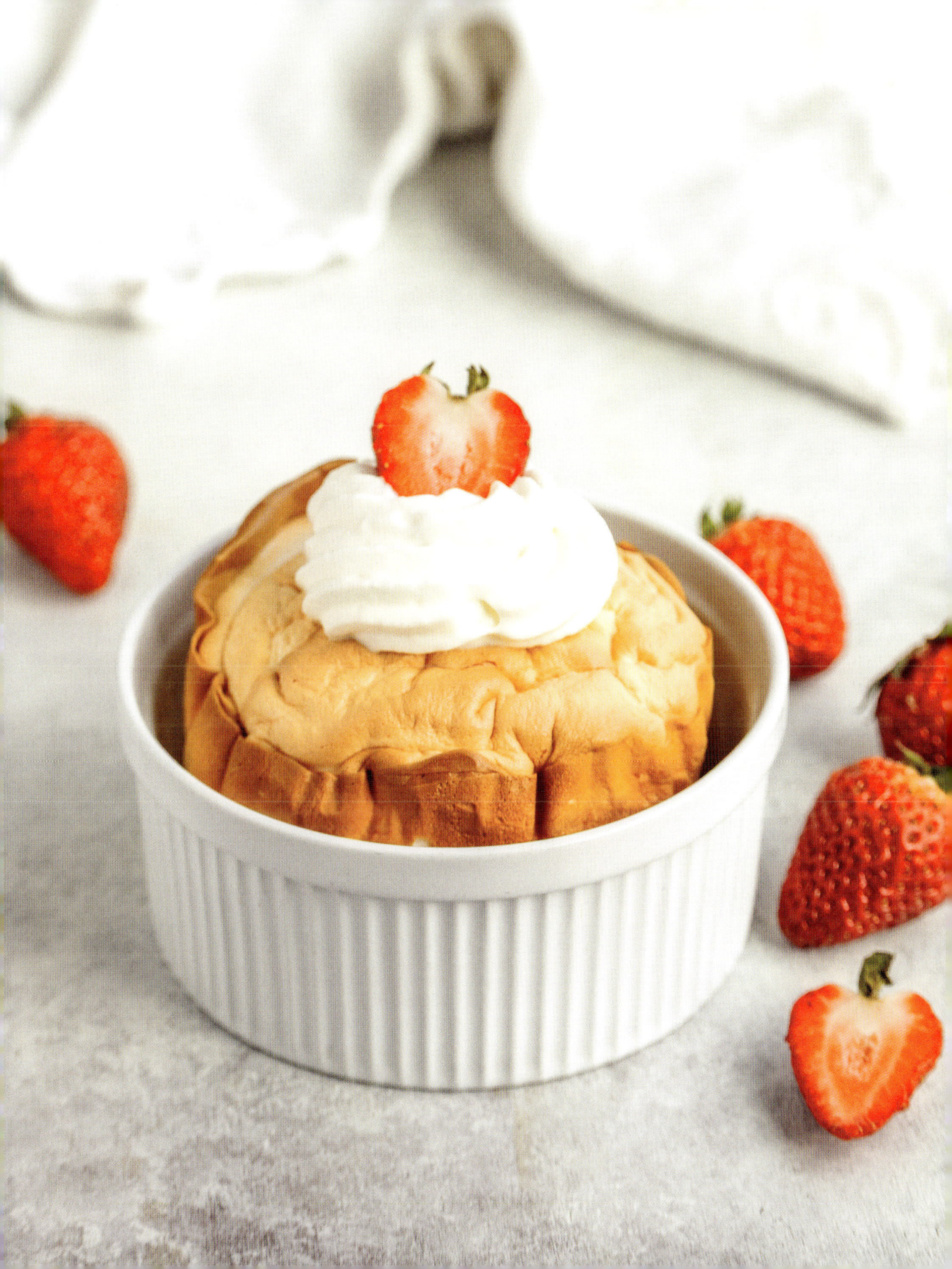

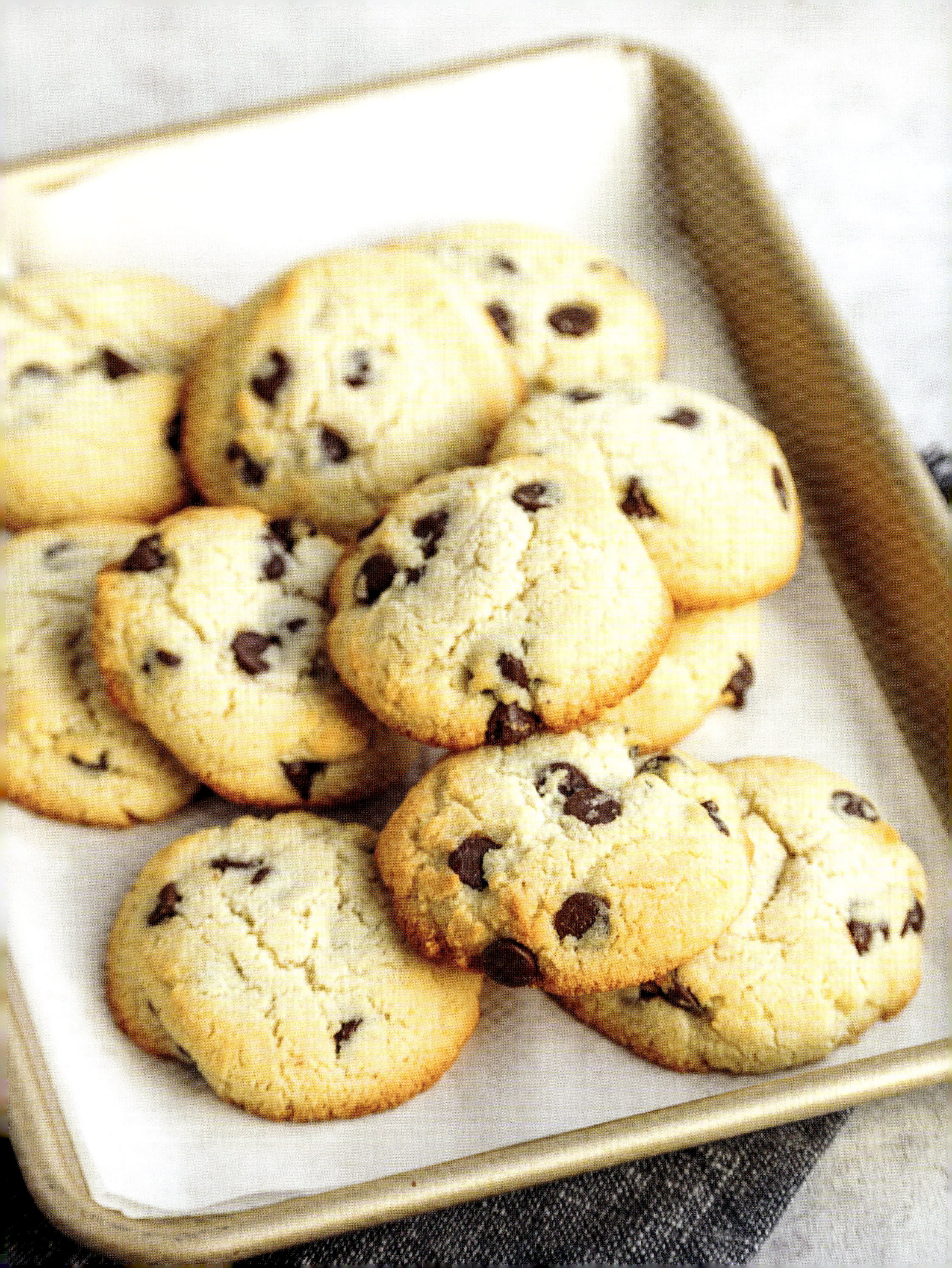

CHOCOLATE CHIP PROTEIN COOKIES

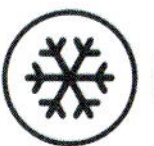

MAKES 18 cookies (2 per serving)

PREP TIME: 10 minutes

COOK TIME: 15 minutes

These cookies are a delicious low-carb treat with 10 grams of protein per serving. Made with almond flour, protein powder, and coconut flour, they're thick and chewy; they remind me of cookies my grandma used to make. For an extra protein boost, add crushed walnuts or pecans.

---

1 cup blanched, super-fine almond flour

2 scoops unflavored or vanilla-flavored protein powder

1½ tablespoons coconut flour

1 teaspoon baking soda

½ teaspoon salt

½ cup (1 stick) unsalted butter, softened

⅓ cup granulated sugar-free sweetener

1 large egg

1 teaspoon vanilla extract

½ cup sugar-free chocolate chips

1. Preheat the oven to 325°F. Line a baking sheet with parchment paper and set aside.
2. In a small bowl, thoroughly combine the almond flour, protein powder, coconut flour, baking soda, and salt. Set aside.
3. In a large bowl, use an electric hand mixer on medium speed to cream the butter and sweetener until light and fluffy. Beat in the egg and vanilla.
4. With the mixer on medium speed, slowly mix the dry ingredients into the wet ingredients. Stir in the chocolate chips.
5. Scoop about 1½ tablespoons of dough onto the prepared pan. Repeat with the rest of the dough, leaving about an inch of space between them. Bake for 14 to 15 minutes, until the cookies are starting to turn golden brown on the edges.
6. Let cool on the pan for 3 to 5 minutes before transferring to a wire rack to cool completely.

(per serving)
CALORIES: **248** | PROTEIN: **10g** | FAT: **21.2g** | TOTAL CARBS: **17.2g** | NET CARBS: **2.1g** | FIBER: **4.5g**
SUGAR ALCOHOLS: **10.6g**

CHOCOLATE PROTEIN MUG CAKE

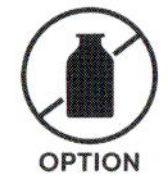

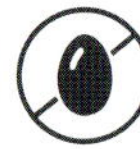
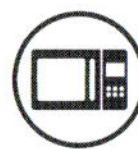

SERVES 1
PREP TIME: 3 minutes
COOK TIME: 75 seconds

This rich, fudgy cake is a favorite single-serve dessert that's packed with more than 30 grams of protein. Baked in a mug or small ramekin, it's a great way to indulge in a chocolate treat without the hassle of a full recipe. Plus, it's easy to double—perfect for you and your partner or when you have a friend over for an afternoon coffee hangout. I think it's best when served with a dollop of whipped cream or a splash of milk.

---

2 tablespoons blanched, super-fine almond flour

1 scoop unflavored protein powder

1½ tablespoons granulated sugar-free sweetener

1 tablespoon unsweetened cocoa powder

¼ teaspoon baking powder

2 tablespoons unsalted butter, softened

¼ cup nut or seed milk of choice

Dollop of whipped cream or a splash of nut or seed milk of choice, for serving (optional)

1. Spray a 6-ounce microwave-safe ramekin or mug with cooking oil. Set aside.
2. In a small bowl, whisk together the almond flour, protein powder, sweetener, cocoa powder, and baking powder.
3. Using a fork, stir in the butter and milk until smooth and evenly combined.
4. Pour into the prepared ramekin or mug. Microwave on high for 60 to 75 seconds, or until the cake is set on top. Let cool for a few minutes. Serve with whipped cream or a splash of milk of choice, if desired.

note

A ramekin is better than a mug for mug cake because it allows for more even cooking due to its wider base. You're less likely to end up with undercooked or overcooked areas.

CALORIES: **412** | PROTEIN: **30.3g** | FAT: **30.6g** | TOTAL CARBS: **24.1g** | NET CARBS: **2.6g** | FIBER: **3.5g** | SUGAR ALCOHOLS: **18g**

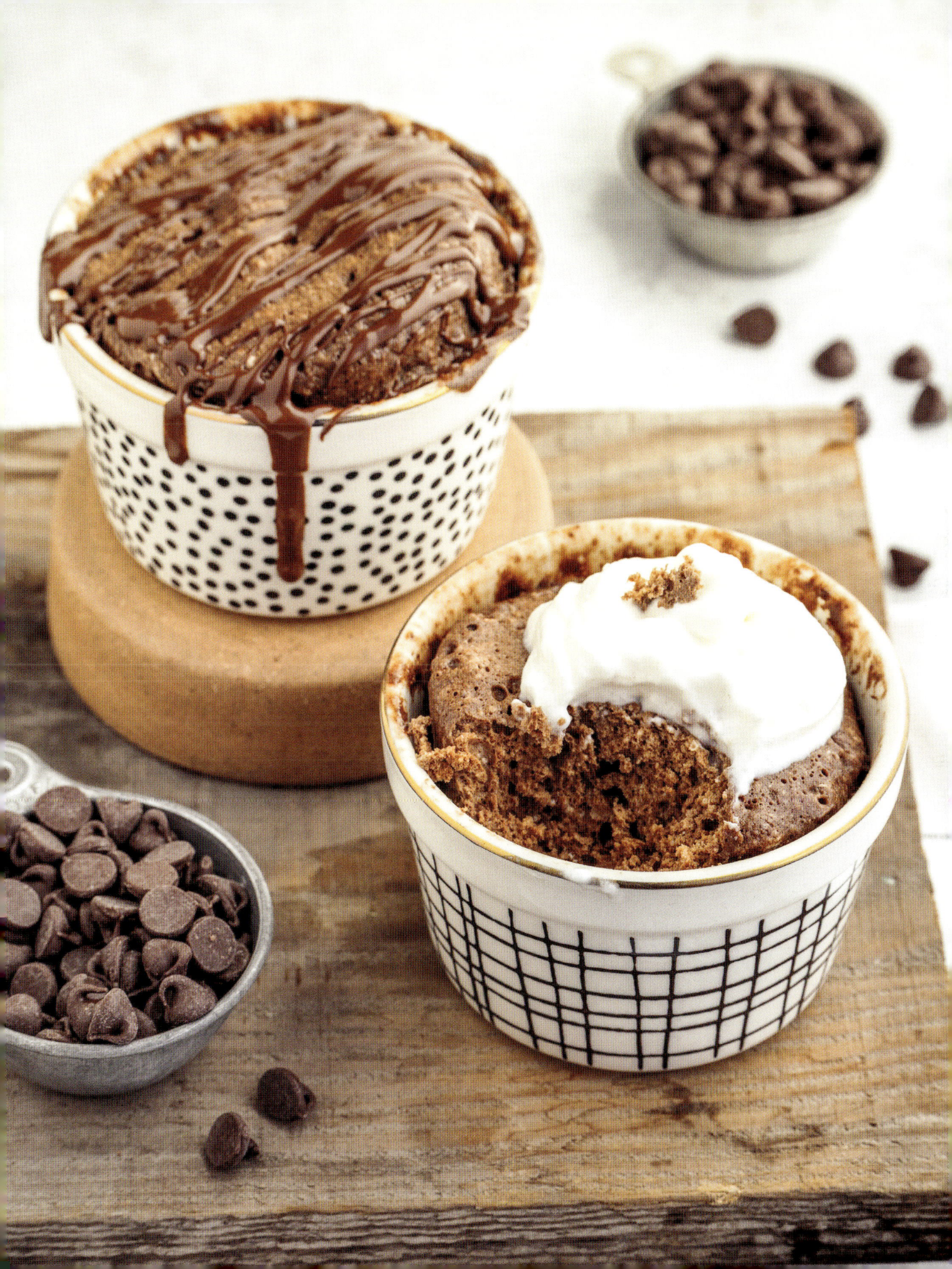

CHOCOLATE PROTEIN PUDDING—2 WAYS

Two easy protein puddings that you can make in just a few minutes! The first is egg free and uses creamy avocado as the thickener and chocolate protein powder for added protein and flavor. The second relies on hard-boiled egg whites for protein and thickness, creating a smooth, silky pudding.

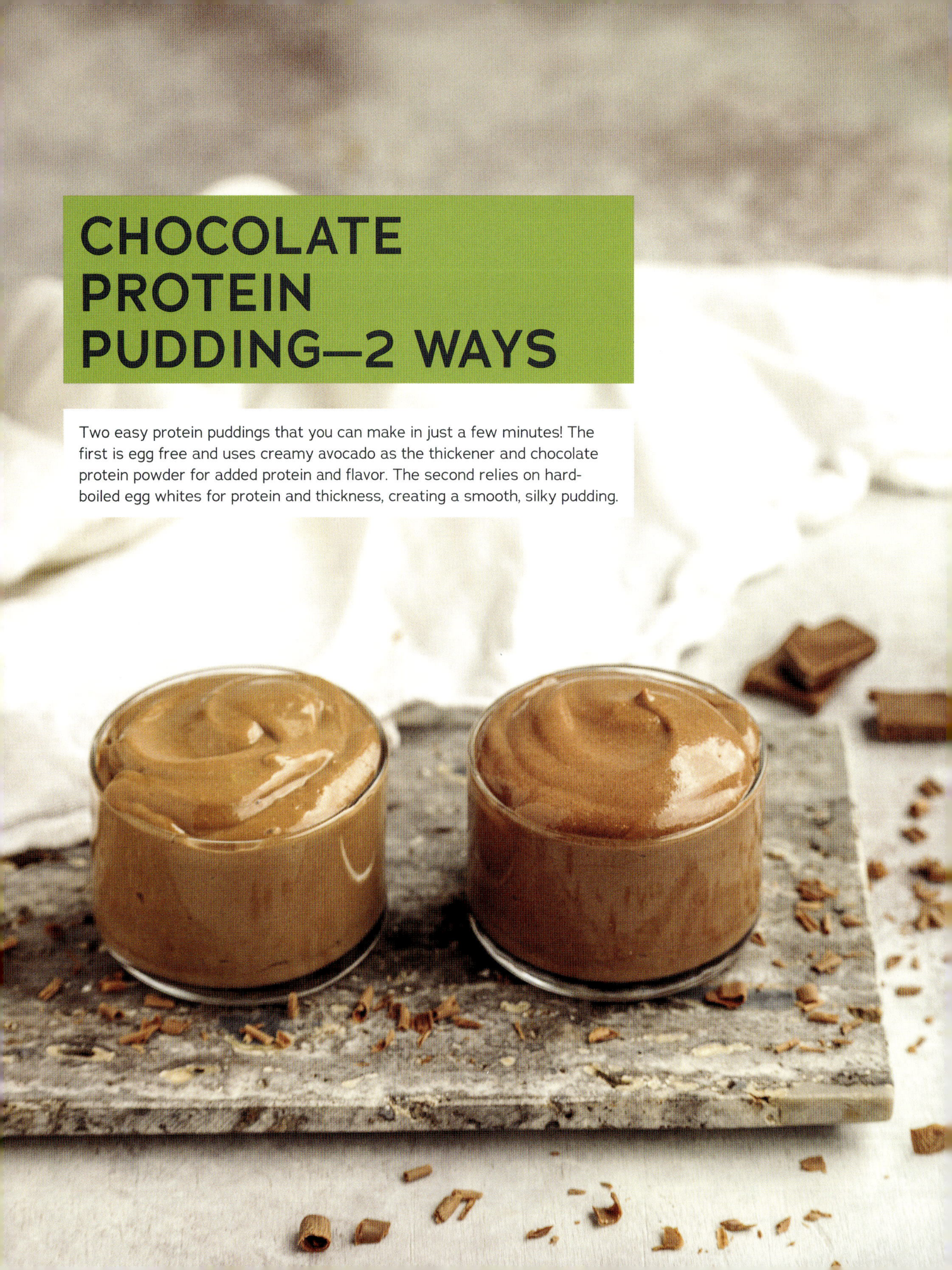

AVOCADO PROTEIN PUDDING

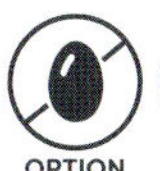
OPTION

OPTION
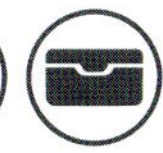

SERVES 1

PREP TIME: 5 minutes

½ medium avocado, pitted and peeled

⅓ cup nut or seed milk of choice

1 scoop chocolate-flavored protein powder

1 to 2 tablespoons granulated sugar-free sweetener (optional)

1. Put all the ingredients in a blender or mini food processor. Blend or puree until smooth and creamy.
2. Enjoy immediately or store in an airtight container in the refrigerator for 2 to 3 days.

note

The sweetener is optional here because chocolate-flavored protein powder is generally sweetened. However, if the pudding is not sweet enough for you, you can add your favorite sugar-free sweetener.

EGG-CELLENT PROTEIN PUDDING

SERVES 1

PREP TIME: 5 minutes (not including time to hard-boil eggs)

3 large hard-boiled egg whites

2½ tablespoons nut or seed milk of choice

1½ to 2 tablespoons granulated sugar-free sweetener

1 tablespoon unsweetened cocoa powder

1. Put all the ingredients in a blender or mini food processor. Blend or puree until smooth and creamy.
2. Enjoy immediately or store in an airtight container in the refrigerator for 2 to 3 days.

(avocado)

CALORIES: **247** | PROTEIN: **29.1g** | FAT: **12g** | TOTAL CARBS: **7.3g** | NET CARBS: **1.3g** | FIBER: **6g**

(egg-cellent)

CALORIES: **71** | PROTEIN: **11.8g** | FAT: **0.5g** | TOTAL CARBS: **21.5g** | NET CARBS: **3.5g** | FIBER: **2g**
SUGAR ALCOHOLS: **16g**

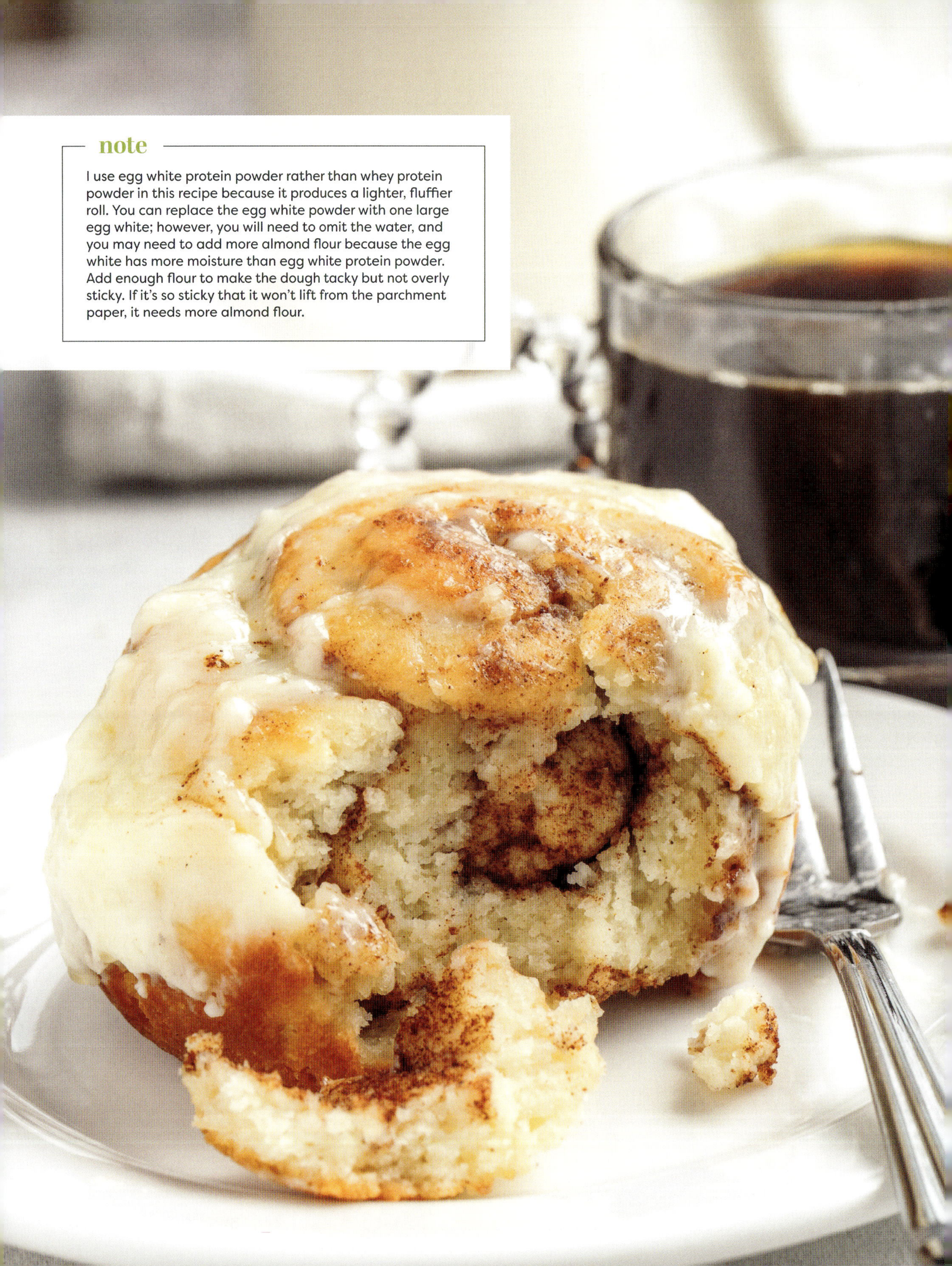

note

I use egg white protein powder rather than whey protein powder in this recipe because it produces a lighter, fluffier roll. You can replace the egg white powder with one large egg white; however, you will need to omit the water, and you may need to add more almond flour because the egg white has more moisture than egg white protein powder. Add enough flour to make the dough tacky but not overly sticky. If it's so sticky that it won't lift from the parchment paper, it needs more almond flour.

CINNAMON ROLL FOR ONE

SERVES 1
PREP TIME: 10 minutes
COOK TIME: 17 minutes

When you're craving a gooey, buttery cinnamon roll but don't want to make a whole batch, this single-serve low-carb cinnamon roll is the perfect solution. Made with a soft, fluffy gluten-free dough and featuring a cinnamon-infused buttery filling, this treat is packed with almost 15 grams of protein. Enjoy as an indulgence at the end of the day or for a cozy breakfast with protein coffee.

FOR THE DOUGH

⅓ cup blanched, super-fine almond flour, plus more if needed

1 tablespoon egg white protein powder (see note)

1 teaspoon granulated sugar-free sweetener

¼ teaspoon baking powder

¼ teaspoon xanthan gum

Pinch of salt

1 tablespoon unsalted butter, melted

1 tablespoon plain Greek or low-carb yogurt or sour cream

1 tablespoon water

FOR THE FILLING

1½ teaspoons unsalted butter, melted

1½ teaspoons brown sugar substitute

½ teaspoon ground cinnamon

Pinch of salt

FOR THE FROSTING

1 tablespoon cream cheese, softened

1½ teaspoons unsalted butter, softened

1 tablespoon powdered sugar-free sweetener

1. Preheat the oven to 325°F. Spray a 4-ounce ramekin with cooking oil. Set aside.
2. To make the dough, whisk together the almond flour, protein powder, sweetener, baking powder, xanthan gum, and salt in a small bowl.
3. Add the melted butter, yogurt, and water. Stir to combine into a tacky dough. If the dough is too wet and sticks to the parchment paper when you mold it, work in 1 to 2 tablespoons more almond flour.
4. Place the dough on top of a sheet of parchment paper. Using your hands, press and mold it into a long, thin strip, 1 to 1½ inches wide and ¼ inch thick. Set aside.
5. To make the filling, combine the melted butter, brown sugar substitute, cinnamon, and salt in a small bowl. Brush the mixture on top of the thin strip of dough.
6. Starting at one narrow end of the dough, roll up the strip until you reach the end.
7. Place in the prepared ramekin and bake for 17 minutes, or until the top is golden brown.
8. Meanwhile, make the frosting. Using a fork, mix the cream cheese, butter, and sweetener until smooth.
9. When the cinnamon roll is done baking, let it cool for a few minutes before spreading the frosting on top.

CALORIES: **516** | PROTEIN: **14.7g** | FAT: **45.9g** | TOTAL CARBS: **33.2g** | NET CARBS: **5.5g** | FIBER: **5.7g**
SUGAR ALCOHOLS: **22g**

KEY LIME CHEESECAKE IN A JAR

SERVES 2

PREP TIME: 10 minutes

This recipe yields two servings in jars for the perfect portion-controlled treat that's easy to prepare and packed with protein. The creamy cheesecake base, made with cottage cheese and yogurt, delivers almost 30 grams of protein per serving! A low-carb vanilla wafer crust adds a satisfying crunch. To change up the flavor, you can easily swap in lemon juice and zest for the lime.

---

1 cup cottage cheese (4% milkfat)

1 cup plain Greek or low-carb yogurt

3 tablespoons granulated sugar-free sweetener

Grated zest and juice of 1 lime

1 teaspoon vanilla extract

1 (2.25-ounce) package HighKey Vanilla Wafers

FOR GARNISH (OPTIONAL)

Whipped cream

Grated lime zest

Thin lime wedges or slices

1. Put the cottage cheese, yogurt, sweetener, lime zest and juice, and vanilla in a blender or food processor. Blend or puree until smooth.
2. Put the cookies in a gallon-size zip-top bag and use a rolling pin to crush them; alternatively, use a food processor to crush the cookies.
3. To assemble, evenly divide the crushed cookies between two 7.4-ounce jars or transparent glass bowls, followed by the lime cheesecake mixture.
4. Top with whipped cream, lime zest, and a lime wedge or slice, if desired.

(per serving)
CALORIES: **298** | PROTEIN: **27.6g** | FAT: **16.5g** | TOTAL CARBS: **38.4g** | NET CARBS: **1.6g** | FIBER: **4.8g**
SUGAR ALCOHOLS: **32g**

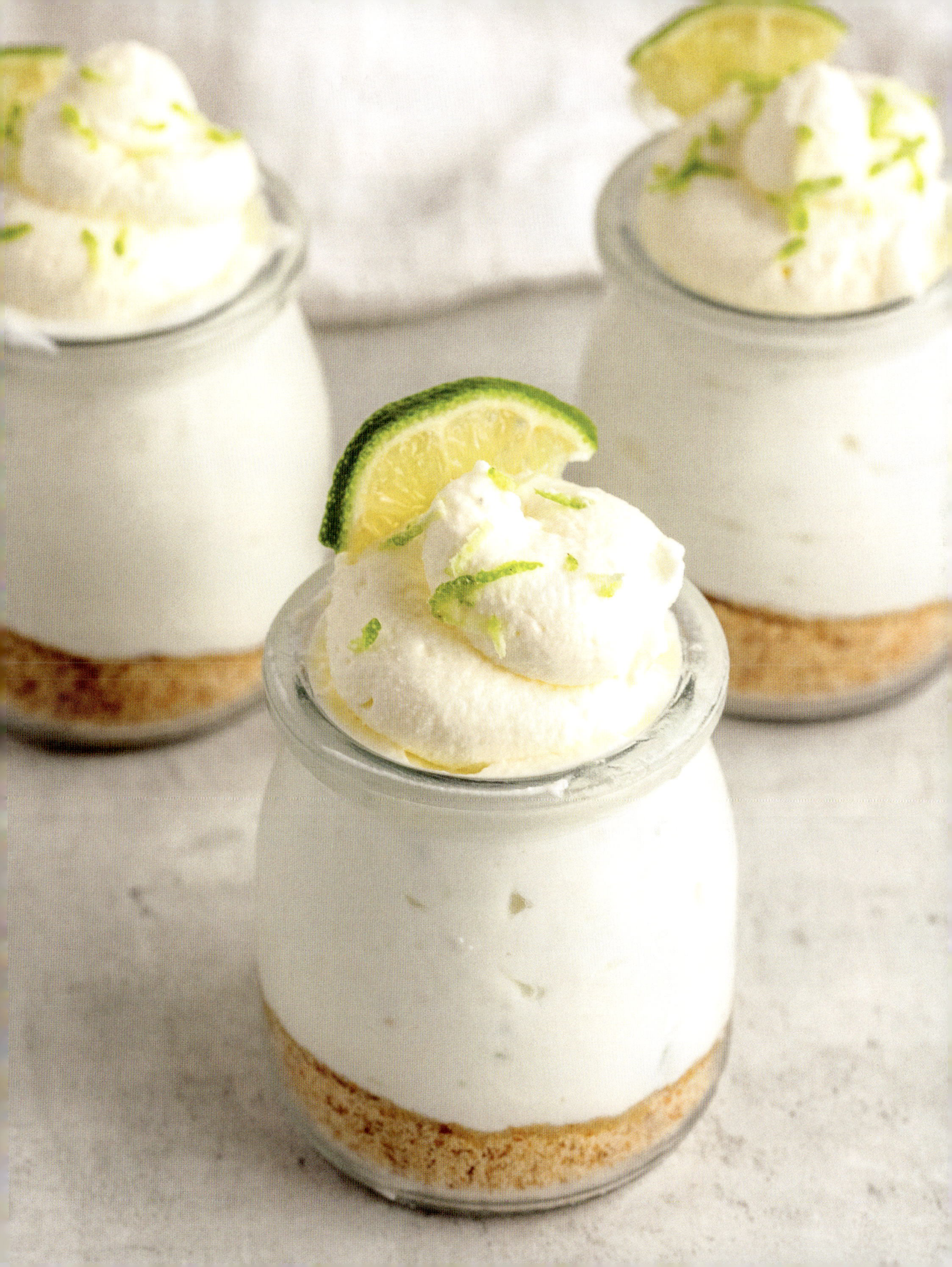

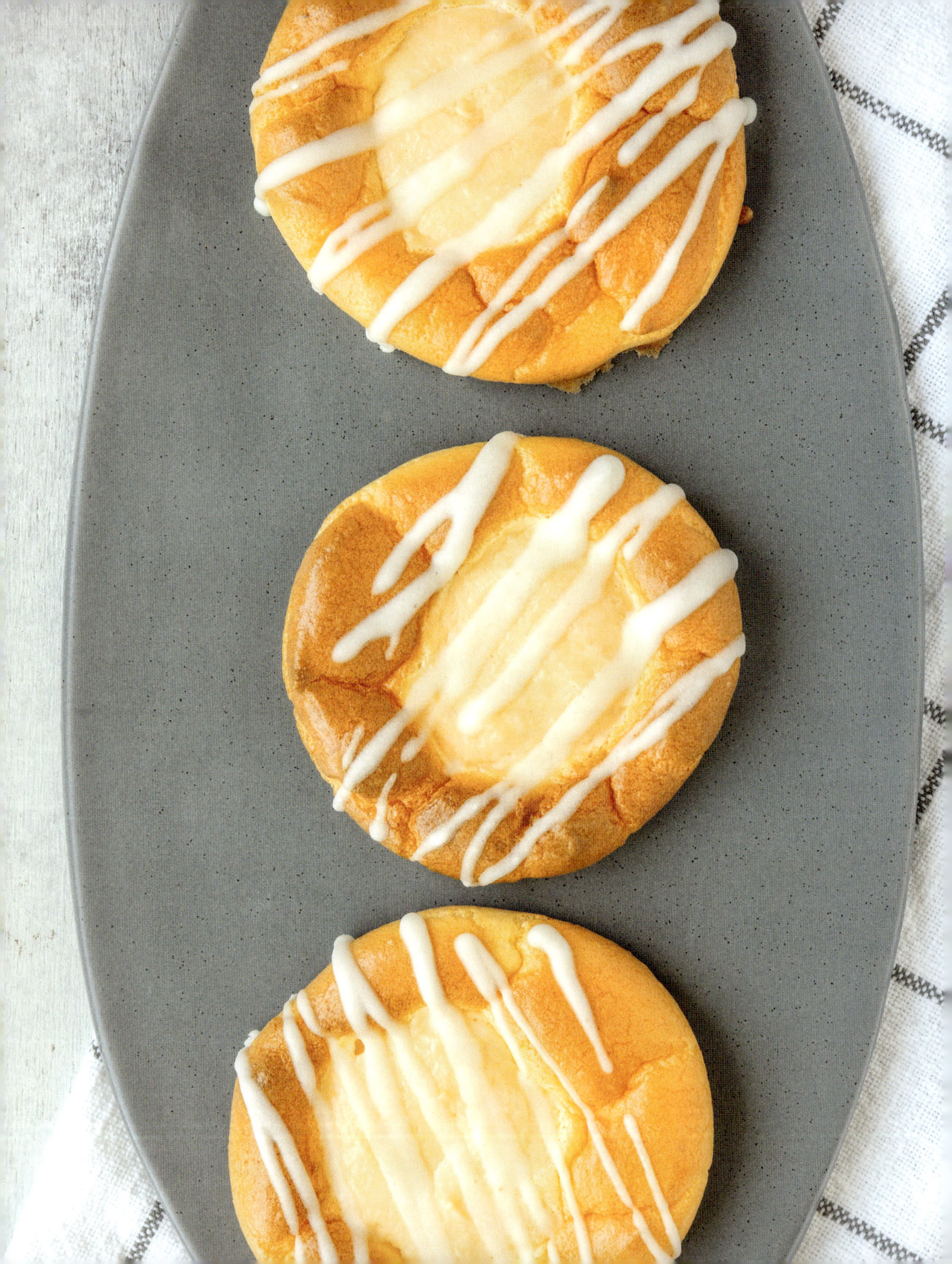

LOW-CARB CREAM CHEESE DANISHES

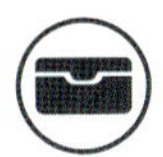

Makes 10 Danishes
PREP TIME: 15 minutes
COOK TIME: 15 minutes

These low-carb Danishes deliver bakery-style deliciousness with only 1 gram of net carbs! Using eggs and protein powder, I was able to achieve a light and airy pastry without the carbs. These ingredients not only boost the protein but also help create a puffed texture. Stuffed in the middle is a sweet, creamy filling, while a sweet lemon icing is drizzled on top to finish. If you like a little sweetness with your breakfast, a Danish is a great accompaniment to savory eggs.

FOR THE FILLING

1 large egg yolk

4 ounces (½ cup) cream cheese, softened

3 tablespoons powdered sugar-free sweetener

½ teaspoon lemon juice

¼ teaspoon vanilla extract

FOR THE DOUGH

3 large eggs

2 tablespoons unflavored protein powder

2 tablespoons blanched, super-fine almond flour

2 ounces (¼ cup) cream cheese, softened

1 tablespoon granulated sugar-free sweetener

½ teaspoon cream of tartar

FOR THE ICING

3 tablespoons powdered sugar-free sweetener

½ teaspoon lemon juice

1 to 2 tablespoons heavy cream

1. Preheat the oven to 325°F. Line a baking sheet with parchment paper.
2. To make the filling, put the egg yolk, cream cheese, powdered sweetener, lemon juice, and vanilla in a medium bowl. Mix on low speed with an electric mixer until smooth and creamy. Set aside.
3. To make the dough, separate the eggs. Put the whites in a clean, dry medium bowl and the yolks in a separate clean, dry bowl. Make sure no yolk gets in the whites or you will have trouble beating the whites to stiff peaks.
4. To the bowl with the egg yolks, add the protein powder, almond flour, cream cheese, and granulated sweetener. Mix on medium speed until smooth. Set aside.
5. Using a clean, dry mixer on medium-low speed, beat the egg whites until they turn frothy. Add the cream of tartar and turn the mixer speed to high. Continue mixing until stiff peaks form. When sufficiently stiff, the foam will be shiny and stand up straight when the beaters are removed.
6. Carefully fold the yolk mixture into the whipped egg whites. Don't mix aggressively. The goal is to keep the airiness of the dough in order to get the pastry to rise.
7. Scoop up about ¼ cup of the dough and place on the prepared baking sheet. Repeat with the remaining dough, spacing the Danishes about 1½ inches apart. You should have a total of ten Danishes. Using the back of a spoon, make a well in the center of each Danish for the filling. Scoop a few tablespoons of the cream cheese filling into each well, distributing the filling evenly among the Danishes. Bake for 15 to 18 minutes, until the Danishes are set and golden brown.
8. Let cool on the pan while you make the icing. In a small bowl, combine the powdered sweetener, lemon juice, and 1 tablespoon of cream. Add up to 1 tablespoon more cream if needed to create a thin icing that can be drizzled. Drizzle the icing over the warm Danishes.

(per Danish)
CALORIES: **106** | PROTEIN: **4.9g** | FAT: **9.2g** | TOTAL CARBS: **7.2g** | NET CARBS: **1g** | FIBER: **0.2g**
SUGAR ALCOHOLS: **6g**

LOW-CARB GINGERBREAD CUPCAKES

Makes 12 cupcakes
PREP TIME: 15 minutes
COOK TIME: 17 minutes

These moist and fluffy spiced cupcakes are the perfect treat for enjoying holiday flavors while getting a little extra protein. Coffee is my secret ingredient to enhance the classic gingerbread flavor!

FOR THE CUPCAKES

1½ cups blanched, super-fine almond flour

½ cup unflavored protein powder

2 teaspoons baking powder

1½ teaspoons ground cinnamon, plus more for topping if desired

1¼ teaspoons ginger powder

½ teaspoon ground cloves

¼ teaspoon salt

6 tablespoons (¾ stick) unsalted butter, softened

½ cup brown sugar substitute

¼ cup cooled brewed coffee

¼ cup plain Greek or low-carb yogurt

3 large eggs

FOR THE FROSTING

4 ounces (½ cup) cream cheese, softened

2 tablespoons unsalted butter, softened

1 teaspoon vanilla extract

Pinch of salt

¾ cup powdered sugar-free sweetener

¾ cup nut or seed milk of choice

1. Preheat the oven to 350°F and line a standard-size 12-cup muffin pan with liners.
2. To make the cupcakes, mix together the almond flour, protein powder, baking powder, cinnamon, ginger, cloves, and salt in a medium bowl. Set aside.
3. In a large bowl, cream the butter and brown sugar substitute using an electric mixer on medium speed until light and fluffy, 3 to 4 minutes.
4. To the butter mixture, add the coffee, yogurt, and eggs and mix until combined. Slowly mix in the dry ingredients on medium speed.
5. Evenly divide the batter among the prepared muffin cups, filling them nearly to the top. Bake for 15 to 17 minutes, until a toothpick inserted in the center of a cupcake comes out clean. Let cool in the pan for several minutes while preparing the frosting. Then remove and let cool completely.
6. To make the frosting, in a medium bowl, use the mixer on medium speed to cream the softened cream cheese and butter until light and fluffy. Mix in the vanilla, salt, and powdered sweetener. Add the milk and mix until smooth and creamy.
7. Spread or pipe the frosting on top of the completely cooled cupcakes.

Pack It with Protein: Add a scoop of unflavored or vanilla-flavored protein powder to the frosting! If necessary, add more milk to thin the frosting.

(per cupcake)
CALIORIES: **227** | PROTEIN: **8.8g** | FAT: **19.6g** | TOTAL CARBS: **19.7g** | NET CARBS: **2g** | FIBER: **1.7g**
SUGAR ALCOHOLS: **16g**

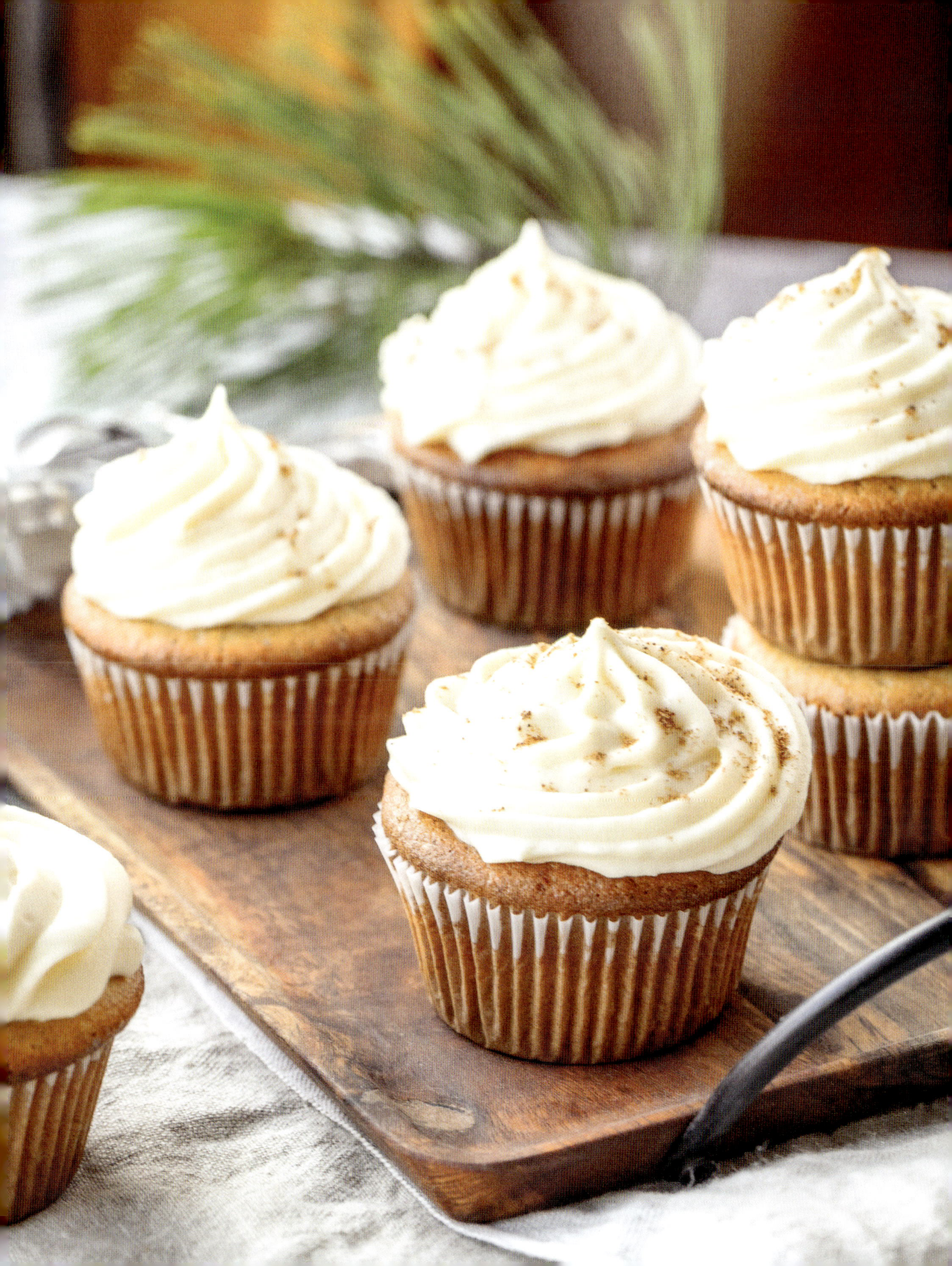

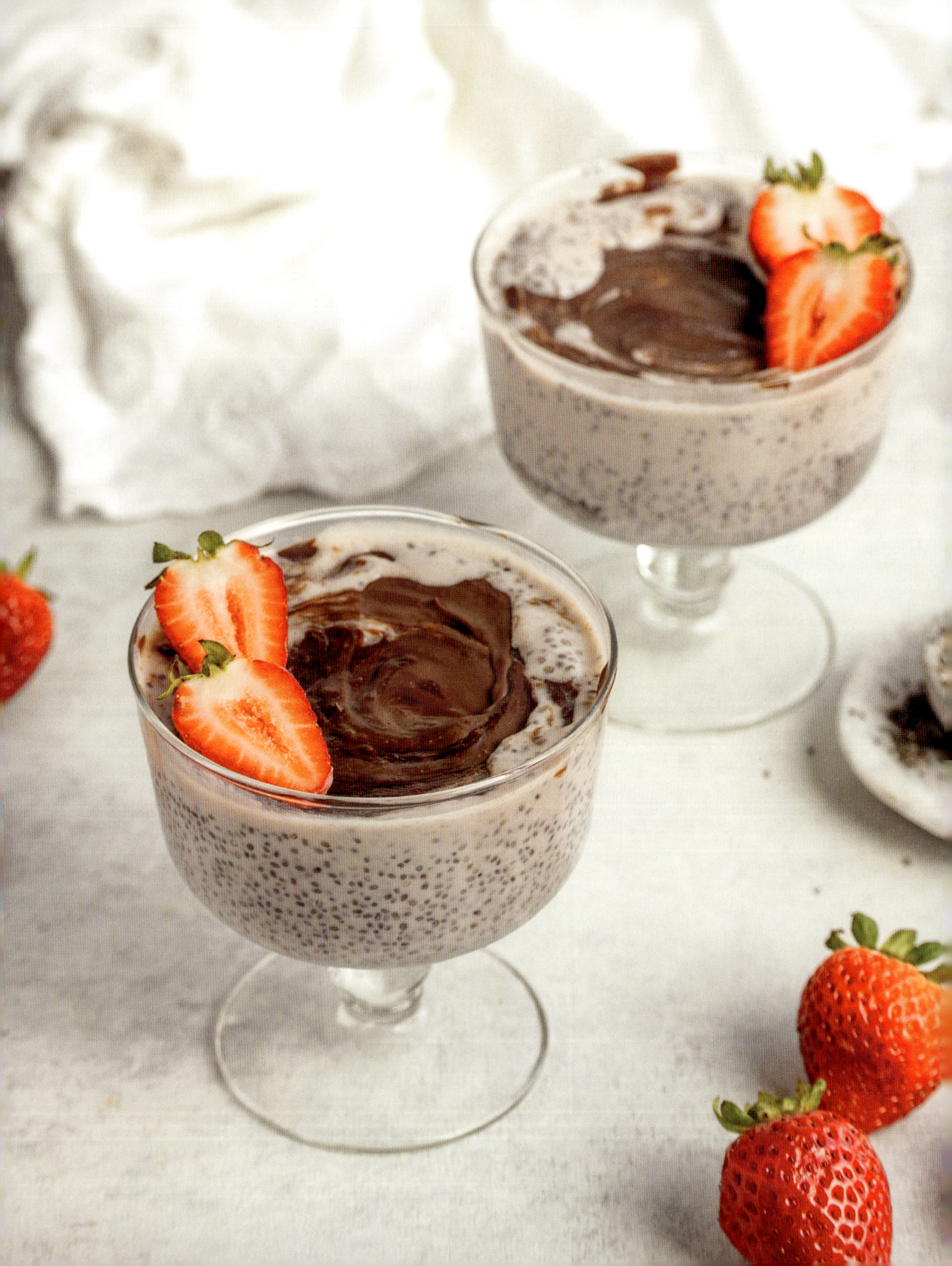

MAGIC SHELL CHIA PUDDING

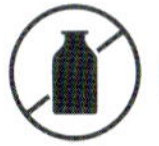 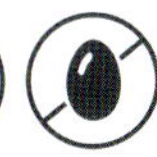 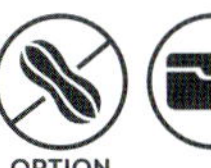 

SERVES 2

PREP TIME: 10 minutes, plus refrigeration time

I make chia pudding for a quick high-protein treat, and sometimes for breakfast. This creamy version is made with fresh strawberries and protein powder. The best part? It's topped with a sugar-free magic shell—a rich chocolate layer that hardens when you drizzle it on top of the chilled pudding. Crack into the chocolate and dig in. You'll get delicious chocolate bits with every bite.

- ½ cup sliced strawberries
- ¾ cup nut or seed milk of choice
- 1 scoop unflavored or vanilla-flavored protein powder
- 1 tablespoon granulated sugar-free sweetener
- ¼ teaspoon vanilla extract
- 5 tablespoons chia seeds
- ½ cup sugar-free chocolate chips
- 2 teaspoons coconut oil
- 2 strawberries, cut in half, for garnish (optional)

1. Put the sliced strawberries, milk, protein powder, sweetener, and vanilla in a blender or food processor. Blend or puree until smooth.
2. Stir in the chia seeds. Evenly divide the mixture between two small glass serving bowls or mason jars. Refrigerate overnight, or until set.
3. Put the chocolate chips and coconut oil in a small microwave-safe bowl. Microwave in 30-second intervals, stirring in between, until the chocolate is melted and smooth.
4. Drizzle the chocolate on top of the chia pudding. Return to the refrigerator to cool until the chocolate hardens. Garnish with halved strawberries, if desired.

note

To vary the flavor, experiment with different berries or flavors of protein powder.

(per serving)
CALORIES: **398** | PROTEIN: **22.3g** | FAT: **26.7g** | TOTAL CARBS: **46.6g** | NET CARBS: **6.8g** | FIBER: **17.8g**
SUGAR ALCOHOLS: **22g**

NO-BAKE COOKIES

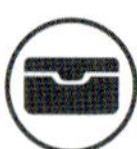

MAKES 2 dozen cookies

PREP TIME: 5 minutes, plus 30 minutes to freeze

COOK TIME: 3 minutes

Many people went crazy for my keto no-bake cookies, so I had to put a high-protein version in this book! Enjoy these quick and easy cookies without turning on the oven; they require only 5 minutes of prep time. They are fudgy, sweet, and crunchy and have all the oaty flavor you'd expect but none of the carbs because I use oat fiber instead of oatmeal!

---

1 cup granulated sugar-free sweetener

½ cup heavy cream

½ cup (1 stick) unsalted butter

¼ cup unsweetened cocoa powder

2 cups unsweetened shredded coconut

1 cup chopped almonds

1 cup no-sugar-added peanut butter

¼ cup oat fiber

2 scoops unflavored or vanilla-flavored protein powder

1 tablespoon vanilla extract

Pinch of salt

1. Line a baking sheet with parchment paper or wax paper.
2. Bring the sweetener, cream, butter, and cocoa powder to a boil in a large saucepan over medium heat, stirring occasionally. Boil for 1 minute, then remove the pan from the heat.
3. Stir in the coconut, almonds, peanut butter, oat fiber, protein powder, vanilla, and salt.
4. Drop heaping tablespoons of the cookie mixture onto the prepared pan. Place the pan in the freezer until the cookies are cooled and hardened, 30 to 60 minutes.
5. To keep their shape and texture, store the cookies in the refrigerator for up to 1 week or in an airtight container or plastic freezer bag in the freezer for 1 to 2 months.

(per cookie)
CALORIES: **183** | PROTEIN: **6.1g** | FAT: **16.2g** | TOTAL CARBS: **14.3g** | NET CARBS: **2.2g** | FIBER: **4.1g**
SUGAR ALCOHOLS: **8g**

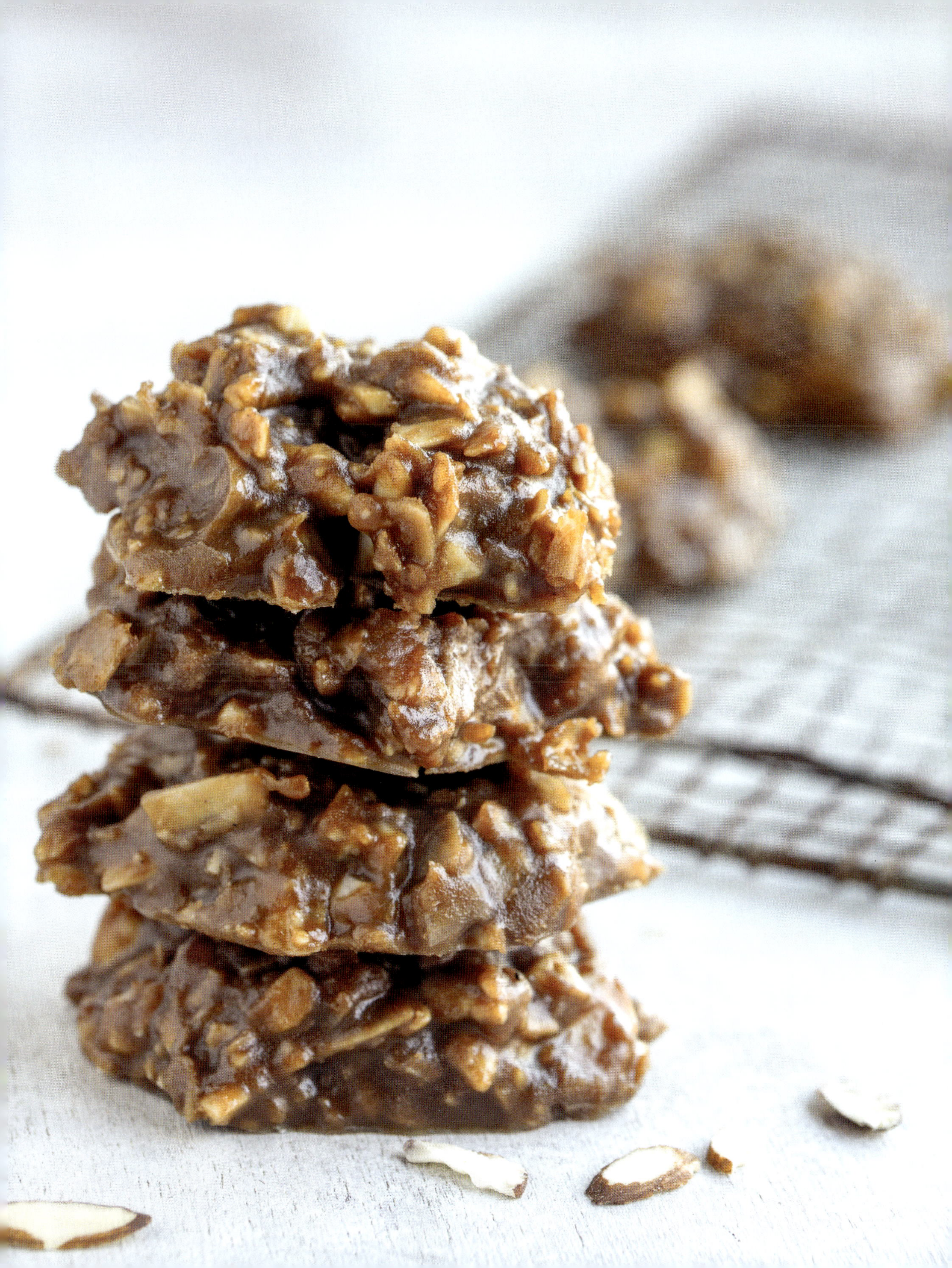

PROTEIN ICE CREAM—3 WAYS

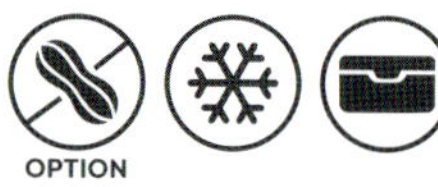

Makes 1 pint (⅔ cup per serving)

PREP TIME: 15 minutes, plus time to churn/freeze

COOK TIME: 10 minutes

These protein-packed ice creams come in three classic flavors and are sweetened with allulose to keep them low carb while delivering over 50 grams of protein per pint. The addition of protein powder not only boosts the protein content but also stabilizes and thickens the ice cream, ensuring a silky texture. You can churn the ice cream in an ice cream maker or make it in a Ninja Creami (my favorite way).

FOR ALL FLAVORS

½ cup heavy cream

½ cup nut or seed milk of choice

⅓ cup powdered allulose

Pinch of salt

3 large eggs

1 scoop vanilla-flavored or unflavored protein powder

FOR VANILLA ICE CREAM

1½ teaspoons vanilla extract

FOR CHOCOLATE ICE CREAM

1 tablespoon unsweetened cocoa powder

2 ounces sugar-free chocolate chips

FOR STRAWBERRY ICE CREAM

1 cup halved strawberries, tops removed

Special equipment: Ice cream maker or Ninja Creami

1. Make the base for the flavor of your choice:
   - Vanilla: Pour the cream and milk into a small saucepan and heat over medium heat. Stir in the allulose and salt. Bring to a simmer, then remove from the heat.
   - Chocolate: Pour the cream and milk into a small saucepan and heat over medium heat. Stir in the allulose, salt, cocoa powder, and chocolate chips. Bring to a simmer. Once the chocolate has melted, remove from the heat.
   - Strawberry: In a food processor or blender, puree the strawberries and allulose until smooth. Pour the strawberry puree into a small saucepan and add the cream, milk, and salt. Bring to a simmer over medium heat, then remove from the heat.
2. Beat the eggs in a small bowl. Stir in the protein powder. The mixture will be lumpy, but don't worry; it will smooth out when you add the cream mixture and reheat it. Temper the eggs by slowly pouring one-third to one-half of the warm cream mixture into the eggs, whisking continuously. Then pour this mixture into the saucepan with the remaining cream. Stir to combine.
3. Return the pan to medium-low heat and gently cook until the mixture has thickened enough to coat the back of a spoon and running a finger down the back of the spoon leaves a clear line. Stir continuously to prevent the eggs from curdling. Don't overheat or leave on the heat for too long or the mixture will curdle. Remove from the heat. If the eggs have curdled, simply strain the curds out of the ice cream base using a fine-mesh sieve.
4. If making vanilla ice cream, stir in the vanilla extract.
5. Pour the ice cream mixture into a medium glass bowl or the pint-size container for the Ninja Creami. Refrigerate for 2 hours before churning or freezing to give the flavors time to deepen. Refrigerating also makes the texture of the finished ice cream softer and creamier.
6. Churn according to the manufacturer's directions for your ice cream maker, or freeze overnight if using a Ninja Creami. Serve right away or store in the freezer for up to 3 months.

notes

To lower the calorie content, swap some of the cream for additional milk.

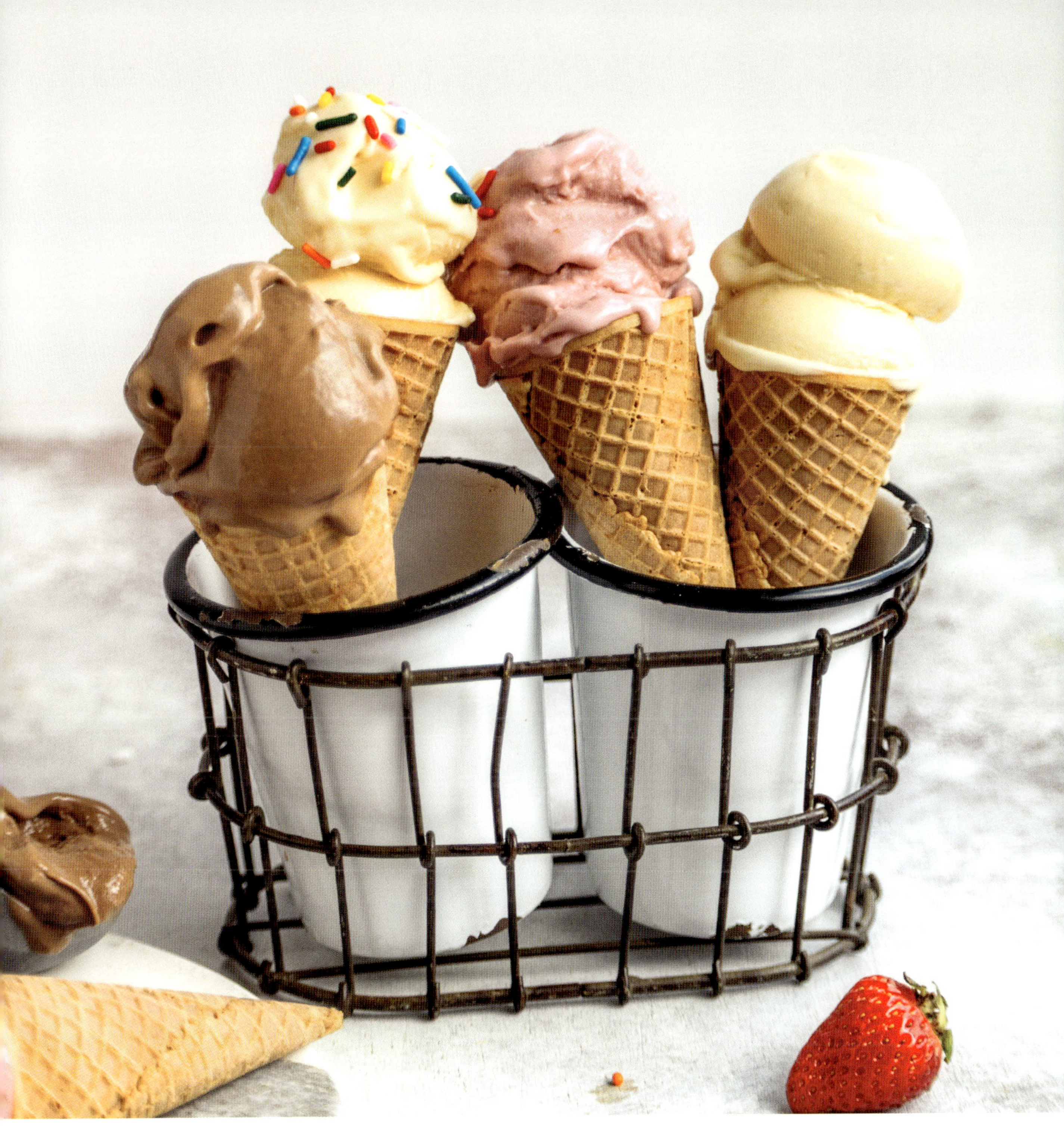

(vanilla, per serving)
CALORIES: **275** | PROTEIN: **16.7g** | FAT: **21.5g** | TOTAL CARBS: **17.4g** | NET CARBS: **1.4g** | FIBER: **0g** | SUGAR ALCOHOLS: **16g**

(chocolate, per serving)
CALORIES: **361** | PROTEIN: **18.4g** | FAT: **29g** | TOTAL CARBS: **31.7g** | NET CARBS: **3.3g** | FIBER: **7.4g** | SUGAR ALCOHOLS: **21g**

(strawberry, per serving)
CALORIES: **291** | PROTEIN: **17g** | FAT: **21.6g** | TOTAL CARBS: **21.3g** | NET CARBS: **4.3g** | FIBER: **1g** | SUGAR ALCOHOLS: **16g**

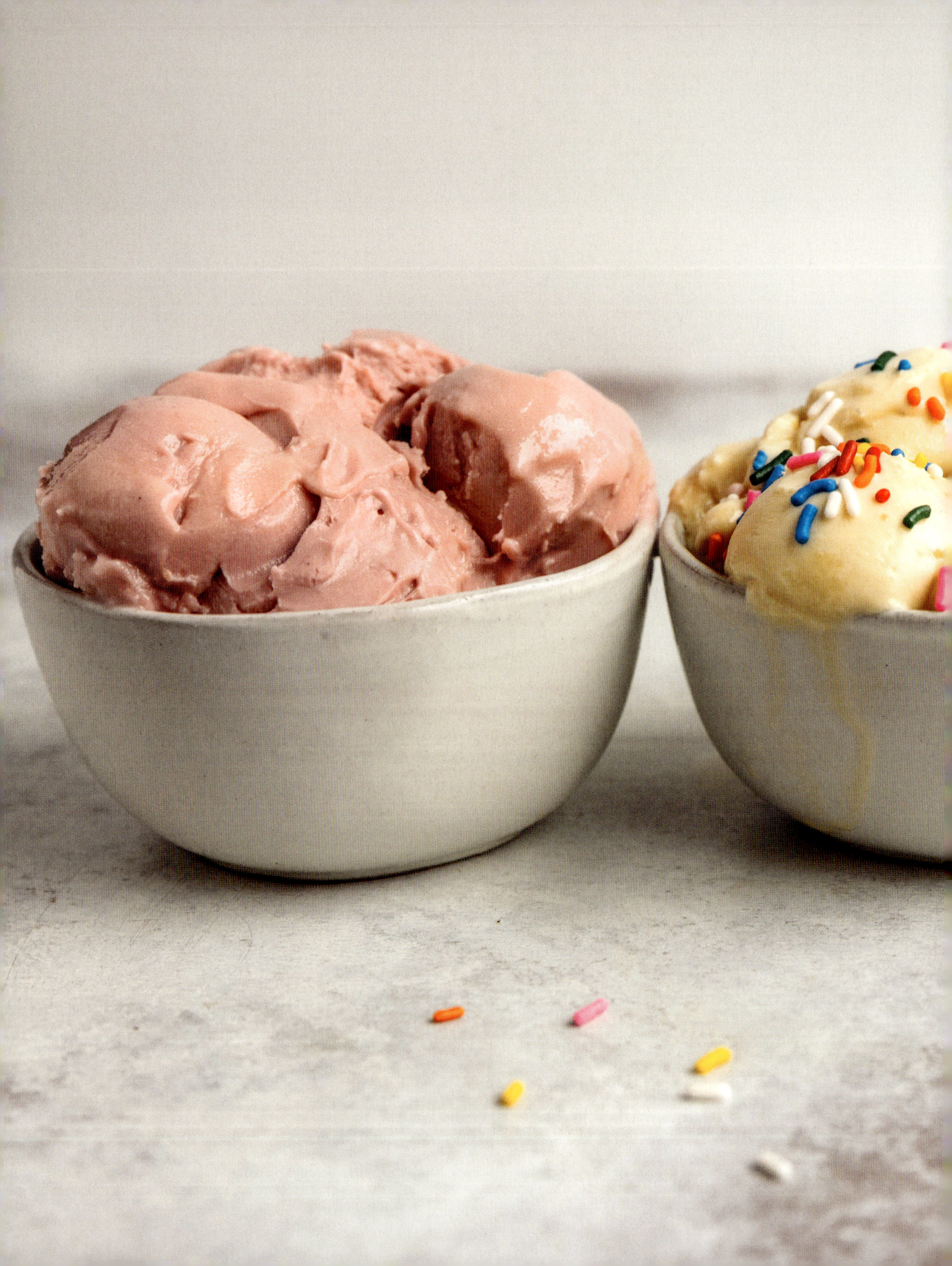

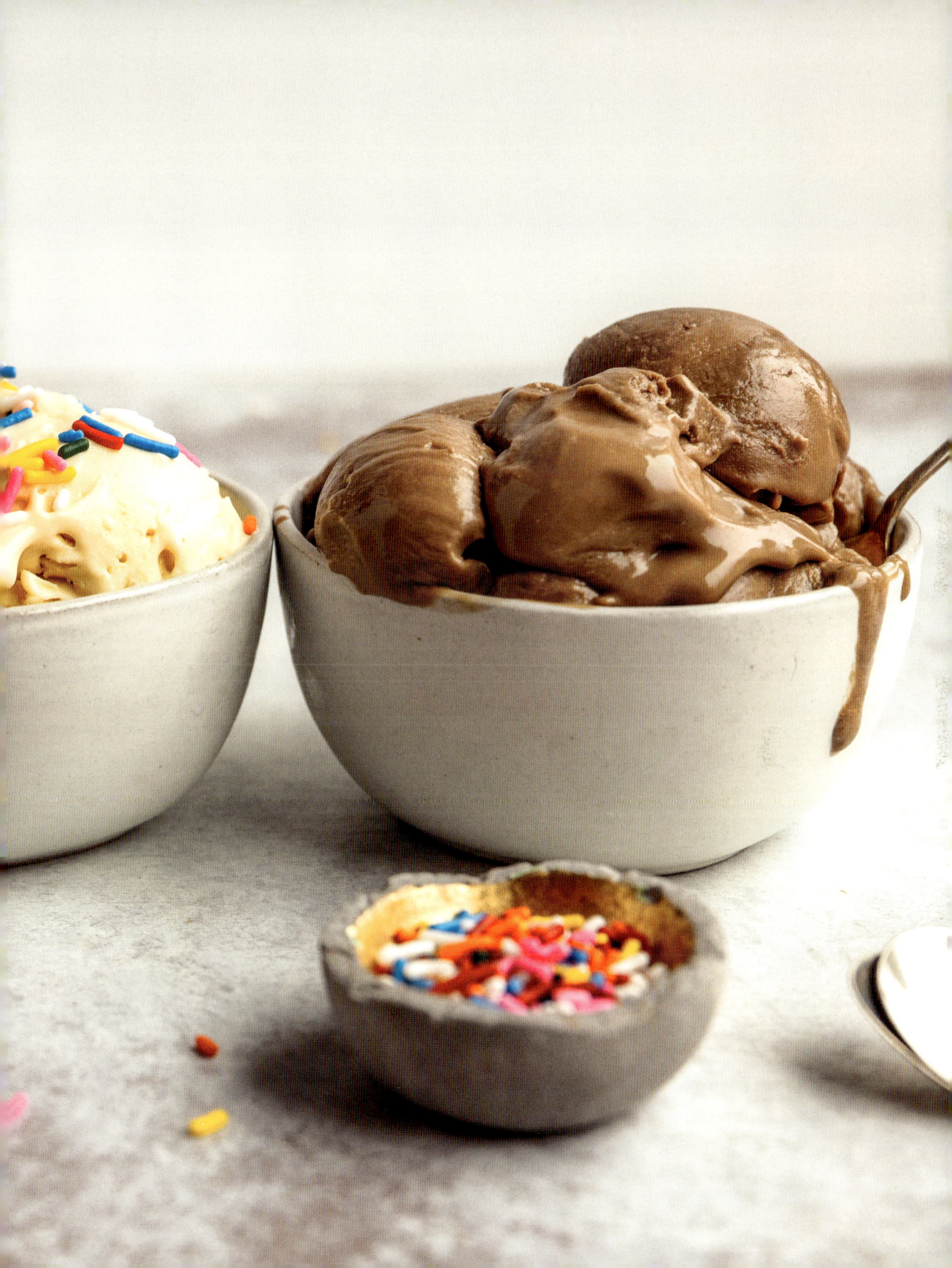

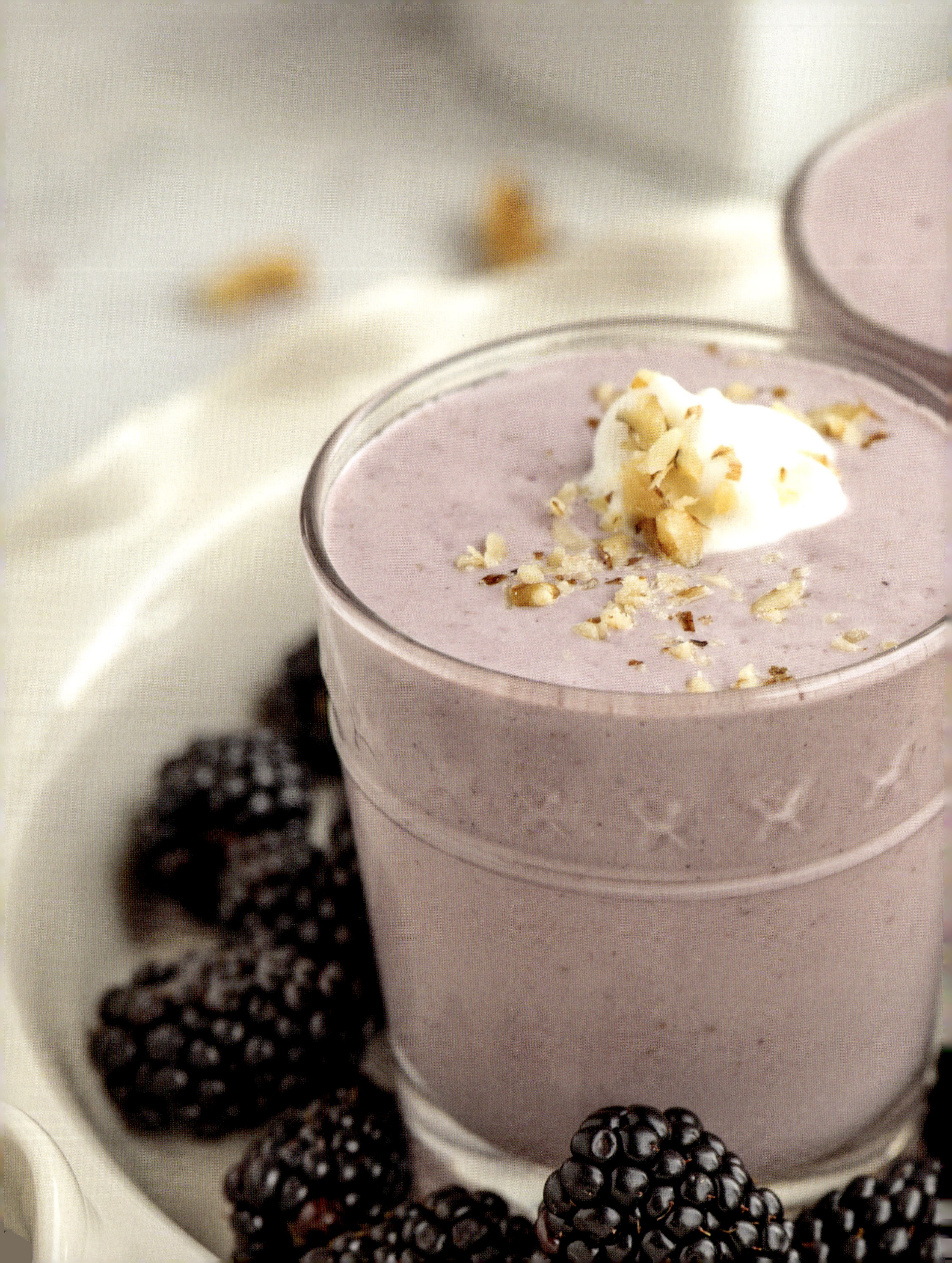

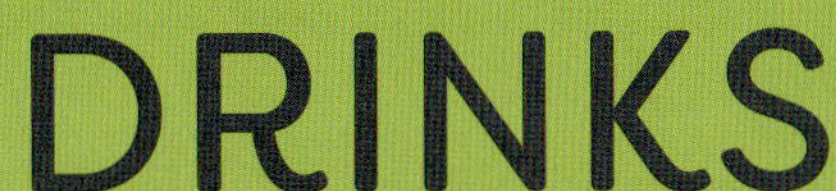

DRINKS

BEEF BONE BROTH

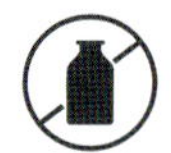
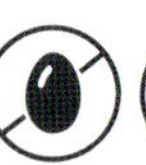
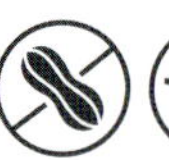
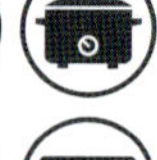
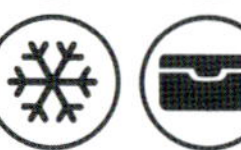

MAKES 4 quarts (1 cup per serving)

PREP TIME: 10 minutes

COOK TIME: 36 to 48 hours

Beef bone broth is packed with collagen, amino acids, gelatin, and essential minerals. I like to use a combination of knuckle, marrow, and oxtail bones, but if I have some leftover bones from a grilled T-bone steak, I throw those in, too. It takes a day or two to pull the nutrients from beef bones because they're big. Slow-cooking the bones for an extended time creates a broth that's golden brown and so gelatinous, you have to scoop it with a spoon when it's cool.

---

5 pounds beef bones (see notes)

1 large onion, quartered

2 celery stalks, roughly chopped

1 medium carrot, roughly chopped

8 cloves garlic, smashed with the side of a knife

3 tablespoons apple cider vinegar

2 teaspoons salt

1½ teaspoons peppercorns

2 bay leaves

A few sprigs of fresh thyme and/or rosemary

1. Put all the ingredients in a 6-quart slow cooker. Add enough water to cover the ingredients and fill the slow cooker.
2. Cover and cook on low for 36 to 48 hours. The longer the broth cooks, the more nutrients get pulled from the bones.
3. Turn off the slow cooker and let the broth cool to room temperature.
4. Strain the broth, discarding the vegetables, herbs, and bones; then transfer the broth to wide-mouth pint- or quart-size jars or other storage containers. Refrigerate for several hours to allow the fat to solidify at the top, then skim off the fat.
5. Store in the refrigerator for up to 1 week or freeze for up to 6 months.

notes

A mix of knuckle bones, shanks, oxtails, and/or marrowbones creates the richest broth, with knuckle bones yielding the most gelatinous results.

I prefer to make bone broth in a slow cooker. Even though the Instant Pot cooks the broth in a fraction of the time, I find that the resulting broth is not as gelatinous, and I worry that I'm not pulling as many nutrients from the bones.

The macros provided are just an estimate. They will vary depending on the type of bones used and how much fat is skimmed off. Plus, it's difficult to determine how much protein, carbs, and fat remain in the broth.

The apple cider vinegar helps leach the nutrients from the bones. Don't skip this ingredient!

(per serving)

CALIORIES: **124** | PROTEIN: **31g** | FAT: **0g** | TOTAL CARBS: **0g** | NET CARBS: **0g** | FIBER: **0g**

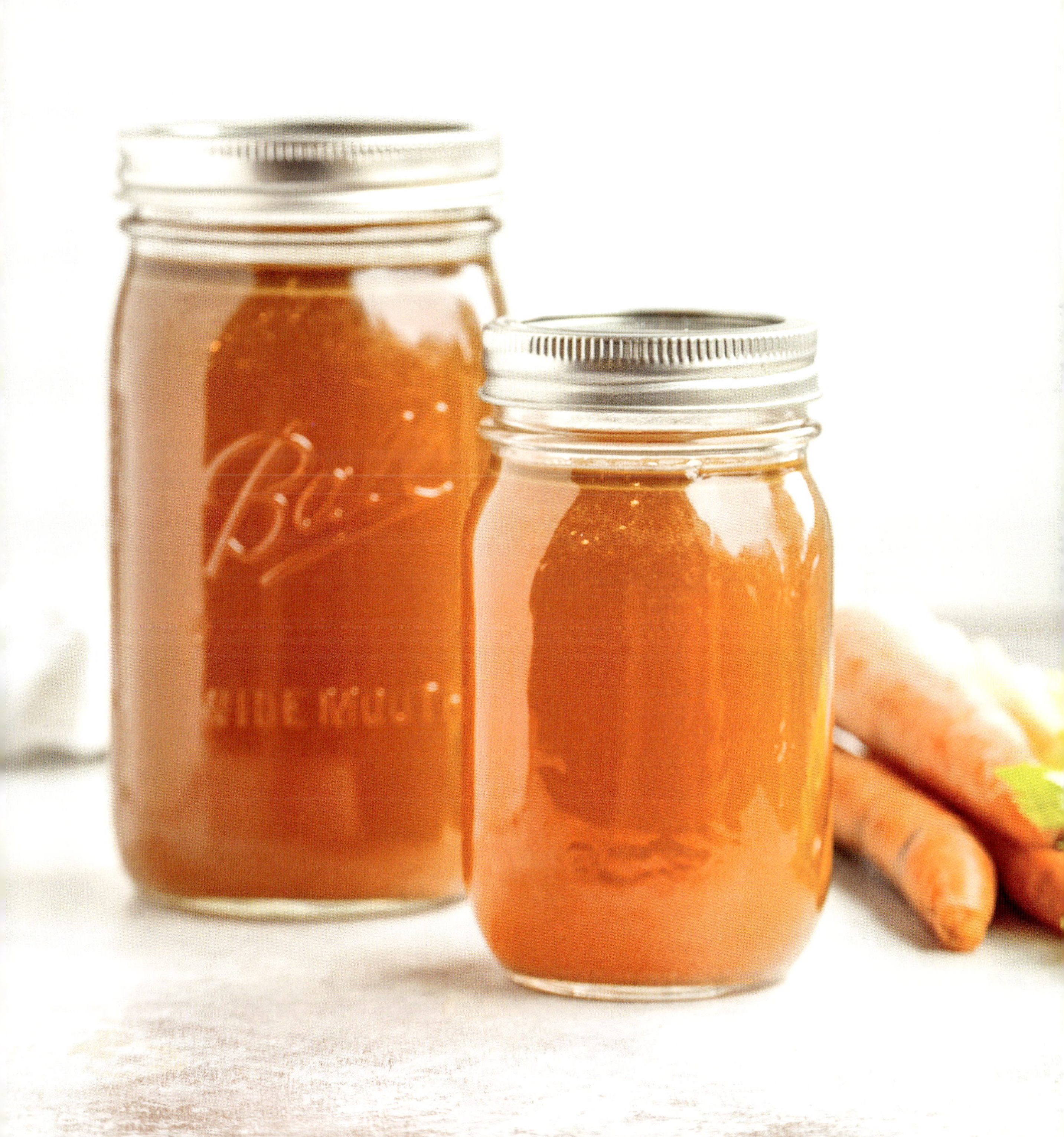

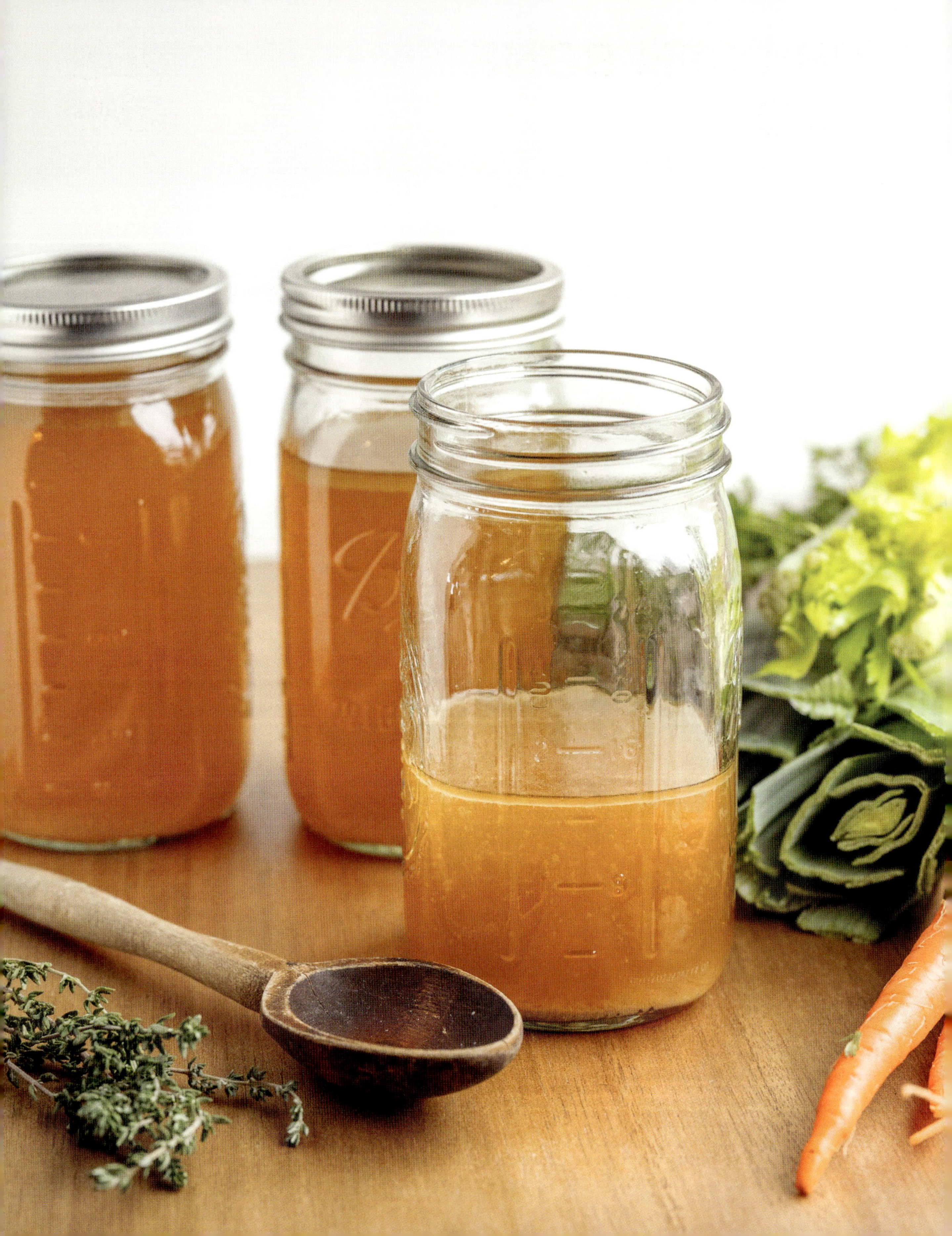

CHICKEN BONE BROTH

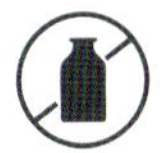
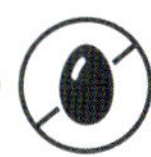

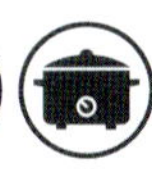
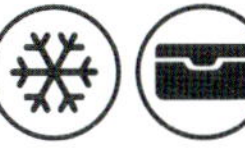

MAKES 4 quarts (1 cup per serving)

PREP TIME: 10 minutes

COOK TIME: 24 to 36 hours

Bone broth is a super nutritious food. Once you make bone broth from scratch, you will never go back to the store-bought stuff that comes in a carton. Not only is there a difference between the two nutritionally, but you can see how homemade bone broth is far superior. The liquid stock is opaque and vibrant yellowish orange in color, so you know it's filled with all the healthy nutrients, minerals, collagen, and vitamins.

- 3 to 5 pounds chicken bones (see notes)
- 4 celery stalks, roughly chopped
- 1 medium leek, ends removed, halved
- 8 cloves garlic, smashed with the side of a knife
- 3 tablespoons apple cider vinegar
- 4 teaspoons salt
- 1 tablespoon anise seeds
- 1 tablespoon ground coriander
- 1½ teaspoons peppercorns
- 2 bay leaves
- A few sprigs of fresh thyme and/or rosemary

1. Put all the ingredients in a 6-quart slow cooker. Add enough water to cover the ingredients and fill the slow cooker.
2. Cover and cook on low for 24 to 36 hours. The longer the broth cooks, the more nutrients get pulled from the bones.
3. Turn off the slow cooker and let the broth cool to room temperature.
4. Strain the broth, discarding the vegetables, herbs, and bones; then transfer the broth to wide-mouth pint- or quart-size jars or other storage containers. Refrigerate for several hours to allow the fat to solidify at the top, then skim off the fat.
5. Store in the refrigerator for up to 1 week or freeze for up to 6 months.

notes

The cheapest way to make chicken broth is to save the carcass from a rotisserie chicken you pick up at the store or a whole chicken you roasted. Just make sure you didn't chew the meat off the bone with your teeth, which would contaminate the broth with bacteria from your mouth.

To get the most gelatinous broth, I recommend using chicken feet. I like to use a combination of feet, necks, and any leftover chicken legs I might have.

See the additional notes on page 284.

(per serving)
CALORIES: **67** | PROTEIN: **16.5g** | FAT: **0g** | TOTAL CARBS: **0.2g** | NET CARBS: **0.2g** | FIBER: **0g**

BLACKBERRY PIE SMOOTHIE

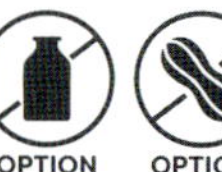

SERVES 1

PREP TIME: 10 minutes (not including time to hard-boil egg)

With this smoothie, you can enjoy pie as a meal! It's a perfect balance of healthy fats, fiber, and nearly 30 grams of protein. You don't even need to add protein powder. The protein comes from an egg, which also acts as a natural thickener, along with creamy yogurt, milk, and a handful of walnuts to mimic the piecrust. If blackberries aren't your favorite, you can easily substitute blueberries, raspberries, or strawberries to create your own version of a fruit pie smoothie. And don't forget the whipped cream! No pie is complete without it.

---

6 ounces fresh or frozen blackberries

1 large hard-boiled egg

¼ cup walnut halves

1½ tablespoons brown sugar substitute

1 cup nut or seed milk of choice (unflavored and unsweetened)

½ cup plain Greek or low-carb yogurt

SUGGESTED TOPPINGS

Dollop of whipped cream

Chopped walnuts

1. Put all the ingredients in a blender and blend until smooth.
2. Pour into a 12-ounce glass and serve. If desired, top with whipped cream and chopped walnuts to complete the "pie."

notes

For a lower-fat, lower-calorie option, decrease the amount of walnuts or omit them altogether.

To make this dairy free, use dairy-free yogurt and omit the whipped cream topping. To make it nut free, use a seed milk and omit the walnut topping.

The nutritional information for this recipe is based on one 12-ounce serving rather than the two smaller servings shown in the photo.

CALORIES: **428** | PROTEIN: **29.7g** | FAT: **29.7g** | TOTAL CARBS: **33.7g** | NET CARBS: **9.2g** | FIBER: **6.5g** SUGAR ALCOHOLS: **18g**

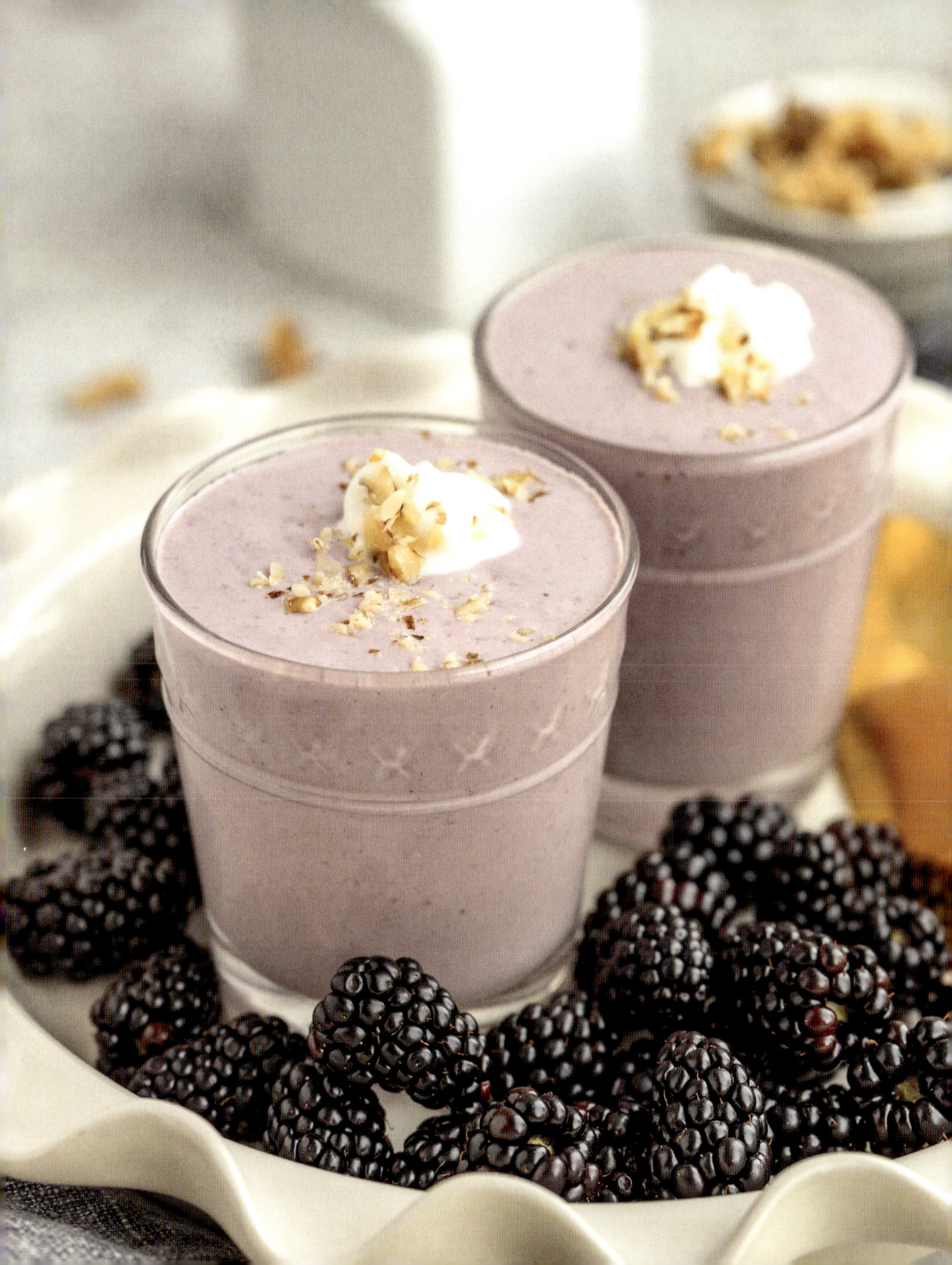

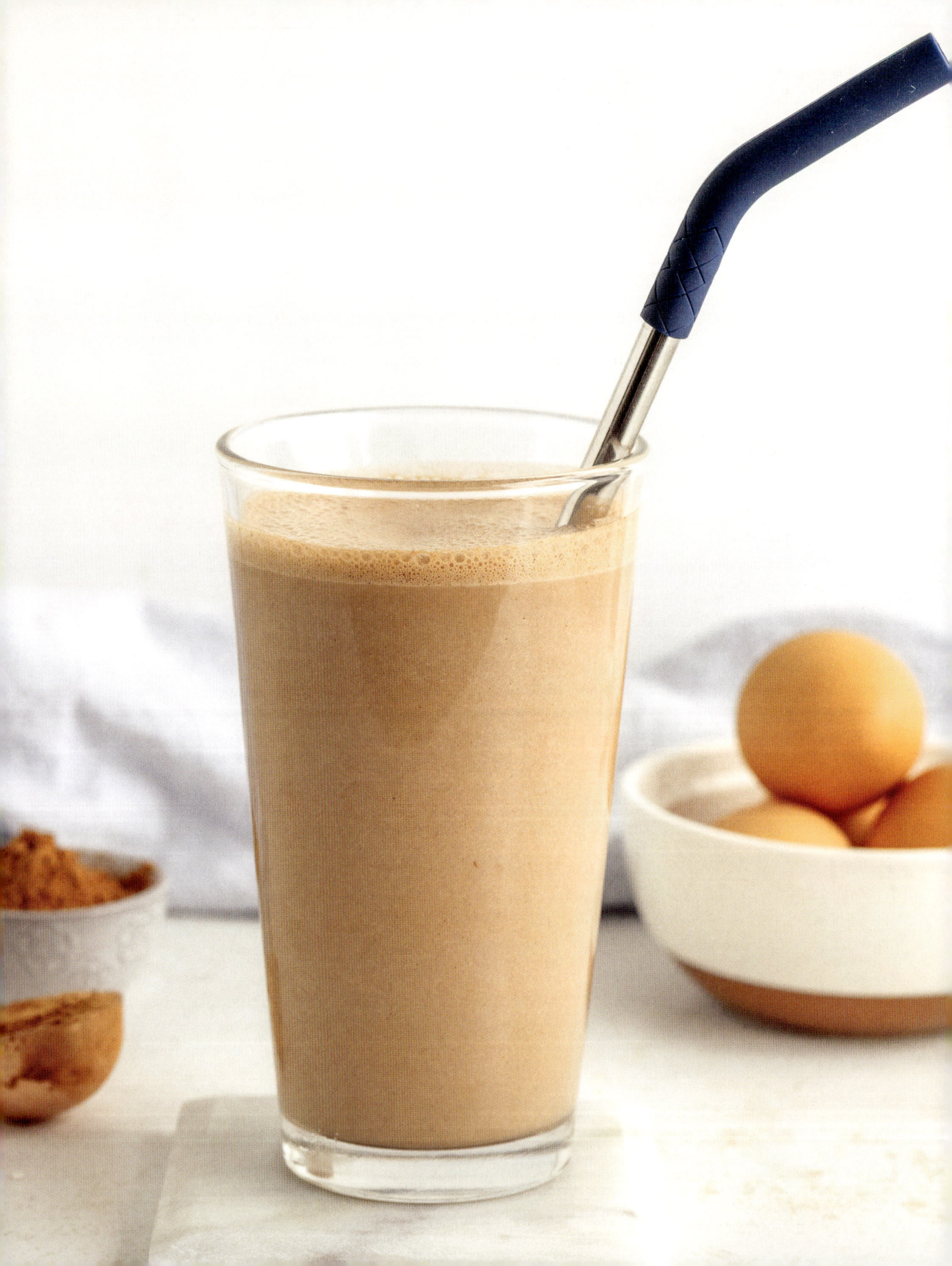

CHOCOLATE PROTEIN SHAKE

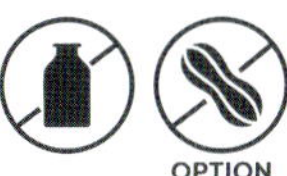

SERVES 1

PREP TIME: 5 minutes (not including time to hard-boil eggs)

Packed with nearly 400 calories and balanced with protein, fat, and fiber, this meal replacement shake will fill you up with the right nutrients. With almost 50 grams of protein from hard-boiled eggs and protein powder, it provides the fuel you need for energy and muscle recovery. The hard-boiled eggs create a thick, creamy texture, eliminating the need for a banana and keeping it low carb. Cauliflower might seem like an unpleasant addition, but it adds bulk and fiber without altering the flavor. Trust me on this one.

---

1 cup nut or seed milk of choice

1 cup frozen cauliflower rice

2 large hard-boiled eggs

2 tablespoons granulated sugar-free sweetener

2 tablespoons unsweetened cocoa powder

1 scoop chocolate-flavored protein powder

1 tablespoon almond butter (optional)

1. Put all the ingredients in a blender and blend until smooth.
2. Pour into a 16-ounce glass and serve.

CALORIES: **370** | PROTEIN: **49.2g** | FAT: **14g** | TOTAL CARBS: **38.1g** | NET CARBS: **6.4g** | FIBER: **7.7g**
SUGAR ALCOHOLS: **24g**

GREEN POWER MEAL-PREP SMOOTHIE

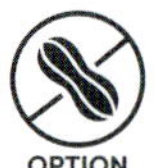

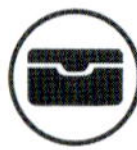

SERVES 2

PREP TIME: 10 minutes (not including time to hard-boil egg)

This power smoothie is packed with more than 40 grams of protein and is brimming with nutrients from all kinds of green foods: spinach, avocado, parsley, and cucumber. Blueberries add a touch of natural sweetness. A hard-boiled egg and the avocado provide creaminess and thicken the smoothie. It's an excellent way to sneak in greens without the smoothie tasting overly healthy. You can double this recipe—which is perfect for meal prepping—to create multiple smoothie bags. In the morning, simply empty a bag into your blender, add the cucumber and milk, and blend!

FOR MEAL PREPPING

3 cups baby spinach

½ avocado, pitted and peeled

½ cup fresh or frozen blueberries

2 handfuls fresh parsley leaves

2 scoops unflavored or vanilla-flavored protein powder

1 large hard-boiled egg, cut in half

FOR 1 SERVING

½ medium English cucumber, or 1 Persian cucumber

1½ cups nut or seed milk of choice

1. Evenly divide the spinach, avocado, blueberries, parsley, protein powder, and egg between two zip-top bags. Refrigerate until ready to make your smoothie, or for up to 3 days.
2. To prepare a serving, put the contents of one bag in a blender. Add the cucumber and milk and blend until smooth.
3. Pour into a 16-ounce glass and serve.

notes

Don't want to use protein powder? Add 1 to 2 more hard-boiled eggs.

To make the smoothie sweeter, use a sweetened nut or seed milk or add 1 to 2 tablespoons sugar-free sweetener.

(per serving)
CALORIES: **325** | PROTEIN: **43.1g** | FAT: **12.5g** | TOTAL CARBS: **13.5g** | NET CARBS: **8.6g** | FIBER: **4.9g**

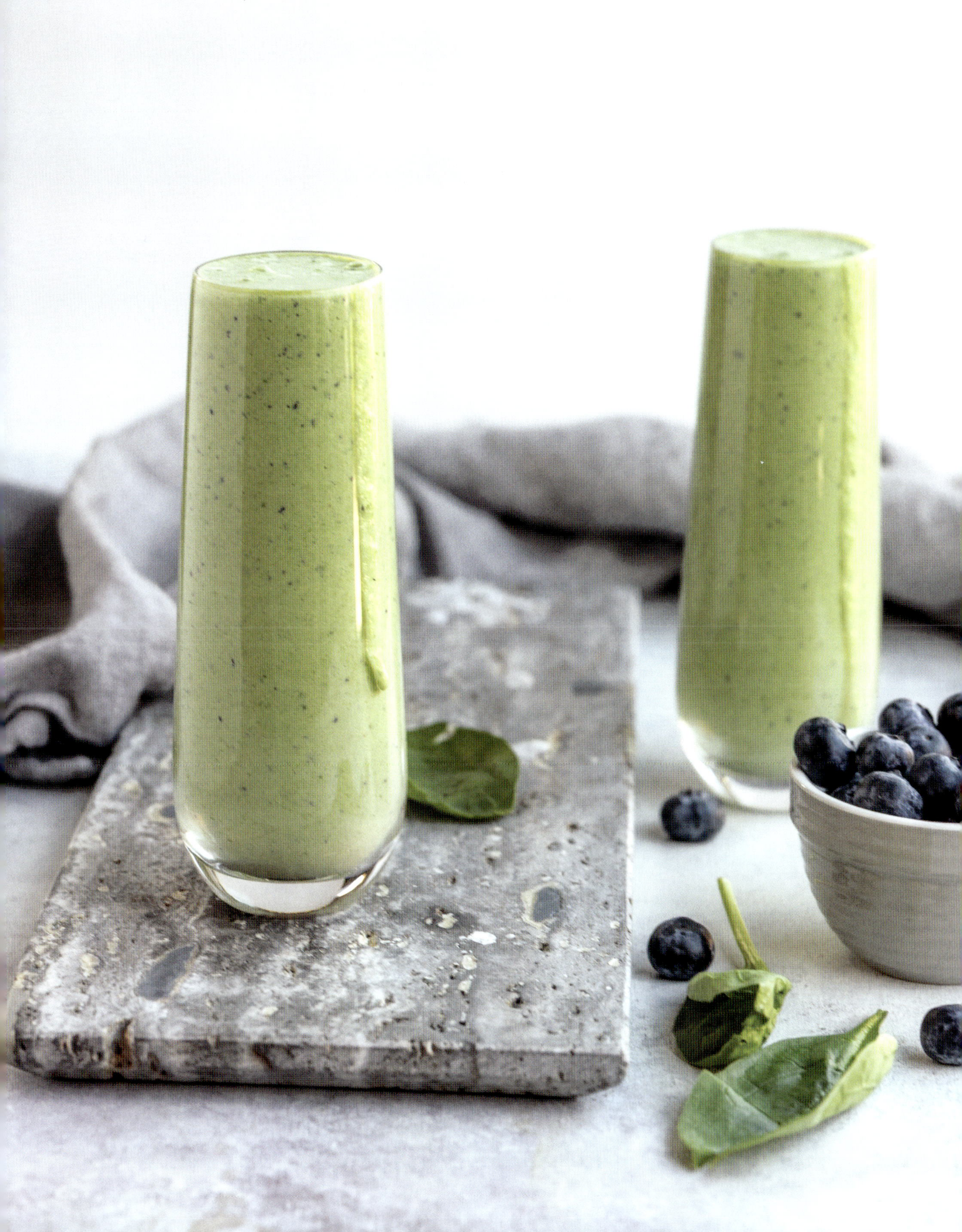

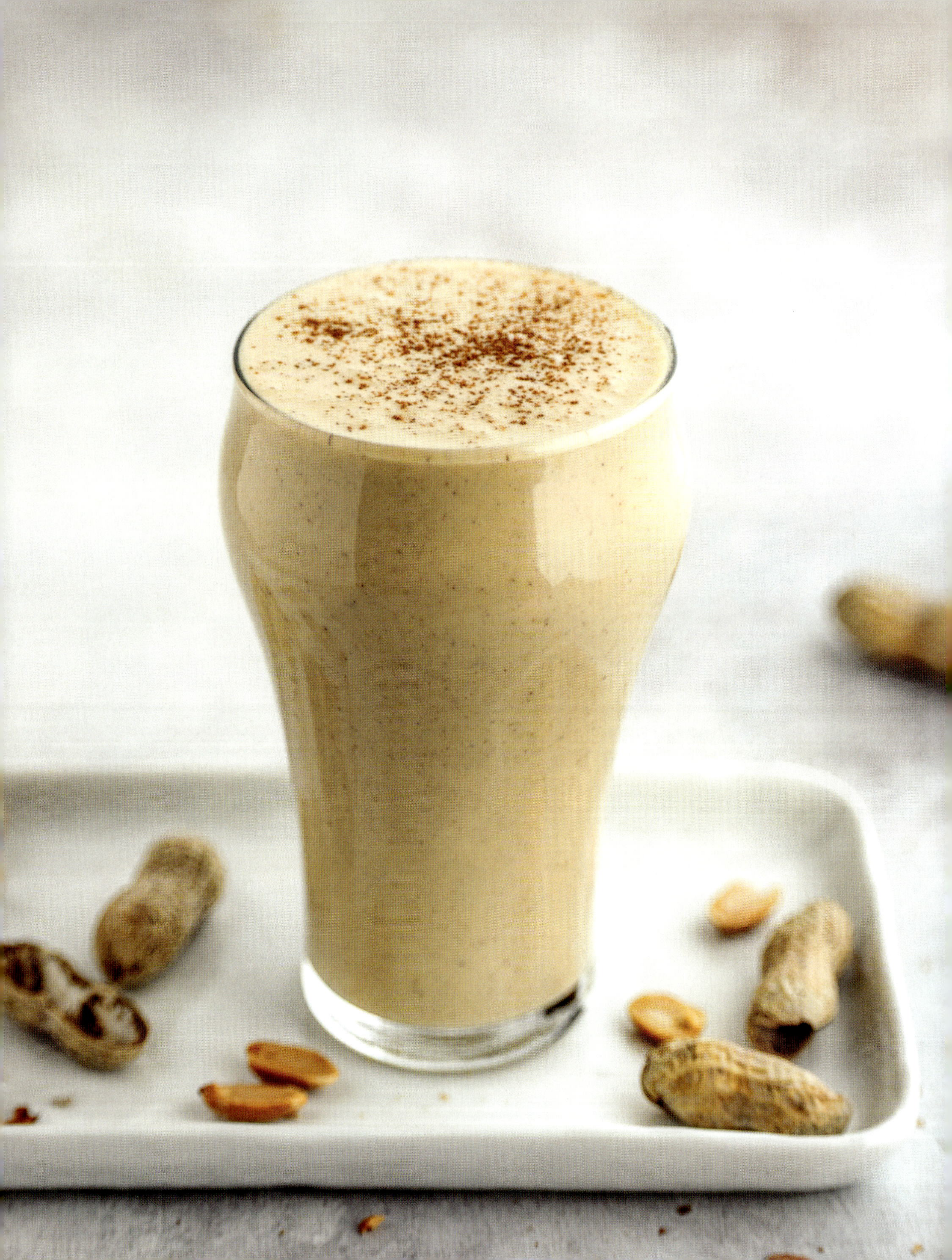

PEANUT BUTTER PROTEIN SMOOTHIE

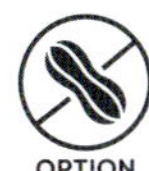

SERVES 1

PREP TIME: 5 minutes (not including time to hard-boil eggs)

This one is for my peanut butter lovers! As a hearty meal replacement, this smoothie is perfect for breakfast, lunch on the go, or a hungry teenager. With over 500 calories, it's balanced with fats and more than 50 grams of protein to keep you full and energized for hours. Two hard-boiled eggs create a thick, creamy texture without the need for a high-carb banana, while the Peanut Butter Cookie protein powder from 1UpNutrition not only boosts the protein content but also delivers incredible flavor. A touch of cinnamon adds a subtle finish that ties everything together.

---

2 large hard-boiled eggs

2 tablespoons no-sugar-added peanut butter

1 scoop peanut butter–flavored protein powder (see notes)

¼ teaspoon ground cinnamon

1 cup nut or seed milk of choice

2 tablespoons plain Greek or low-carb yogurt

1. Put all the ingredients in a blender and blend until smooth and creamy.
2. Pour into a 12-ounce glass and serve.

notes

Peanut Butter Cookie ISO Protein by 1UpNutrition is phenomenal in this recipe. If you don't want to purchase a peanut butter–flavored protein powder, use unflavored or vanilla flavored and add more peanut butter or a few tablespoons of dry-roasted peanuts for more flavor and 1 to 2 tablespoons sugar-free sweetener for sweetness.

For a lower-fat, lower-calorie option, use a powdered peanut butter such as PB2 in place of the peanut butter.

CALORIES: **529** | PROTEIN: **55.8g** | FAT: **30.3g** | TOTAL CARBS: **11g** | NET CARBS: **7.7g** | FIBER: **3.3g**

PROTEIN COFFEE

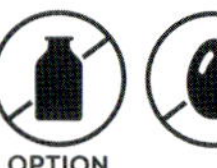 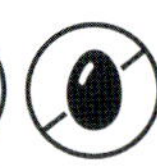 

SERVES 1

PREP TIME: 5 minutes (not including time to brew coffee)

Coffee is a must for me in the mornings—my day doesn't truly start without it. Adding protein to my coffee is a great way to kick off the day with an energy boost, and now it's become a part of my routine. I wouldn't have it any other way.

This protein coffee starts with a homemade creamer made from your choice of milk (nut, flax, coconut, or dairy), heavy cream for extra creaminess, and protein powder. You can customize the creamer by adding a flavor extract like vanilla or peppermint, you can make a frappé by blending the ingredients, or you can make an iced version. When I need a quick option, I use a store-bought caramel- or vanilla-flavored protein shake as my creamer, adding ¼ cup of the shake to my coffee.

FOR THE PROTEIN CREAMER

¼ cup nut or seed milk of choice

2 tablespoons heavy cream

½ to 1 scoop unflavored or vanilla-flavored protein powder

1 to 2 teaspoons granulated sugar-free sweetener (optional)

10 to 12 ounces hot brewed coffee

1. To make the creamer, pour the milk, cream, protein powder, and sweetener into a tall glass or liquid measuring cup. Whisk with a fork or use a stick frother to mix.
2. Pour the creamer into a 16-ounce mug, then pour in the hot coffee. Stir to combine.

VARIATIONS:

- **Iced Protein Coffee.** Complete Step 1 above, using 1 scoop of protein powder. Fill a tall pint glass with 1 cup ice and pour in 10 to 12 ounces chilled brewed coffee, leaving 1 to 1¼ inches of room at the top for the creamer. Pour in the protein creamer and stir to combine.
- **Protein Frappé.** To make a frappé, put all the ingredients, including 10 to 12 ounces chilled brewed coffee and about 1 cup ice, in a blender. Blend for about 30 seconds, until smooth. Pour into a pint glass and enjoy!

notes

To make this dairy free, use coconut cream instead of heavy cream, or just add more nut or seed milk.

If you have an espresso machine, you can make a protein latte. Pour the creamer into your mug, brew espresso over the creamer, and then pour frothed milk over the espresso to the top. Stir to combine.

NUTRITIONAL INFORMATION:

Based on 10 ounces coffee, ½ scoop protein powder in the creamer, and Good Karma Flaxmilk + Protein for the milk in the creamer

CALORIES: **188** | PROTEIN: **15.5g** | FAT: **12.8g** | TOTAL CARBS: **0.9g** | NET CARBS: **0.9g** | FIBER: **0g**

(iced protein coffee)
CALORIES: **237** | PROTEIN: **27.8g** | FAT: **12.8g** | TOTAL CARBS: **0.9g** | NET CARBS: **0.9g** | FIBER: **0g**

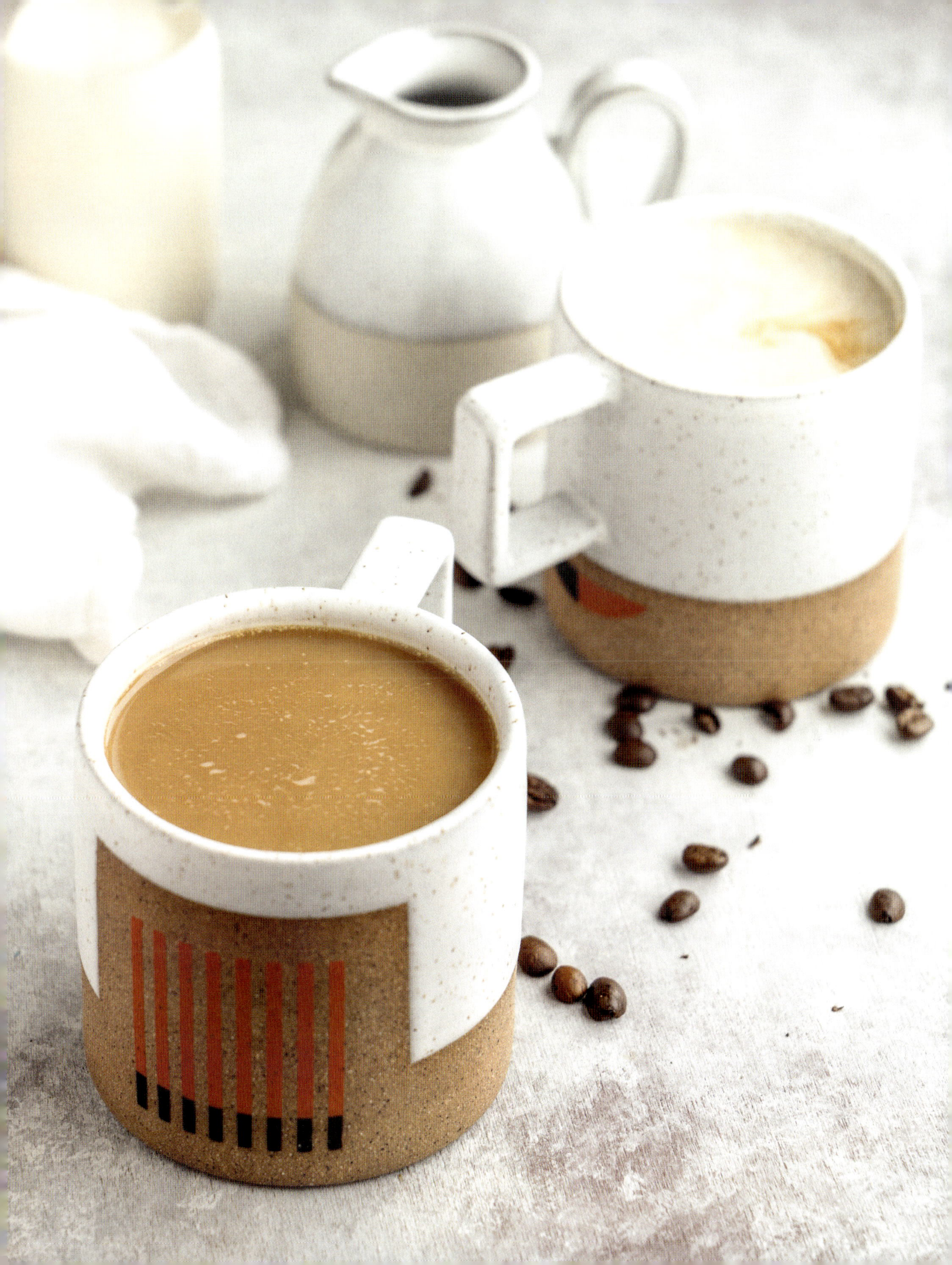

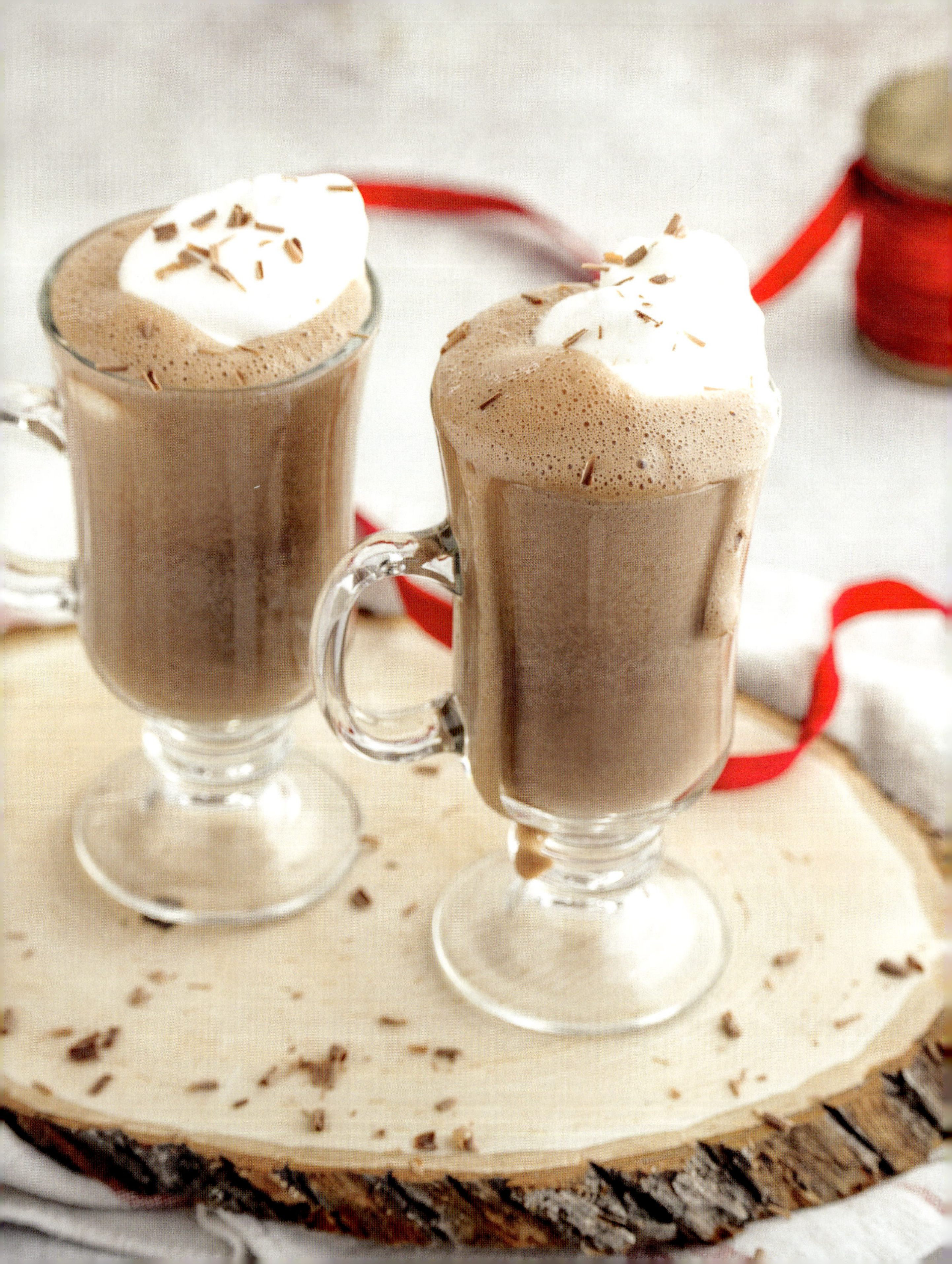

PROTEIN HOT CHOCOLATE

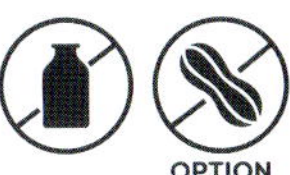

SERVES 4

PREP TIME: 10 minutes

COOK TIME: 5 minutes

I like to sneak extra protein in wherever I can, and hot chocolate is no exception. This protein-packed hot cocoa is a creamy, velvety treat with a rich chocolate flavor. The secret to its smooth texture and protein boost is the addition of eggs, which also enhances the creaminess. Instead of whipped cream, top your hot chocolate with a sweet meringue—one more way to get extra protein.

FOR THE HOT CHOCOLATE

¼ cup unsweetened cocoa powder

⅓ cup boiling water

2 cups nut or seed milk of choice

¼ cup granulated sugar-free sweetener

Pinch of salt

4 large eggs (see note)

1 teaspoon vanilla extract

FOR TOPPING

2 large egg whites

¼ cup powdered sugar-free sweetener

Shaved sugar-free or dark chocolate, for topping (optional)

1. In a small bowl, whisk together the cocoa powder and boiling water until the cocoa powder has dissolved. Set aside.
2. Pour the milk into a medium saucepan. Stir in the sweetener and salt. Bring to a simmer over medium heat. Whisk in the cocoa mixture and stir to combine. Remove the pan from the heat.
3. Prepare the meringue topping: Pour the egg whites into a medium bowl. Beat the whites using an electric mixer on medium speed until they start to foam. Slowly sprinkle in the powdered sweetener, beating at medium speed until incorporated. Then beat on high speed until soft peaks form. Set aside.
4. Crack the eggs into a blender. Pour in the chocolate cream mixture and vanilla and blend until smooth.
5. Pour into four 8-ounce mugs and top with the meringue and shaved chocolate, if desired.

Pack It with Protein: Add a scoop of collagen or protein powder to the blender in Step 4.

note

If the idea of consuming raw eggs is concerning to you, you can use pasteurized eggs for this recipe.

(per serving)
CALORIES: **120** | PROTEIN: **12g** | FAT: **6.5g** | TOTAL CARBS: **25.4g** | NET CARBS: **2.4g** | FIBER: **2g**
SUGAR ALCOHOLS: **21g**

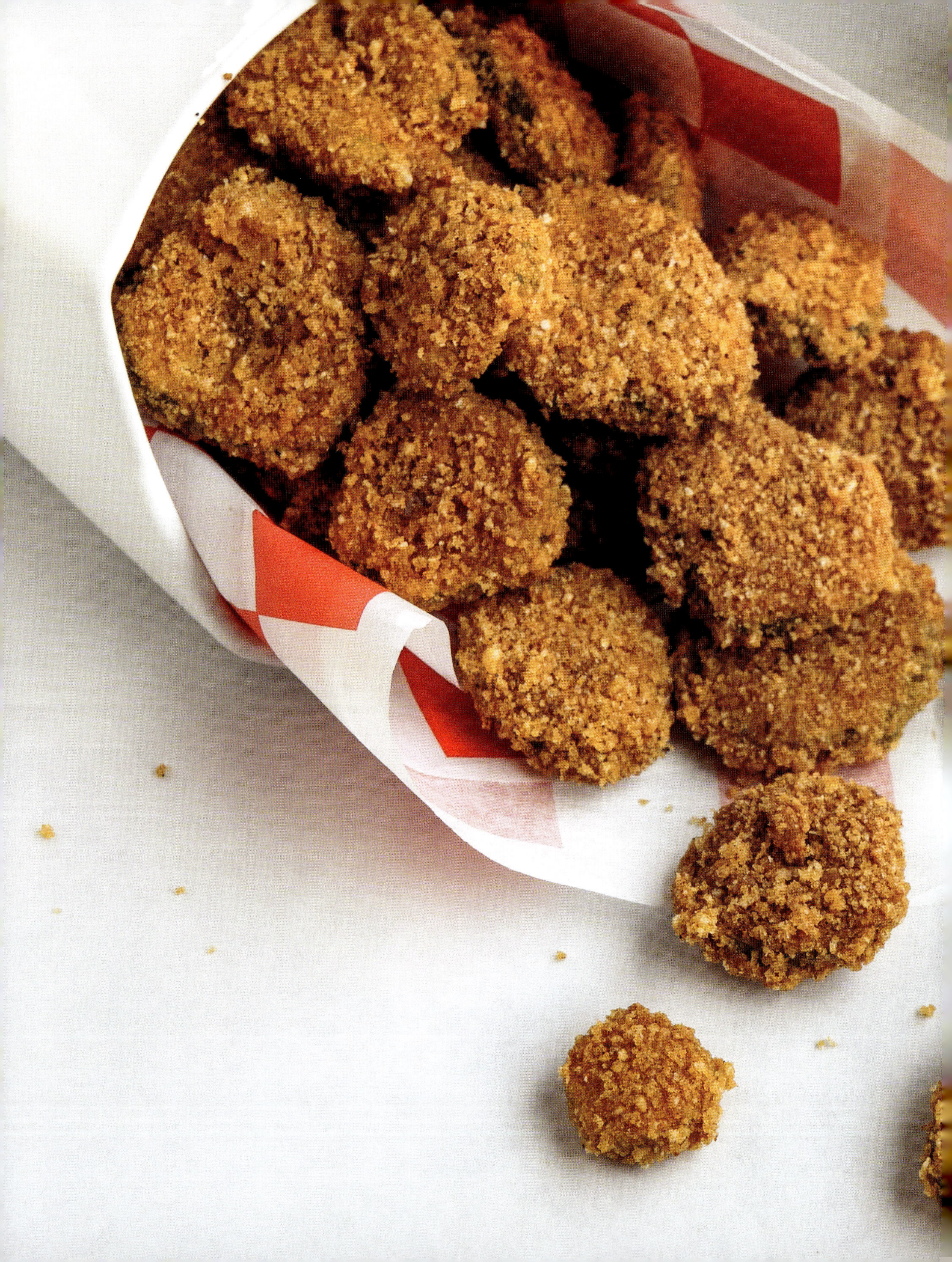

SNACKS & APPS

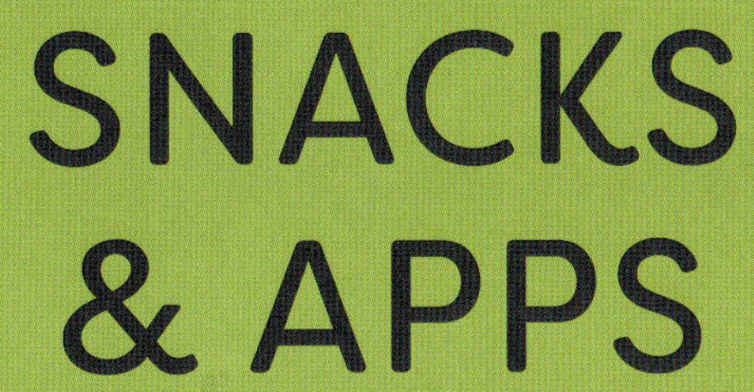

BUFFALO CHICKEN DIP

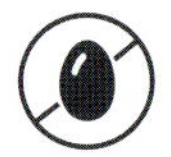  

OPTION

SERVES 8

PREP TIME: 5 minutes (not including time to cook chicken)

COOK TIME: 15 minutes or 4 hours, depending on method

This high-protein, crowd-pleasing appetizer has nearly 20 grams of protein per serving. It features shredded chicken swimming in a creamy, cheesy, spicy sauce. It's easy to make, and I've included both oven and slow cooker instructions, making it perfect for any occasion. Serve it as an appetizer with celery sticks, sliced mini bell peppers, pork rinds, or tortilla chips at your next party, or enjoy it as a meal on its own!

---

1 tablespoon salted butter

2 cups shredded cooked chicken

½ cup Buffalo sauce

¼ cup plain Greek or low-carb yogurt or sour cream

½ teaspoon lemon juice

6 ounces (¾ cup) cream cheese, softened and cubed

½ cup shredded Monterey Jack cheese, divided

⅓ cup crumbled blue cheese, plus more for garnish if desired

2 tablespoons sliced chives or green onions, for garnish

OVEN INSTRUCTIONS:

1. Preheat the oven to 375°F.
2. Melt the butter in an 8-inch cast-iron or other oven-safe skillet over medium heat. Add the shredded chicken and Buffalo sauce. Cook until the sauce is heated through. Remove the pan from the heat.
3. Stir in the yogurt, lemon juice, cream cheese, and 2 tablespoons of the Monterey Jack. Top with the remaining Monterey Jack and the blue cheese.
4. Bake for 10 minutes, or until the cheese is melted and bubbly. Sprinkle with the chives and/or more crumbled blue cheese.

SLOW COOKER INSTRUCTIONS:

Put all the ingredients in the slow cooker. Cook on low for 3 to 4 hours. Stir to combine, then lower the heat to the warm setting until ready to enjoy. Before serving, sprinkle with the chives and/or more crumbled blue cheese.

(per serving)
CALORIES: **202** | PROTEIN: **17.9g** | FAT: **13.6g** | TOTAL CARBS: **1.6g** | NET CARBS: **1.4g** | FIBER: **0.2g**

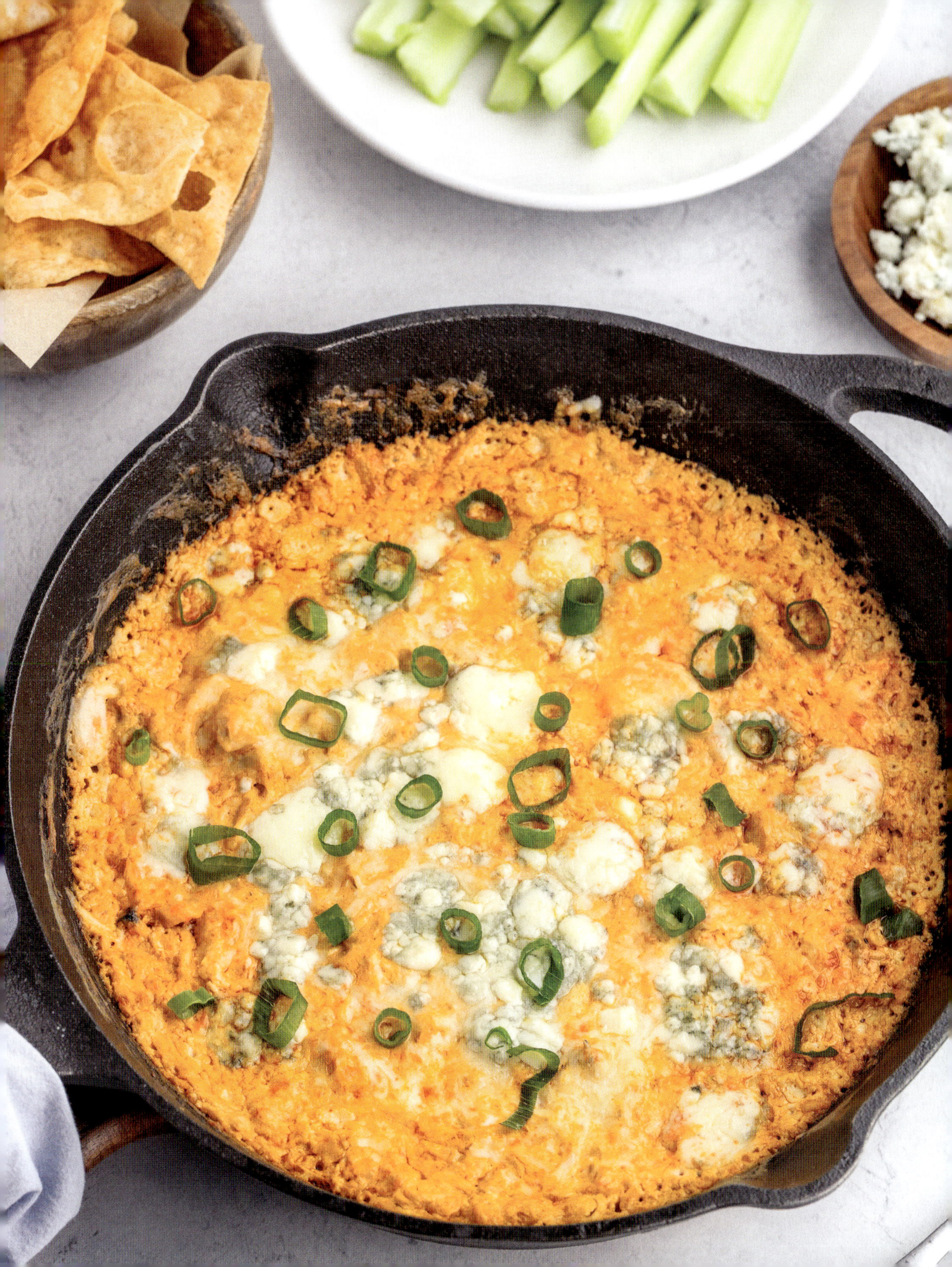

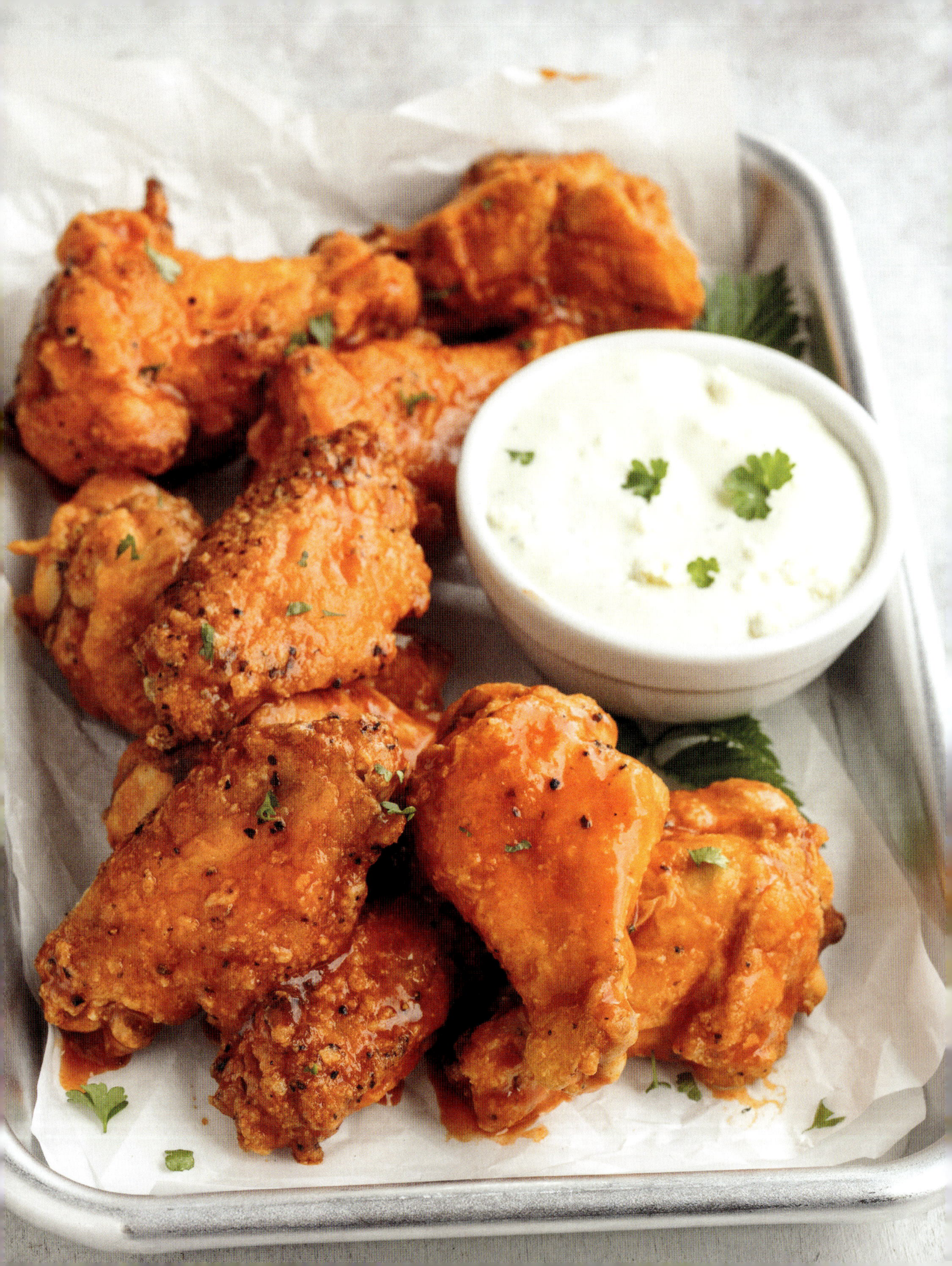

BUFFALO WINGS

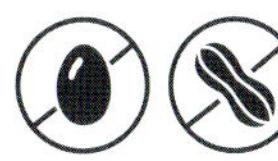

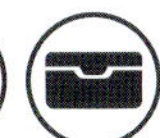

SERVES 6
PREP TIME: 10 minutes
COOK TIME: 35 minutes

Get restaurant-worthy wings right at home with this recipe. These Buffalo wings are coated with a delicious seasoning blend and baked in the oven to create a crispy wing, then generously coated with an easy Buffalo sauce for a fiery kick. I like to make these as an appetizer for parties and serve them with blue cheese dressing, but they make for a tasty lunch or dinner as well.

- 2½ pounds split (aka party) chicken wings (see note)
- 1 tablespoon baking powder
- 1 teaspoon salt, divided
- 1 teaspoon garlic powder
- ½ teaspoon ground black pepper
- ⅓ cup Frank's RedHot Sauce
- ¼ cup unsalted butter, melted
- 2 tablespoons minced garlic
- 1 tablespoon sherry vinegar or distilled white vinegar
- Chopped parsley and/or crumbled blue cheese, for garnish (optional)
- Blue cheese dressing or ranch dressing, for serving (optional)

1. Preheat the oven to 450°F.
2. Pat the wings dry with a paper towel and place in a large bowl.
3. In a small bowl, stir together the baking powder, ½ teaspoon of the salt, the garlic powder, and pepper.
4. Sprinkle half of the baking powder mixture on the wings and toss. Sprinkle with the remaining mixture and toss again until evenly coated.
5. Cover a rimmed baking sheet with foil and set a wire rack on top. Spray the rack with cooking oil. Evenly space the wings on top of the wire rack. Bake for 28 to 35 minutes, until the internal temperature is 165°F and the wings are crispy on the outside. Flip the wings halfway through cooking to cook both sides evenly.
6. Meanwhile, combine the hot sauce, melted butter, garlic, vinegar, and remaining ½ teaspoon of salt in a large bowl.
7. Add the cooked wings to the sauce bowl and stir to coat. Garnish with parsley and/or crumbled blue cheese, if desired. Serve with blue cheese dressing or ranch dressing, if desired.

STORAGE INSTRUCTIONS: Store in an airtight container in the refrigerator for up to 4 days or in the freezer for up to 3 months.

REHEATING INSTRUCTIONS:

- **Oven:** Preheat the oven to 350°F. Place refrigerated or thawed wings on a foil-lined rimmed baking sheet and reheat for 10 to 15 minutes.
- **Air fryer:** Place refrigerated or thawed wings in a single layer in the air fryer tray or basket and air-fry at 350°F for 5 to 8 minutes.
- Remember, the wings may not be as crispy as they were when first baked.

note

Split chicken wings are sold precut into the two main parts: the drumette and the flat (aka wingette), with the tips removed. This saves you the time of breaking down whole wings at home.

(per serving)
CALORIES: **490** | PROTEIN: **35.3g** | FAT: **37.4g** | TOTAL CARBS: **1.9g** | NET CARBS: **1.8g** | FIBER: **0.1g**

CHILI GARLIC WINGS 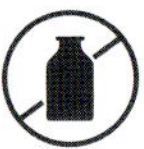 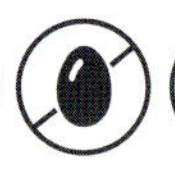 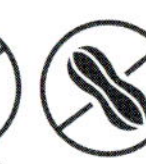 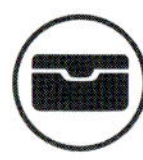

OPTION

SERVES 6

PREP TIME: 10 minutes, plus 1 hour to marinate

COOK TIME: 65 minutes

A few years ago, I filmed a YouTube video that features different flavors of party wings. This is my family's favorite flavor, so I had to share it with you. These juicy oven-baked wings with their deliciously sticky, sweet, spicy glaze make the best snack or appetizer.

2 pounds split (aka party) chicken wings (see note, page 305)

FOR THE MARINADE AND GLAZE

⅓ cup avocado oil

⅓ cup soy sauce or tamari

¼ cup plus 1 tablespoon sugar-free or regular honey, divided

¼ cup chili garlic sauce

4 cloves garlic, minced

1 teaspoon ginger powder

FOR GARNISH (OPTIONAL)

Thinly sliced green onions

Sesame seeds

1. Pat the wings dry with a paper towel. Put them in a large bowl and set aside.
2. To make the marinade, combine the avocado oil, soy sauce, ¼ cup of the honey, the chili garlic sauce, garlic, and ginger powder in a small bowl.
3. Reserve ¼ cup of the marinade for later. Pour the rest of the marinade into the bowl with the chicken. Toss the wings to coat. Cover with plastic wrap and refrigerate for 1 to 2 hours.
4. Preheat the oven to 400°F. Line a rimmed baking sheet with foil, then set a wire rack on top.
5. Arrange the wings on the rack, spacing them evenly; discard the leftover marinade. Bake for 25 minutes. Flip the wings, then bake for another 25 to 30 minutes, until the internal temperature reaches 165°F.
6. To make the glaze, pour the reserved ¼ cup of marinade into a small saucepan and add the remaining tablespoon of honey. Bring to a boil over medium heat, then reduce the heat to medium-low and simmer until thickened, 3 to 5 minutes.
7. Brush the glaze all over the wings. Place under the broiler for 1 to 2 minutes to caramelize the glaze.
8. Garnish with sliced green onions and/or sesame seeds, if desired.

STORAGE INSTRUCTIONS: Store in an airtight container in the refrigerator for up to 4 days or in the freezer for up to 3 months.

REHEATING INSTRUCTIONS:

- **Oven:** Preheat the oven to 350°F. Place refrigerated or thawed wings on a foil-lined rimmed baking sheet and reheat for 10 to 15 minutes.
- **Air fryer:** Set the temperature to 350°F, place refrigerated or thawed wings in a single layer in the air fryer tray or basket, and air-fry for 4 to 5 minutes.
- To get the wings crispy again, it's best to use an air fryer, or you can finish the wings under the oven broiler for a couple of minutes.

(per serving, using sugar-free honey)
CALORIES: **415** | PROTEIN: **28.6g** | FAT: **31.1g** | TOTAL CARBS: **16.1g** | NET CARBS: **2.7g** | FIBER: **5.1g**
SUGAR ALCOHOLS: **8.3g**

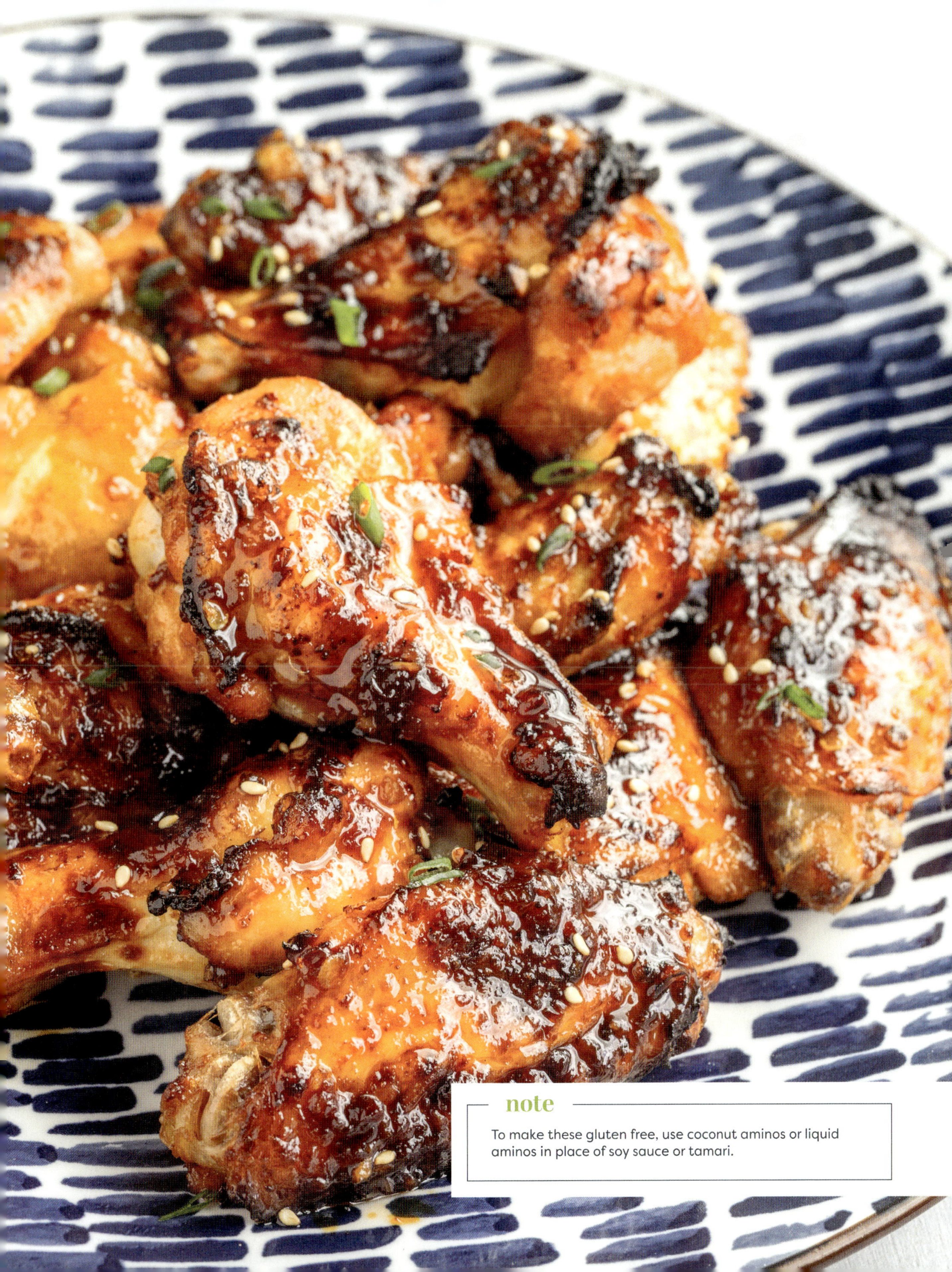

note

To make these gluten free, use coconut aminos or liquid aminos in place of soy sauce or tamari.

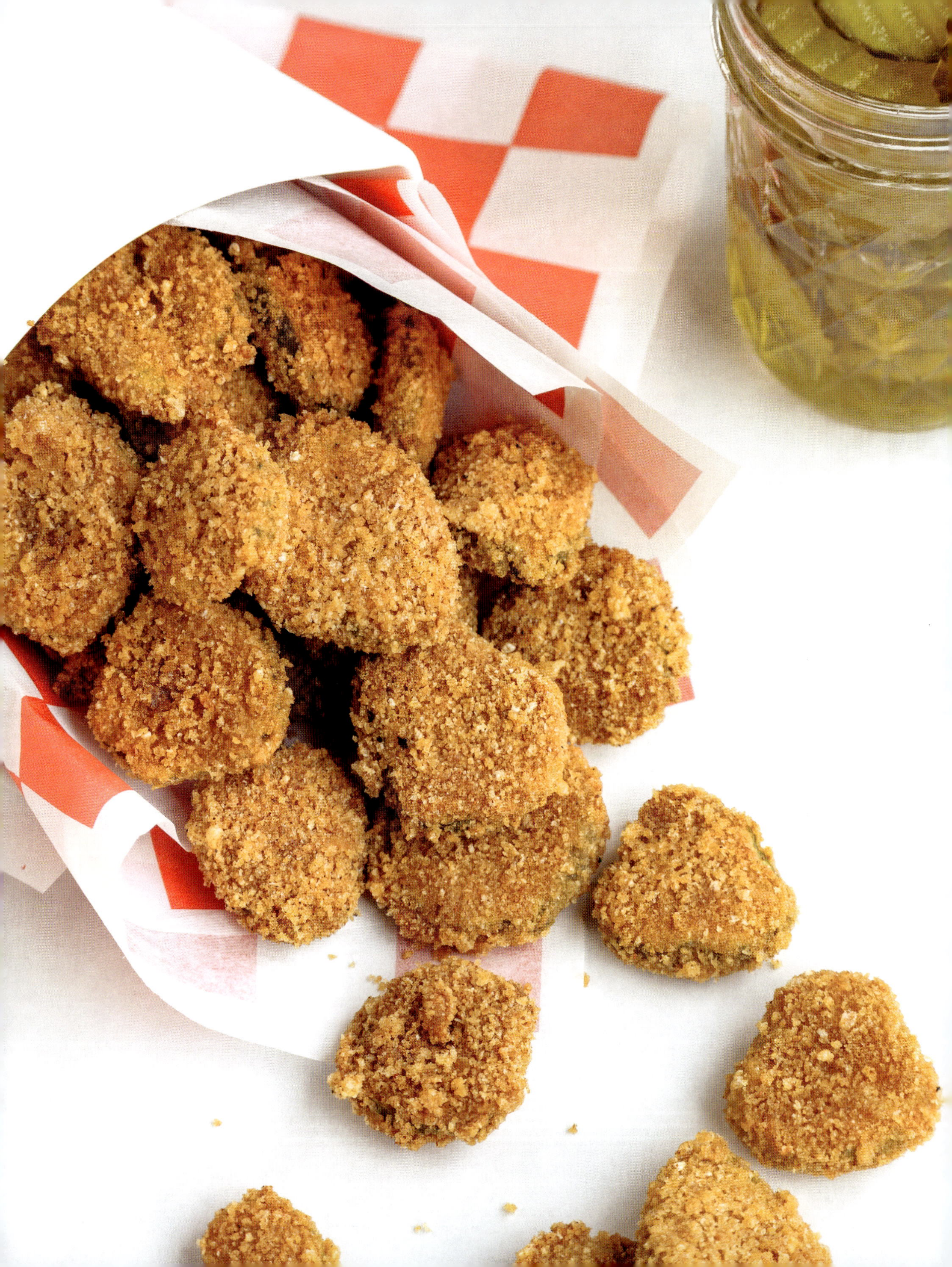

AIR-FRIED PICKLE CHIPS

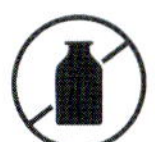
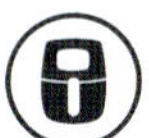

SERVES 6 (about 12 chips per serving)

PREP TIME: 25 minutes

COOK TIME: 24 minutes

These crispy pickle chips have nearly 20 grams of protein per serving. The flavorful breading made from almond flour, eggs, pork panko, and seasoning makes them a perfectly crunchy snack, appetizer for your next tailgating party, or side to serve alongside my Low-Carb Fish and Chips (page 188). Fried pickle chips don't reheat well and are best enjoyed right away.

- 1 (16-ounce) jar dill pickle chips
- ½ cup blanched, super-fine almond flour
- 1 teaspoon Cajun seasoning (optional)
- ½ teaspoon salt
- 3 large eggs
- 2 tablespoons pickle juice (from the jar of pickles)
- 2 cups pork panko
- 1 teaspoon garlic powder
- ½ teaspoon cayenne pepper
- Ranch dressing or other dipping sauce of choice, for serving (optional)

1. Place the pickle chips in between two paper towels to absorb most of the liquid.
2. Prepare the breading station using three bowls. In the first bowl, mix together the almond flour, Cajun seasoning (if using), and salt. In the second bowl, whisk together the eggs and pickle juice. In the third bowl, mix together the pork panko, garlic powder, and cayenne.
3. Dip a pickle chip into the almond flour mixture and toss to fully coat. Then dip it into the egg wash. Finally, dredge the pickle chip in the pork panko mixture, pressing the mixture into the chip. Set aside on a paper towel–lined plate and repeat with the remaining pickle chips and breading.
4. Preheat the air fryer to 400°F. Working in batches, place a layer of breaded pickles in the air fryer basket or tray, leaving ¼ inch of space between them. Spray the breaded pickles with cooking oil. Air-fry for 6 minutes, flip over each slice, and air-fry for an additional 6 minutes, or until the chips are browned and crispy. Remove from the basket and repeat with the remaining breaded pickles.
5. Serve with ranch dressing or your favorite dipping sauce, if desired.

(per serving)
CALORIES: **261** | PROTEIN: **19.5g** | FAT: **18g** | TOTAL CARBS: **5.9g** | NET CARBS: **4.3g** | FIBER: **1.6g**

LOW-CARB HUMMUS

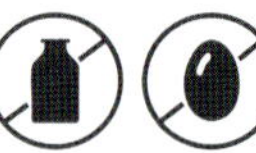
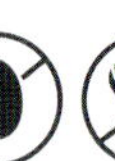

SERVES 8

PREP TIME: 10 minutes

How about a low-carb hummus that tastes and looks like real hummus? This recipe ingeniously substitutes chickpeas with lupini beans—the low-carb legume—resulting in a dip that mimics the flavor and texture of traditional hummus. Serve with your favorite low-carb chips and vegetables.

1 cup jarred lupini beans (see note, page 227)

⅓ cup tahini

2 tablespoons extra-virgin olive oil, divided

1 large clove garlic, peeled

1 teaspoon ground cumin

½ teaspoon salt

Juice of ½ lime

2 to 5 tablespoons cold water

FOR GARNISH (OPTIONAL)

Chopped fresh parsley

Paprika

1. Put the lupini beans, tahini, 1 tablespoon of the olive oil, the garlic clove, cumin, salt, lime juice, and 2 tablespoons of cold water in a food processor. Process until smooth. If the hummus is too thick, add another 1 to 3 tablespoons of cold water to thin it out to the proper consistency. Taste and adjust the seasoning if needed, adding more cumin, salt, and/or lime juice.
2. Transfer the hummus to a serving bowl or platter. Drizzle the remaining tablespoon of olive oil on top and garnish with chopped parsley and/or paprika, if desired.

(per serving)
CALORIES: **123** | PROTEIN: **5.2g** | FAT: **10g** | TOTAL CARBS: **3.4g** | NET CARBS: **1.2g** | FIBER: **2.2g**

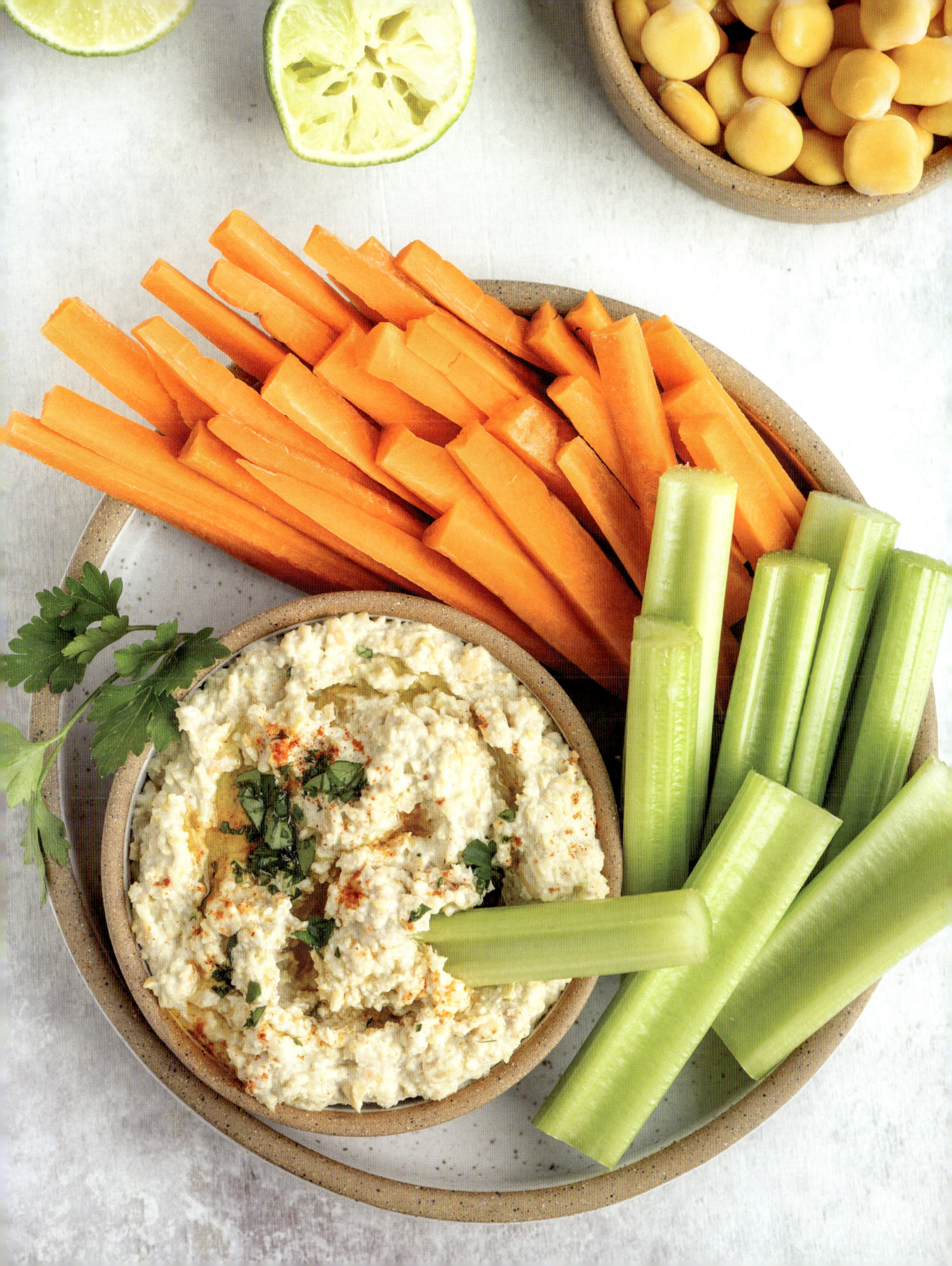

LOW-CARB TORTILLA CHIPS

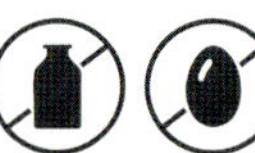
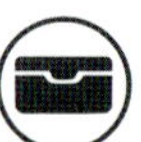

SERVES 5
PREP TIME: 15 minutes
COOK TIME: 15 minutes

Say goodbye to chip aisle cravings with this easy low-carb tortilla chip recipe! Made with just a few ingredients, these crispy chips are ready in 30 minutes. The secret to their irresistible crunch lies in the protein powder, which gives them that classic texture and a boost of protein, while xanthan gum keeps the dough pliable for rolling and frying. They even look like authentic fried tortilla chips with their signature bumps!

⅔ cup blanched, super-fine almond flour

1 tablespoon unflavored protein powder

1 tablespoon xanthan gum

½ teaspoon salt

3 tablespoons hot water

1 dropperful corn flavor extract (see notes)

Avocado oil, for the pan

1. In a medium bowl, whisk together the almond flour, protein powder, xanthan gum, and salt. Pour in the hot water and add the corn flavor extract. Mix with a fork until a tacky dough forms.
2. Form the dough into a ball and place between two 16-inch sheets of parchment paper. Press the dough with your hand to flatten it. Using a rolling pin, roll out in all directions (attempting to form a rectangle shape) until the dough is very thin (⅛ inch or less). The thinner it is, the crispier the chips will be. (A tortilla press works even better for flattening the dough; see notes, opposite.) To remove the tortilla from the parchment paper, carefully peel off one side of the paper, place that piece of parchment back on the tortilla rectangle, and flip the whole thing over. Now carefully peel off the top piece of parchment. Remove the tortilla from the bottom piece of parchment. The dough will release easily when you cut your triangles.
3. Using a pizza cutter or knife, cut the dough into triangles and pull them apart to let air circulate between them. Let the dough dry for several minutes—the time it takes to prep and heat the oil is sufficient.
4. Pour enough avocado oil into a large skillet to cover the dough triangles as they fry (about ½ inch). Heat the oil over medium heat. To test if the oil is hot enough, pinch off a tiny piece of dough and place it in the hot oil. If it sizzles, the oil is ready. Working in batches, add an even layer of triangles to the oil and fry until golden brown on both sides, about 1 minute. You can flip the chips or lightly press them into the oil with a spatula to make sure they're submerged.
5. Once the chips start to turn golden brown, remove them using a slotted spatula or spoon and place on a paper towel–lined plate or baking sheet. Lightly season with salt. The chips will continue to crisp up as they sit. Store in a brown paper bag at room temperature for up to 3 days.

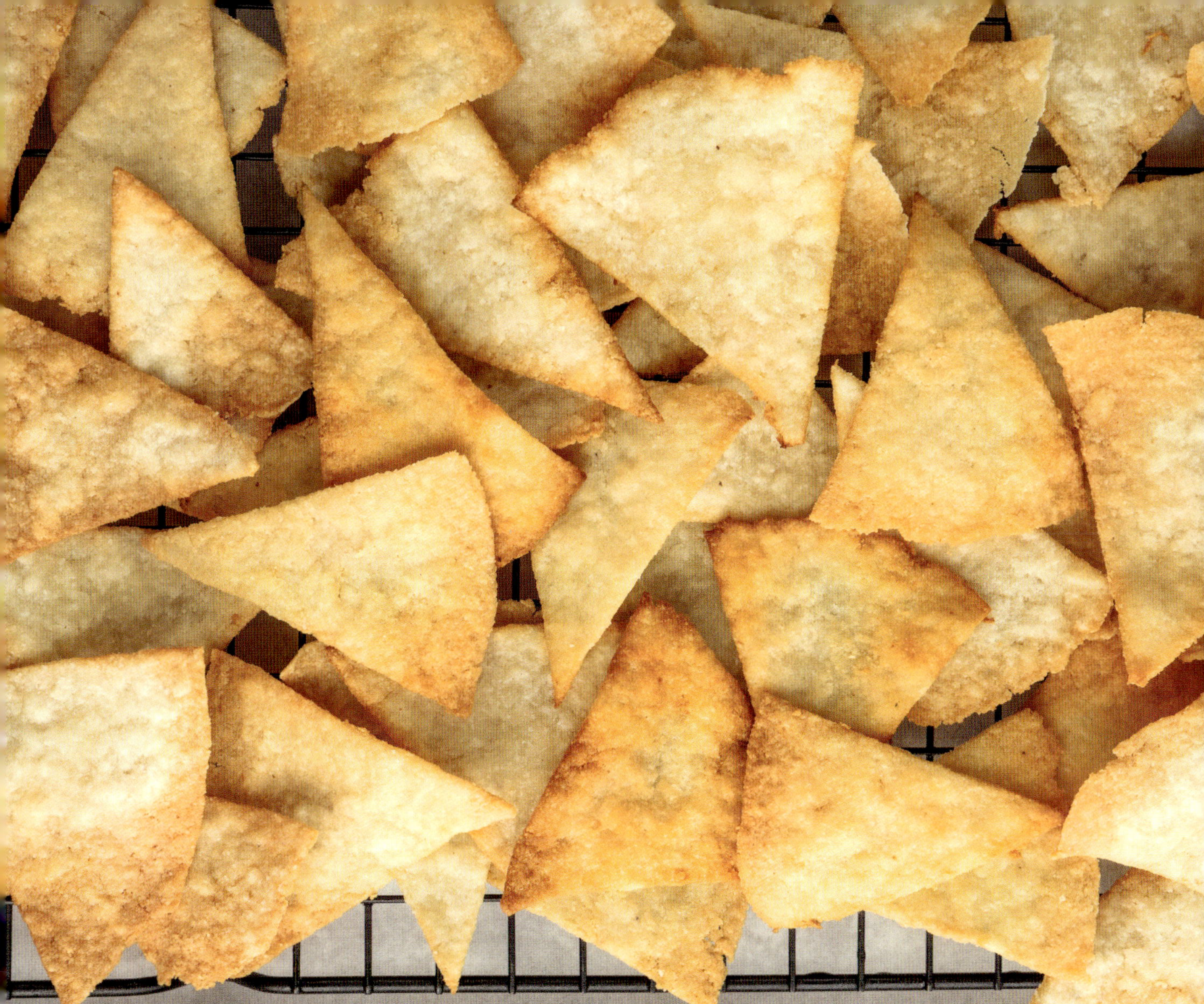

notes

For this recipe, I use the Corn Tortilla Flavoring from One on One Flavors. You can use another corn flavor extract if you prefer.

Instead of rolling it out with a rolling pin, you can divide the dough into eight equal-size balls and use a tortilla press to flatten each ball between two parchment paper circles. Use a knife or pizza cutter to cut the flattened dough into triangles as you would a pizza.

VARIATIONS:

- **Cool Ranch Tortilla Chips:** In a small bowl, mix together 1 tablespoon powdered ranch dressing mix, ¼ teaspoon smoked paprika, ⅛ teaspoon garlic powder, and ⅛ teaspoon onion powder. Put the fried chips in a zip-top bag or bowl. Pour in the seasoning mixture and toss to coat evenly.
- **Nacho Cheese Tortilla Chips:** In a small bowl, mix together 1 tablespoon cheddar cheese powder, ½ teaspoon chili powder, and ¼ teaspoon smoked paprika. Put the fried chips in a zip-top bag or bowl. Pour in the seasoning mixture and toss to coat evenly.

(per serving)
CALORIES: **100** | PROTEIN: **3.9g** | FAT: **7.5g** | TOTAL CARBS: **5.6g** | NET CARBS: **1.6g** | FIBER: **4g**

PROTEIN BENTO BOX—2 WAYS

Bento boxes are like Lunchables for adults. They are also the ultimate Girl Meal—you know, the kind you eat when you are by yourself and want to graze on a variety of small, satisfying bites without committing to a full, structured meal that requires cooking or a lot of effort. I've included some of my favorite high-protein options, but you can make it your own by mixing in your go-to protein-packed cheeses, nuts, veggies, and fruits. Whether you're meal prepping or packing to eat on the go, it's a fun way to stay fueled. Check out my list of snacks on page 318 for even more inspiration.

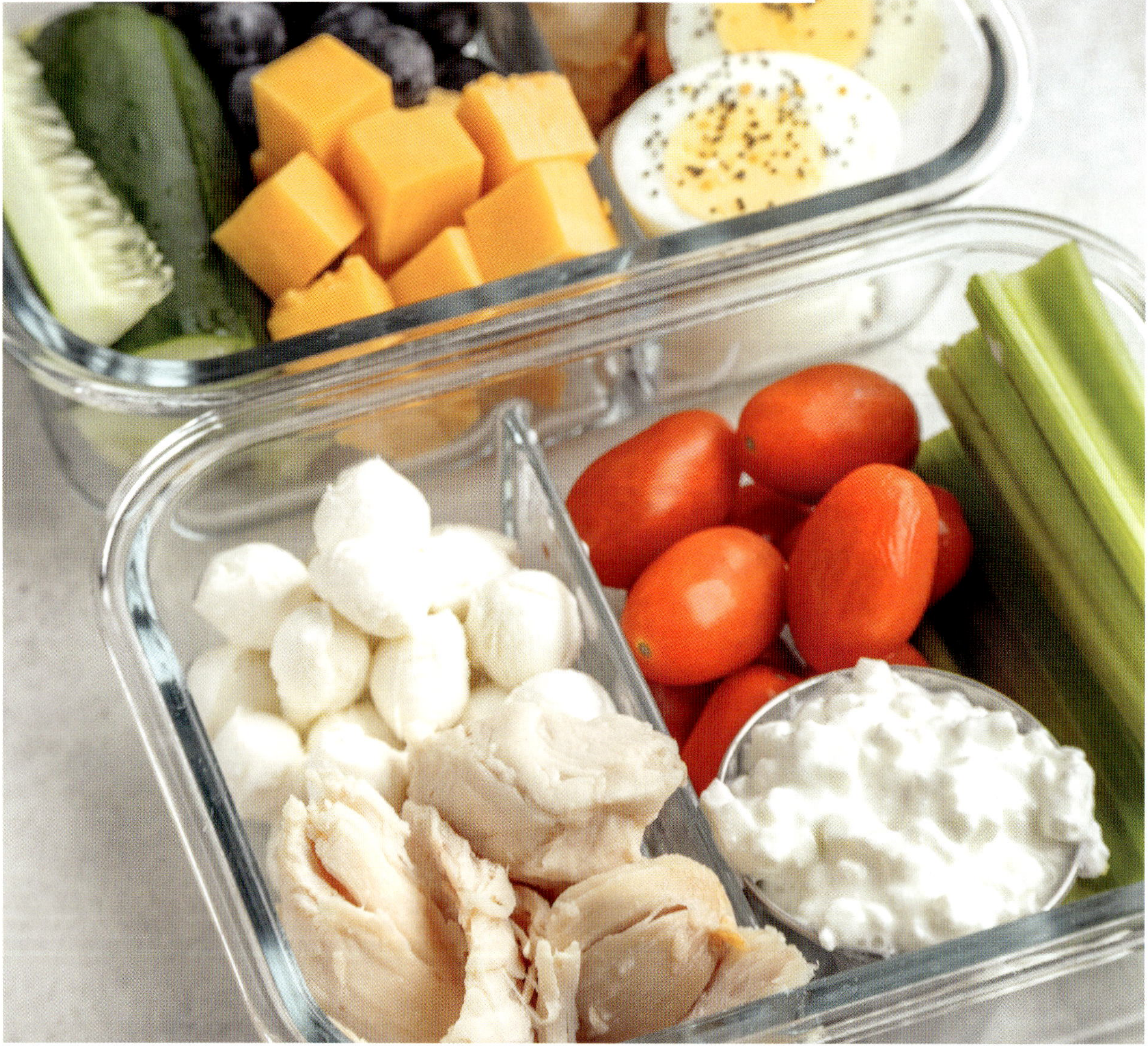

CHICKEN BENTO BOX

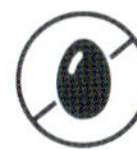
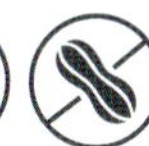
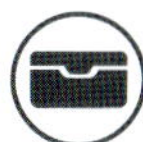

SERVES 1

PREP TIME: 10 minutes (not including time to cook chicken)

---

4 ounces cooked chicken, shredded or cubed

2½ ounces fresh mini mozzarella balls

¼ cup cottage cheese (4% milkfat)

8 or 9 grape tomatoes

1 celery stalk, ends trimmed, sliced in half

1. Assemble the ingredients in a bento box or meal prep container with dividers.
2. Store in the refrigerator for up to 4 days.

CALORIES: **415** | PROTEIN: **48.7g** | FAT: **18.8g** | TOTAL CARBS: **10.4g** | NET CARBS: **7.5g** | FIBER: **2.9g**

TURKEY & EGG BENTO BOX

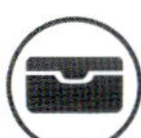

SERVES 1

PREP TIME: 10 minutes (not including time to boil eggs)

---

4 ounces sliced deli turkey

2 large hard-boiled eggs

2 ounces cheddar cheese, cubed

2 ounces fresh blueberries

½ medium cucumber, cut lengthwise into quarters

Everything bagel seasoning

1. Assemble the ingredients in a bento box or meal prep container with dividers. Before serving, cut the eggs in half and sprinkle with everything bagel seasoning.
2. Store in the refrigerator for up to 4 days.

CALORIES: **506** | PROTEIN: **46.9g** | FAT: **29.3g** | TOTAL CARBS: **15.8g** | NET CARBS: **13.9g** | FIBER: **1.9g**

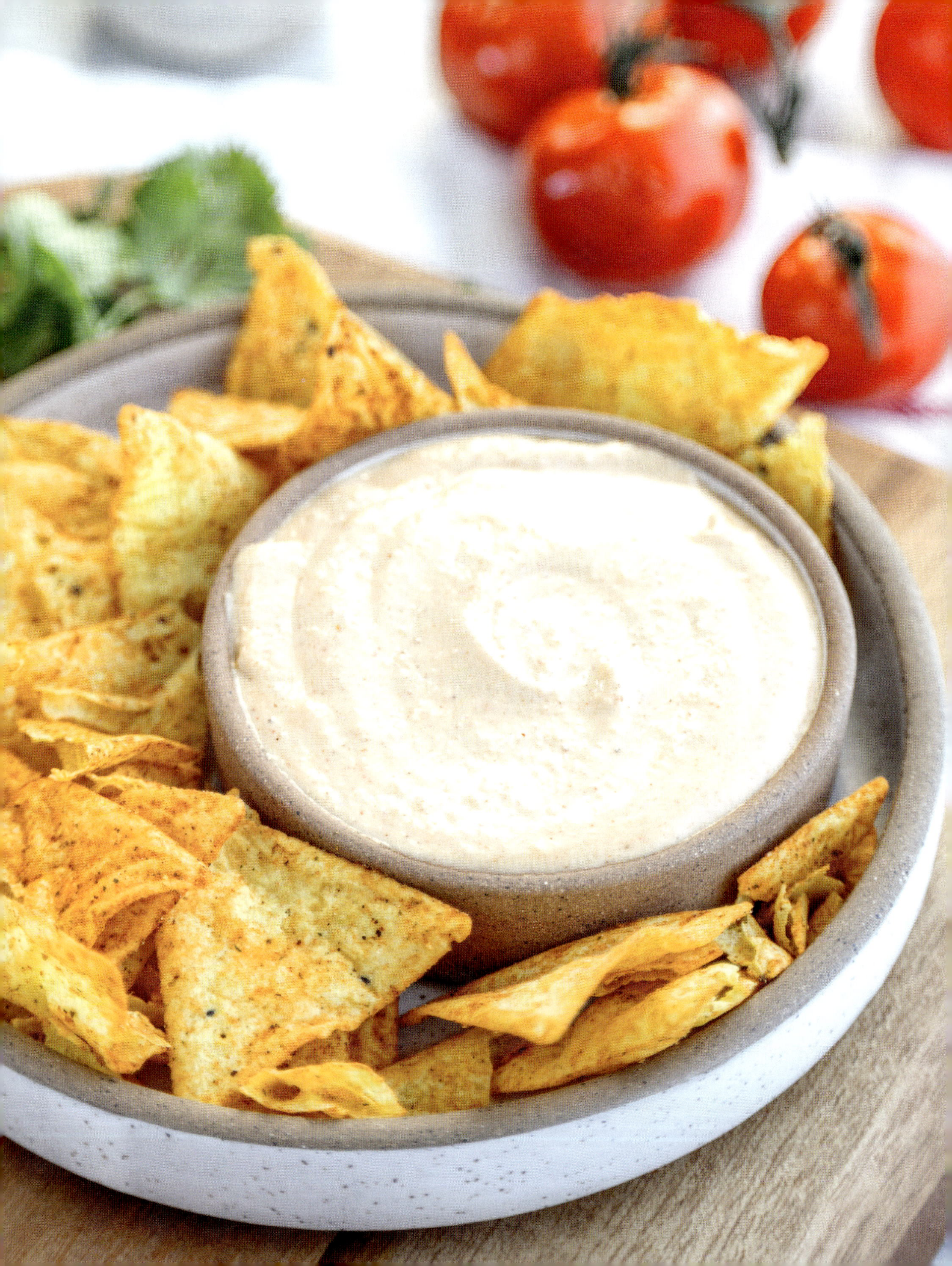

PROTEIN NACHO CHEESE SAUCE

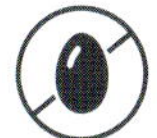

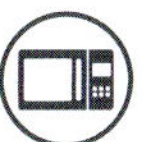
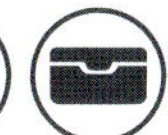

MAKES 2 cups (¼ cup per serving)

PREP TIME: 5 minutes

COOK TIME: 1 minute

This creamy sauce is a protein-packed option made with cottage cheese and cheddar cheese, with an optional touch of chili powder for a hint of spice. It's perfect for my Carne Asada Nachos (page 97) or as a dip for my Low-Carb Tortilla Chips (page 312). I love to make a batch of this sauce for the week because it can be stored in the refrigerator and reheated when needed.

---

1 cup cottage cheese (4% milkfat)

2 cups shredded sharp cheddar cheese

1½ teaspoons chili powder (optional)

½ cup water

1. Put the cottage cheese, cheddar, and chili powder, if using, in a blender or food processor. Pour in the water and blend until smooth.
2. Pour the sauce into a microwave-safe bowl. Microwave for 30 to 60 seconds, just until warmed. Overheating the dip can cause the cheese to separate.
3. Store leftover sauce in an airtight container in the refrigerator for up to 5 days. Reheat in the microwave for 30 to 60 seconds.

(per serving)
CALORIES: **148** | PROTEIN: **9.5g** | FAT: **11.1g** | TOTAL CARBS: **1.8g** | NET CARBS: **1.8g** | FIBER: **0g**

HIGH-PROTEIN SNACKS

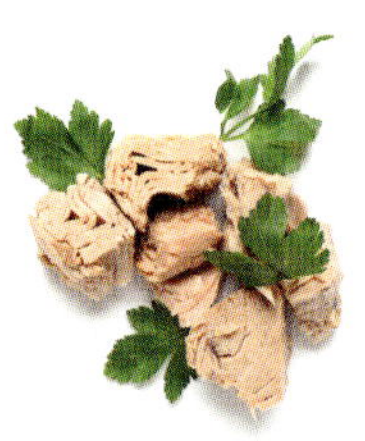

CANNED TUNA

5 oz ~ 38g protein

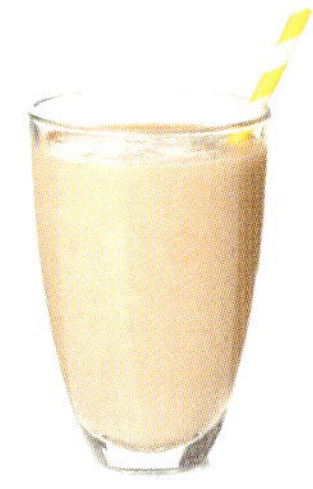

PROTEIN SHAKE

11 oz ~ 30g protein

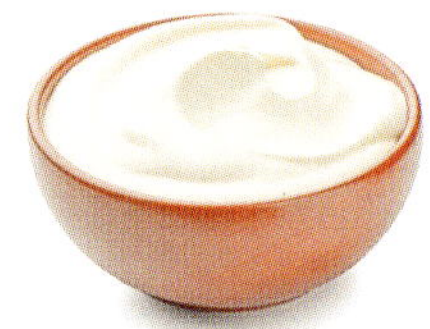

GREEK YOGURT

¾ cup ~ 17g protein

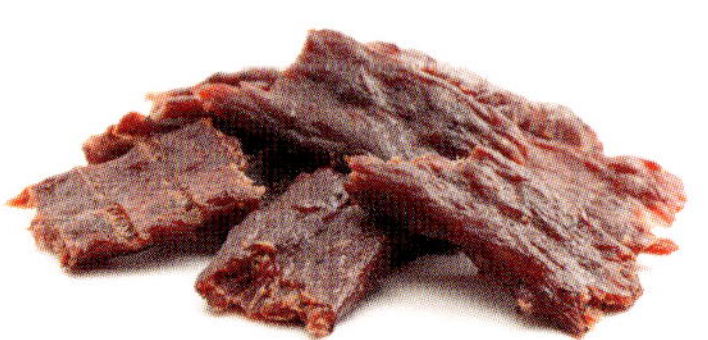

BEEF JERKY

1 oz ~ 15g protein

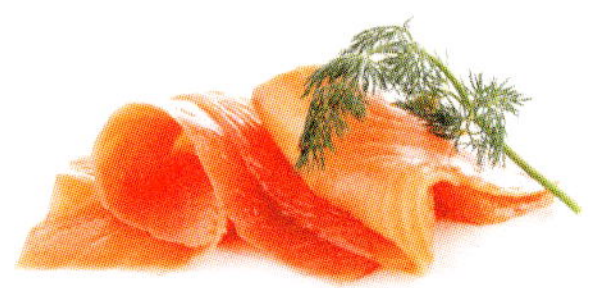

SMOKED SALMON

3 oz ~ 15g protein

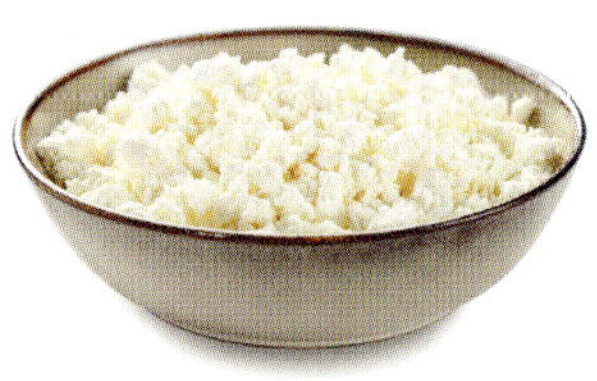

COTTAGE CHEESE

½ cup ~ 14g protein

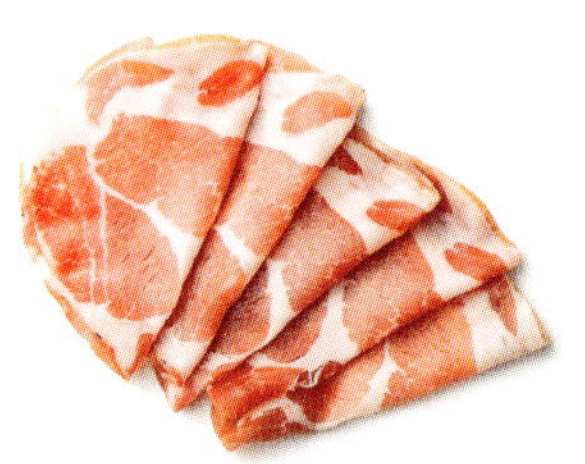

DELI MEAT

2 oz ~ 13g protein

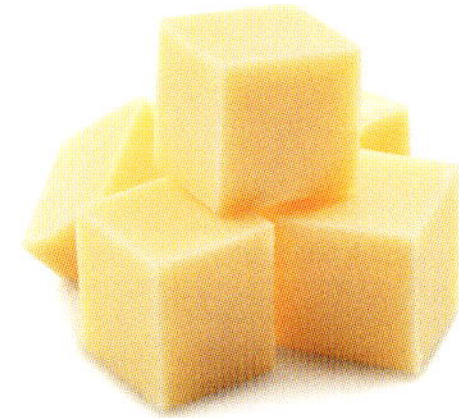

CHEDDAR CHEESE CUBES

2 oz ~ 12g protein

HARD-BOILED EGGS

2 eggs ~ 12g protein

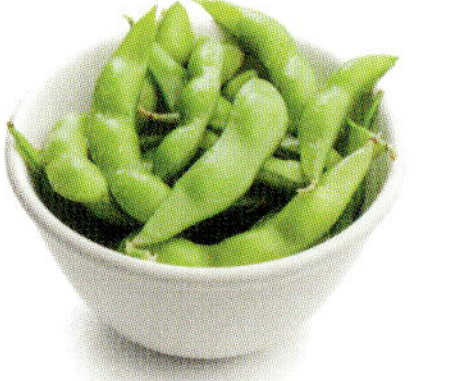

EDAMAME

½ cup ~ 8g protein

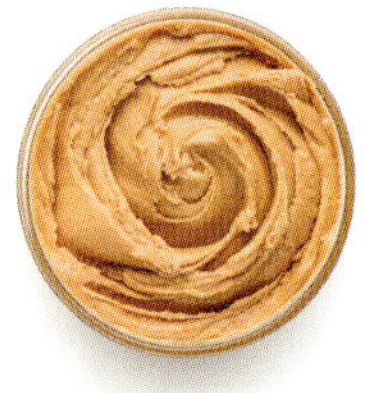

PEANUT BUTTER

2 tablespoons ~ 8g protein

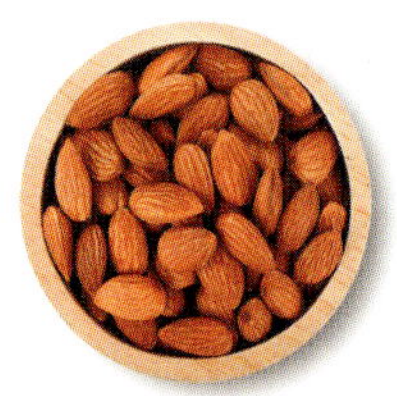

ALMONDS

¼ cup ~ 7.5g protein

ACKNOWLEDGMENTS

First and foremost, thank you to my amazing audience and the low-carb community. Your support, encouragement, and shared excitement for this way of eating are what keep me inspired to keep creating. I love hearing your stories about your success. You've turned sharing recipes into something so much more—a connection, a lifestyle, and a collective path.

To the entire Victory Belt crew—thank you for believing in this book, for your patience in its creation, and for helping shape it into what it is today. I'm so thankful for your guidance and all the work that brought this vision to life.

To my husband and kids—thank you for your love and support, and for being my taste testers through every phase of this process. You kept me grounded and reminded me what really matters.

To my mom—your spirit is in every part of this book. I wish you could be here to hold it. You were the queen of effortless no-recipe dinners, and you made magic out of simple ingredients. Thank you for teaching me to cook with confidence and love. I miss you every day.

To my dad and brother—thank you for your steadfast support and for always cheering me on.

To Margie and Gary, my in-laws and the best next-door neighbors a girl could ask for—thank you for the cupcake liners, the fresh herbs, the spare oven, and your unwavering support throughout this whole process.

To my photographers—Eva, thank you for beautifully capturing so many of the dishes in this book. And Miranda Kelton, thank you for photographing me in my element and helping me feel at ease in front of the camera.

To Elena, my recipe tester—you helped me fine-tune so many of these recipes, and your thoughtful feedback gave me confidence throughout the process.

To Jenner Family Beef—thank you for raising me on wholesome pasture-raised beef and for all those summer visits to the ranch. So many of the meals in this book were inspired by memories made around your table.

And to my girls, Deanna, Crystal, Sarah, April, Lindsay, Renee, Danielle, and more—thank you for being my constant cheerleaders, my hype squad, and my sounding board. Your support means the world to me.

END NOTES

Chapter 1: What Is Protein?

1. M. J. Lopez and S. S. Mohiuddin, "Biochemistry, Essential Amino Acids," *StatPearls*, April 2024, https://www.statpearls.com/articlelibrary/viewarticle/36202#ref_26041391.
2. Yongqing Hou and Guoyao Wu, "Nutritionally Essential Amino Acids," *Advances in Nutrition* 9, no. 6 (2018): 849–851. https://www.sciencedirect.com/science/article/pii/S216183132201273X?via%3Dihub.
3. Yongqing Hou, Yulong Yin, and Guoyao Wu, "Dietary Essentiality of 'Nutritionally Non-Essential Amino Acids' for Animals and Humans," *Experimental Biology and Medicine* 240, no. 8 (2015): 997–1007. https://journals.sagepub.com/doi/10.1177/1535370215587913.
4. Peng Li, Yu-Long Yin, Defa Li, Sung Woo Kim, and Guoyao Wu, "Amino Acids and Immune Function," *British Journal of Nutrition* 98, no. 2 (2007): 237–252. https://www.cambridge.org/core/journals/british-journal-of-nutrition/article/amino-acids-and-immune-function/B1A9C1587A8602613F6447BA8404D8E1.
5. Kaya Teh, *Principles of Nutrition* (Sierra College, 2024), chap. 6.5, 190.
6. Hugo Juárez Olguín, David Calderón Guzmán, Ernestina Hernández García, and Gerardo Barragán Mejía, "The Role of Dopamine and Its Dysfunction as a Consequence of Oxidative Stress," *Oxidative Medicine and Cellular Longevity* (2016): Article ID 9730467, 13 pages. https://onlinelibrary.wiley.com/doi/10.1155/2016/9730467.
7. Alice Callahan, Heather Leonard, and Tamberly Powell, *Nutrition: Science and Everyday Application* (Open Oregon Educational Resources, 2020), 282, https://openoregon.pressbooks.pub/nutritionscience2e/.
8. "Health Lesson: Learning About Bones," National Institute of Arthritis and Musculoskeletal and Skin Diseases, https://www.niams.nih.gov/health-topics/educational-resources/health-lesson-learning-about-bones.
9. Kara Rogers, "Keratin," Britannica, https://www.britannica.com/science/keratin.
10. R. I. Litvinov and J. W. Weisel, "What Is the Biological and Clinical Relevance of Fibrin?" *Seminars in Thrombosis and Hemostasis* 42, no. 4 (2016): 333–43, https://doi.org/10.1055/s-0036-1571342.

Chapter 2: Protein Considerations and Requirements

1. Institute of Medicine (US) Subcommittee on Interpretation and Uses of Dietary Reference Intakes; Institute of Medicine (US) Standing Committee on the Scientific Evaluation of Dietary Reference Intakes, *DRI Dietary Reference Intakes: Applications in Dietary Assessment* (Washington, DC: National Academies Press, 2000), chap. 2, "Current Uses of Dietary Reference Standards," https://www.ncbi.nlm.nih.gov/books/NBK222870/.
2. National Institutes of Health, *Dietary Reference Intakes: Energy, Carbohydrates, Fiber, Fat, Fatty Acids, Cholesterol, Protein, and Amino Acids* (Washington, DC: National Academies Press, 2005), chap. 10, "Protein and Amino Acids," 589–768, and chap. 1, 21–37.
3. *Dietary Reference Intakes: Energy, Carbohydrates, Fiber, Fat, Fatty Acids, Cholesterol, Protein, and Amino Acids* (Washington, DC: National Academies Press, 2005).
4. Dr. Peter Attia and Dr. Don Layman, "#224—Dietary Protein: Amount Needed, Ideal Timing, Quality, and More," *The Drive*, podcast, September 26, 2022, https://peterattiamd.com/donlayman/.
5. Robert R. Wolfe, Andrea M. Cifelli, Georgia Kostas, and Il-Young Kim, "Optimizing Protein Intake in Adults: Interpretation and Application of the Recommended Dietary Allowance Compared with the Acceptable Macronutrient Distribution Range," *Advances in Nutrition* 8, no. 2 (2017): 266–275, https://doi.org/10.3945/an.116.013821.
6. Tyler Stokes, Andrew J. Hector, Robert W. Morton, Christopher McGlory, and Stuart M. Phillips, "Recent Perspectives Regarding the Role of Dietary Protein for the Promotion of Muscle Hypertrophy with Resistance Exercise Training," *Nutrients* 10 (2018): 180, https://doi.org/10.3390/nu10020180.

7. Jonathan W. Carbone, James P. McClung, and Stefan M. Pasiakos, "Recent Advances in the Characterization of Skeletal Muscle and Whole-Body Protein Responses to Dietary Protein and Exercise during Negative Energy Balance," *Advances in Nutrition* 10 (2019): 70–79, https://doi.org/10.1093/advances/nmy087.

8. Cameron J. Mitchell, Amna M. Milan, Sara M. Mitchell, Ning Zeng, Farah Ramzan, et al., "The Effects of Dietary Protein Intake on Appendicular Lean Mass and Muscle Function in Elderly Men: A 10-Week Randomized Controlled Trial," *American Journal of Clinical Nutrition* 106 (2017): 1375–1383, https://doi.org/10.3945/ajcn.117.160325.

9. Rajavel Elango, Muhammad A. Humayun, Ronald O. Ball, and Peter B. Pencharz, "Evidence That Protein Requirements Have Been Significantly Underestimated," *Current Opinion in Clinical Nutrition and Metabolic Care* 13 (2010): 52–57, https://doi.org/10.1097/MCO.0b013e328332f9b7.

10. D. T. Thomas, K. A. Erdman, and L. M. Burke, "Position of the Academy of Nutrition and Dietetics, Dietitians of Canada, and the American College of Sports Medicine: Nutrition and Athletic Performance," *Journal of the Academy of Nutrition and Dietetics* 116 (2016): 501–528, https://doi.org/10.1016/j.jand.2015.12.006.

11. Robert Jäger, Chad M. Kerksick, Bill I. Campbell, Paul J. Cribb, Shawn D. Wells, et al., "International Society of Sports Nutrition Position Stand: Protein and Exercise," *Journal of the International Society of Sports Nutrition* 14 (2017): 20, https://doi.org/10.1186/s12970-017-0177-8.

12. G. B. Forbes, M. R. Brown, S. L. Welle, and B. A. Lipinski, "Deliberate Overfeeding in Women and Men: Energy Cost and Composition of the Weight Gain," *British Journal of Nutrition* 56, no. 1 (1986): 1–9, https://doi.org/10.1079/bjn19860080.

13. Peter Attia and Bill Gifford, *Outlive: The Science & Art of Longevity* (London: Vermilion, 2023).

14. R. Jäger, C. M. Kerksick, B. I. Campbell, et al., "International Society of Sports Nutrition Position Stand: Protein and Exercise," *Journal of the International Society of Sports Nutrition* 14, no. 1 (2017): 20, https://doi.org/10.1186/s12970-017-0177-8.

15. Robert W. Morton, Kieran T. Murphy, Sean R. McKellar, Brad J. Schoenfeld, Menno Henselmans, et al., "A Systematic Review, Meta-Analysis and Meta-Regression of the Effect of Protein Supplementation on Resistance Training-Induced Gains in Muscle Mass and Strength in Healthy Adults," *British Journal of Sports Medicine* 52, no. 6 (2018): 376–384, https://doi.org/10.1136/bjsports-2017-097608.

16. Brandon M. Roberts, Eric R. Helms, Eric T. Trexler, and Patrick J. Fitschen, "Nutritional Recommendations for Physique Athletes," *Journal of Human Kinetics* 71 (2020): 79–108, https://doi.org/10.2478/hukin-2019-0096.

17. Daniel A. Traylor, Stefan H. M. Gorissen, and Stuart M. Phillips, "Perspective: Protein Requirements and Optimal Intakes in Aging: Are We Ready to Recommend More Than the Recommended Daily Allowance?" *Advances in Nutrition* 9, no. 3 (2018): 171–182, https://doi.org/10.1093/advances/nmy003.

18. Harvard Health Publishing, "Preserve Your Muscle Mass," *Harvard Health*, February 19, 2016, https://www.health.harvard.edu/staying-healthy/preserve-your-muscle-mass.

19. Elena Volpi, Reza Nazemi, and Shinya Fujita, "Muscle Tissue Changes with Aging," *Current Opinion in Clinical Nutrition and Metabolic Care* 7, no. 4 (2004): 405–410, https://doi.org/10.1097/01.mco.0000134362.76653.b2.

20. Steven W. Lamberts, Anne W. van den Beld, and Aart J. van der Lely, "The Endocrinology of Aging," *Science* 278 (1997): 419–424, https://doi.org/10.1126/science.278.5337.419.

21. Jeffrey S. Tenover, "Effects of Testosterone Supplementation in the Aging Male," *Journal of Clinical Endocrinology and Metabolism* 75 (1992): 1092–1098, https://doi.org/10.1210/jcem.75.4.1400877.

22. Brian C. Collins, Eija K. Laakkonen, and Dawn A. Lowe, "Aging of the Musculoskeletal System: How the Loss of Estrogen Impacts Muscle Strength," *Bone* 123 (2019): 137–144, https://doi.org/10.1016/j.bone.2019.03.033.

23. Julia L. Krok-Schoen, Archdeacon Price, Min Luo, Olivia J. Kelly, and Carolyn A. Taylor, "Low Dietary Protein Intakes and Associated Dietary Patterns and Functional Limitations in an Aging Population: A NHANES Analysis," *Journal of Nutrition, Health & Aging* 23, no. 4 (2019): 338–347, https://doi.org/10.1007/s12603-019-1174-1.

24. Ana Sandoiu, "US Adults Do Not Consume Enough Protein, Study Warns," *Medical News Today*, February 25, 2019, https://www.medicalnewstoday.com/articles/324533.

25. Chiara Tezze, Marco Sandri, and Paolo Tessari, "Anabolic Resistance in the Pathogenesis of Sarcopenia in the Elderly: Role of Nutrition and Exercise in Young and Old People," *Nutrients* 15, no. 18

(September 20, 2023): 4073, https://doi.org/10.3390/nu15184073.

26. Eric A. Nunes, Laura Colenso-Semple, Sean R. McKellar, Allison Yau, Muhammad U. Ali, et al., "Systematic Review and Meta-Analysis of Protein Intake to Support Muscle Mass and Function in Healthy Adults," *Journal of Cachexia, Sarcopenia and Muscle* 13, no. 2 (2022): 795–810, https://doi.org/10.1002/jcsm.12922.

27. Trevor V. Stephens, Megan Payne, Ronald O. Ball, Peter B. Pencharz, and Rajavel Elango, "Protein Requirements of Healthy Pregnant Women during Early and Late Gestation Are Higher than Current Recommendations," *Journal of Nutrition* 145, no. 1 (2015): 73–78, https://doi.org/10.3945/jn.114.198622.

28. Kathleen J. Motil, Caroline M. Montandon, Mary Thotathuchery, and Cutberto Garza, "Dietary Protein and Nitrogen Balance in Lactating and Nonlactating Women," *American Journal of Clinical Nutrition* 51, no. 3 (1990): 378–384, https://doi.org/10.1093/ajcn/51.3.378.

29. Betina Rasmussen, Madeleine Ennis, Paul Pencharz, Ronald Ball, Glenda Courtney-Martin, et al., "Protein Requirements of Healthy Lactating Women Are Higher Than the Current Recommendations," *Current Developments in Nutrition* 4, Supplement 2 (2020): nzaa049_046, https://doi.org/10.1093/cdn/nzaa049_046.

30. Rajavel Elango, Muhammad A. Humayun, Ronald O. Ball, and Peter B. Pencharz, "Protein Requirement of Healthy School-Age Children Determined by the Indicator Amino Acid Oxidation Method," *American Journal of Clinical Nutrition* 94, no. 6 (2011): 1545–52, https://doi.org/10.3945/ajcn.111.012815.

31. Jonathan W. Carbone and Stefan M. Pasiakos, "Dietary Protein and Muscle Mass: Translating Science to Application and Health Benefit," *Nutrients* 11, no. 5 (2019): 1136, https://doi.org/10.3390/nu11051136.

32. Ga Won Ko, Csaba M. Rhee, Kamyar Kalantar-Zadeh, and Shivam Joshi, "The Effects of High-Protein Diets on Kidney Health and Longevity," *Journal of the American Society of Nephrology* 31, no. 8 (2020): 1667–1679, https://doi.org/10.1681/ASN.2020010028.

33. Shawn M. Arent, Heather P. Cintineo, Brandon A. McFadden, Alexandria J. Chandler, and Melissa A. Arent, "Nutrient Timing: A Garage Door of Opportunity?" *Nutrients* 12, no. 7 (2020): 1948, https://doi.org/10.3390/nu12071948.

34. Sarah Katz, "Fact or Fiction: The Anabolic Window," *Georgia State University*, October 13, 2021, https://lewis.gsu.edu/2021/10/13/fact-or-fiction-the-anabolic-window/.

35. Nicholas A. Burd, Daniel W. West, Daniel R. Moore, Philip J. Atherton, Adam W. Staples, et al., "Enhanced Amino Acid Sensitivity of Myofibrillar Protein Synthesis Persists for up to 24 Hours after Resistance Exercise in Young Men," *Journal of Nutrition* 141, no. 4 (2011): 568–573, https://doi.org/10.3945/jn.110.135038.

36. B. J. Schoenfeld and A. A. Aragon, "Is There a Postworkout Anabolic Window of Opportunity for Nutrient Consumption? Clearing up Controversies," *Journal of Orthop Sports Physical Therapy* 48, no. 12 (2018): 911–914. doi: 10.2519/jospt.2018.0615. PMID: 30702982.

37. Melissa M. Mamerow, Jamie A. Mettler, Kirk L. English, Sarah L. Casperson, Emily Arentson-Lantz, Melinda Sheffield-Moore, Donald K. Layman, and Douglas Paddon-Jones, "Dietary Protein Distribution Positively Influences 24-Hour Muscle Protein Synthesis in Healthy Adults," *Journal of Nutrition* 144, no. 6 (2014): 876–880, https://doi.org/10.3945/jn.113.185280.

38. Peter J. Arciero, Michael J. Ormsbee, Christopher L. Gentile, Bradley C. Nindl, Jonathan R. Brestoff, and Brian C. Ruby, "Increased Protein Intake and Meal Frequency Reduces Abdominal Fat during Energy Balance and Energy Deficit," *Obesity* 21, no. 7 (2013): 1357–1366, https://doi.org/10.1002/oby.20135.

39. Brad Jon Schoenfeld and Alan Albert Aragon, "How Much Protein Can the Body Use in a Single Meal for Muscle-Building? Implications for Daily Protein Distribution," *Journal of the International Society of Sports Nutrition* 15 (2018): 10, https://doi.org/10.1186/s12970-018-0215-1.

40. Daniel R. Moore, Tyler A. Churchward-Venne, Oliver Witard, Leigh Breen, Nicholas A. Burd, Kevin D. Tipton, and Stuart M. Phillips, "Protein Ingestion to Stimulate Myofibrillar Protein Synthesis Requires Greater Relative Protein Intakes in Healthy Older versus Younger Men," *Journal of Gerontology: Series A, Biological Sciences and Medical Sciences* 70, no. 1 (2015): 57–62, https://doi.org/10.1093/gerona/glu103.

41. Brad J. Schoenfeld and Alan A. Aragon, "How Much Protein Can the Body Use in a Single Meal for Muscle-Building? Implications for Daily Protein Distribution," *Journal of the International Society of Sports Nutrition* 15 (2018): 10, https://doi.org/10.1186/s12970-018-0215-1.

42. Jorn Trommelen, Gijs A. A. van Lieshout, Jeremiah Nyakayiru, Anne M. Holwerda, Joris S. J. Smeets, et al., "The Anabolic Response to Protein Ingestion During Recovery from Exercise Has No Upper Limit in Magnitude and Duration In Vivo in Humans," *Cell Reports Medicine* 4, no. 12 (2023): 101324, https://doi.org/10.1016/j.xcrm.2023.101324.

43. Emily Williamson and Daniel R. Moore, "A Muscle-Centric Perspective on Intermittent Fasting: A Suboptimal Dietary Strategy for Supporting Muscle Protein Remodeling and Muscle Mass?" *Frontiers in Nutrition* 8 (2021): 640621, https://doi.org/10.3389/fnut.2021.640621.

44. Alex E. Mohr, Karen L. Sweazea, Devin A. Bowes, Paniz Jasbi, Corrie M. Whisner, et al., "Gut Microbiome Remodeling and Metabolomic Profile Improves in Response to Protein Pacing with Intermittent Fasting versus Continuous Caloric Restriction," *Nature Communications* 15 (2024): 4155, https://doi.org/10.1038/s41467-024-48355-5.

Chapter 3: Protein Sources

1. Julie Floyd Jones, "Chicken vs. Fish: Which Is Healthier? Here's What Science Says," *EatingWell*, July 3, 2024, https://www.eatingwell.com/chicken-vs-fish-which-is-healthier-8673831.

2. N. Roohani, R. Hurrell, R. Kelishadi, and R. Schulin, "Zinc and Its Importance for Human Health: An Integrative Review," *Journal of Research in Medical Sciences* 18, no. 2 (2013): 144–157, https://www.ncbi.nlm.nih.gov/pmc/articles/PMC3724376/.

3. E. Dolan, B. Gualano, and E. S. Rawson, "Beyond Muscle: The Effects of Creatine Supplementation on Brain Creatine, Cognitive Processing, and Traumatic Brain Injury," *European Journal of Sport Science* 19, no. 1 (2018): 1–14, https://doi.org/10.1080/17461391.2018.1500644.

4. A. J. Aguiar Bonfim Cruz et al., "Creatine Improves Total Sleep Duration Following Resistance Training Days versus Non-Resistance Training Days among Naturally Menstruating Females," *Nutrients* 16 (2024): 2772, https://doi.org/10.3390/nu16162772.

5. Darren G. Candow et al., "Current Evidence and Possible Future Applications of Creatine Supplementation for Older Adults," *Nutrients* 13 (2021): 745, https://doi.org/10.3390/nu13030745.

6. Arunabh Bhattacharya et al., "Biological Effects of Conjugated Linoleic Acids in Health and Disease," *The Journal of Nutritional Biochemistry* 17, no. 12 (2006): 789–810, https://doi.org/10.1016/j.jnutbio.2006.02.009.

7. Natalie A. Suedekum et al., "Iron and the Athlete," *Current Sports Medicine Reports* 4, no. 4 (2005): 199–202.

8. U.S. Department of Agriculture, "Beef, Rib Eye Steak, Boneless, Lip-On, Separable Lean and Fat, Trimmed to 1/8" Fat, All Grades, Cooked, Grilled," *FoodData Central*, April 1, 2019, https://fdc.nal.usda.gov/food-details/173392/nutrients.

9. Michael J. Puglisi and Maria L. Fernandez, "The Health Benefits of Egg Protein," *Nutrients* 14, no. 14 (2022): 2904, https://doi.org/10.3390/nu14142904.

10. Maria L. Fernandez and Catherine J. Andersen, "Eggs, Composition and Health," in *Encyclopedia of Food and Health*, ed. P. M. Finglas, F. Toldrá, and B. Caballero (Amsterdam: Elsevier, 2015), 470–475.

11. Matt Pikosky, "What Is the Difference Between Whey and Casein Protein?" *Undeniably Dairy*, July 6, 2016, https://www.usdairy.com/news-articles/whats-the-difference-between-casein-and-whey.

12. Patrick J. M. Pinckaers, Jorn Trommelen, Tim Snijders, and Luc J. C. van Loon, "The Anabolic Response to Plant-Based Protein Ingestion," *Sports Medicine* 51, Supplement 1 (2021): 59–74, https://doi.org/10.1007/s40279-021-01540-8.

13. U.S. Department of Agriculture, *FoodData Central*, accessed Dec 2024, https://fdc.nal.usda.gov/.

14. Nutritionix, accessed Dec 2024, https://www.nutritionix.com/.

15. CalorieKing, accessed Dec 2024, https://www.calorieking.com/us/en/.

16. Jay R. Hoffman and Michael J. Falvo, "Protein—Which Is Best?" *Journal of Sports Science and Medicine* 3 (2004): 118–130.

17. Elena Volpi, Hiroshi Kobayashi, Melinda Sheffield-Moore, Bettina Mittendorfer, and Robert R. Wolfe, "Essential Amino Acids Are Primarily Responsible for the Amino Acid Stimulation of Muscle Protein Anabolism in Healthy Elderly Adults," *American Journal of Clinical Nutrition* 78, no. 2 (2003): 250–258, https://doi.org/10.1093/ajcn/78.2.250.

18. Robert R. Wolfe, "Branched-Chain Amino Acids and Muscle Protein Synthesis in Humans: Myth or Reality?" *Journal of the International Society of Sports Nutrition* 14 (2017): 30, https://doi.org/10.1186/s12970-017-0184-9.
19. Stephen B. Wilkinson, Mark A. Tarnopolsky, Michael J. Macdonald, Jennifer R. Macdonald, Donald Armstrong, et al., "Consumption of Fluid Skim Milk Promotes Greater Muscle Protein Accretion after Resistance Exercise Than Does Consumption of an Isonitrogenous and Isoenergetic Soy-Protein Beverage," *American Journal of Clinical Nutrition* 85, no. 4 (2007): 1031–1040, https://doi.org/10.1093/ajcn/85.4.1031.
20. Patrick J. M. Pinckaers, Jorn Trommelen, Tim Snijders, and Luc J. C. van Loon, "The Anabolic Response to Plant-Based Protein Ingestion," *Sports Medicine* 51, Supplement 1 (2021): 59–74, https://doi.org/10.1007/s40279-021-01540-8.
21. Sindhu Kashyap, Nirupama Shivakumar, Aneesia Varkey, Rajendran Duraisamy, Tinku Thomas, et al., "Ileal Digestibility of Intrinsically Labeled Hen's Egg and Meat Protein Determined with the Dual Stable Isotope Tracer Method in Indian Adults," *American Journal of Clinical Nutrition* 108, no. 5 (2018): 980–987, https://doi.org/10.1093/ajcn/nqy178.
22. Sindhu Kashyap, Aneesia Varkey, Nirupama Shivakumar, Sarita Devi, B. H. Rajashekar Reddy, et al., "True Ileal Digestibility of Legumes Determined by Dual-Isotope Tracer Method in Indian Adults," *American Journal of Clinical Nutrition* 110, no. 4 (2019): 873–882, https://doi.org/10.1093/ajcn/nqz159.
23. Nathalie Gausserès, Séverine Mahé, Robert Benamouzig, Claude Luengo, Fabienne Ferriere, et al., "[15N]-Labeled Pea Flour Protein Nitrogen Exhibits Good Ileal Digestibility and Postprandial Retention in Humans," *Journal of Nutrition* 127, no. 6 (1997): 1160, https://doi.org/10.1093/jn/127.6.1160.
24. Nicholas A. Burd, Joseph W. Beals, Ingrid G. Martinez, Ana F. Salvador, and Sarah K. Skinner, "Food-First Approach to Enhance the Regulation of Post-Exercise Skeletal Muscle Protein Synthesis and Remodeling," *Sports Medicine* 49, Supplement 1 (2019): 59–68, https://doi.org/10.1007/s40279-018-1009-y.

Chapter 4: Protein Myths and Controversies

1. Rafaela de Miranda, Patricia Weimer, and Ricardo Rossi, "Effects of Hydrolyzed Collagen Supplementation on Skin Aging: A Systematic Review and Meta-Analysis," *International Journal of Dermatology* (2021).
2. Carole Paul, Stefanie Leser, and Stephan Oesser, "Significant Amounts of Functional Collagen Peptides Can Be Incorporated in the Diet While Maintaining Indispensable Amino Acid Balance," *Nutrients* 11, no. 5 (2019): 1079, https://doi.org/10.3390/nu11051079.
3. Katie McCallum, "Are Egg Whites Healthy?" *Houston Methodist*, June 8, 2023, https://www.houstonmethodist.org/blog/articles/2023/jun/are-egg-whites-healthy-healthier-than-whole-eggs/.
4. Jonathan W. Carbone and Stefan M. Pasiakos, "Dietary Protein and Muscle Mass: Translating Science to Application and Health Benefit," *Nutrients* 11, no. 5 (2019): 1136, https://doi.org/10.3390/nu11051136.
5. Cassandra E. Berryman, Sonya Agarwal, Harris R. Lieberman, Victor L. Fulgoni, and Stefan M. Pasiakos, "Diets Higher in Animal and Plant Protein Are Associated with Lower Adiposity and Do Not Impair Kidney Function in US Adults," *American Journal of Clinical Nutrition* 104 (2016): 743–749, https://doi.org/10.3945/ajcn.116.133819.
6. Mark C. Devries, Arjuna Sithamparapillai, Krista S. Brimble, Laura Banfield, Robert W. Morton, et al., "Changes in Kidney Function Do Not Differ between Healthy Adults Consuming Higher- Compared with Lower- or Normal-Protein Diets: A Systematic Review and Meta-Analysis," *Journal of Nutrition* 148 (2018): 1760–1775, https://doi.org/10.1093/jn/nxy197.
7. Vivek Panwar, Aishwarya Singh, Manini Bhatt, Rajiv K. Tonk, Shavkatjon Azizov, et al., "Multifaceted Role of mTOR (Mammalian Target of Rapamycin) Signaling Pathway in Human Health and Disease," *Signal Transduction and Targeted Therapy* 8 (2023): 375, https://doi.org/10.1038/s41392-023-01608-z.
8. Peter Attia and Bill Gifford, *Outlive: The Science & Art of Longevity* (London: Vermilion, 2023).
9. Dr. Peter Attia and Dr. Layne Norton, "#205—Dispelling myths that excess protein intake increases cancer risk," *The Drive*, podcast, May 2, 2022, https://peterattiamd.com/dispelling-myths-protein-increases-cancer-risk/.

10. Leandro F. M. Rezende, Dong Hoon Lee, NaNa Keum, Kana Wu, José Eluf-Neto, et al., "Resistance Training and Total and Site-Specific Cancer Risk: A Prospective Cohort Study of 33,787 US Men," *British Journal of Cancer* 123 (2020): 666–672, https://doi.org/10.1038/s41416-020-0921-8.

11. Kelly M. Mazzilli, Charles E. Matthews, Emily A. Salerno, and Steven C. Moore, "Weight Training and Risk of 10 Common Types of Cancer," *Medicine & Science in Sports & Exercise* 51, no. 9 (2019): 1845–1851, https://doi.org/10.1249/MSS.0000000000001987.

12. Andrew Huberman and Layne Norton, "Is mTOR Signaling Bad?" *Huberman Lab*, https://ai.hubermanlab.com/c/52474c34-bbed-11ef-a70a-cf526bf3165e.

13. Heather Cooan, "Gluconeogenesis: Does Too Much Protein Convert to Sugar?" *Heather Cooan*, June 9, 2024, https://heathercooan.com/gluconeogenesis/.

14. Corentin Fromentin, Didier Tomé, Françoise Nau, Louis Flet, Claude Luengo, Dalila Azzout-Marniche, et al., "Dietary Proteins Contribute Little to Glucose Production, Even under Optimal Gluconeogenic Conditions in Healthy Humans," *Diabetes* 62, no. 5 (2013): 1435–1442, https://doi.org/10.2337/db12-1208.

15. Dr. Peter Attia and Dr. Don Layman, "#224—Dietary Protein: Amount Needed, Ideal Timing, Quality, and More," *The Drive*, podcast, September 26, 2022, https://peterattiamd.com/donlayman/.

Chapter 5: Low-Carb, High-Protein Basics

1. Michael W. Brands and Melaku M. Manhiani, "Sodium-Retaining Effect of Insulin in Diabetes," *American Journal of Physiology: Regulatory, Integrative and Comparative Physiology* 303, no. 11 (2012): R1101–R1109, https://doi.org/10.1152/ajpregu.00390.2012.

2. Saima Faruque, Jing Tong, Vera Lacmanovic, Charles Agbonghae, David M. Minaya, et al., "The Dose Makes the Poison: Sugar and Obesity in the United States—A Review," *Polish Journal of Food and Nutrition Sciences* 69, no. 3 (2019): 219–233, https://doi.org/10.31883/pjfns/110735.

3. P. A. Dyson, S. Beatty, and D. R. Matthews, "A Low-Carbohydrate Diet Is More Effective in Reducing Body Weight Than Healthy Eating in Both Diabetic and Non-Diabetic Subjects," *Diabetic Medicine* 24, no. 12 (2007): 1430–1435, https://doi.org/10.1111/j.1464-5491.2007.02290.x.

4. Timothy P. Wycherley, Lisa J. Moran, Peter M. Clifton, Manny Noakes, and Grant D. Brinkworth, "Effects of Energy-Restricted High-Protein, Low-Fat Compared with Standard-Protein, Low-Fat Diets: A Meta-Analysis of Randomized Controlled Trials," *American Journal of Clinical Nutrition* 96 (2012): 1281–1298, https://doi.org/10.3945/ajcn.112.044321.

5. Nancy Santesso, Elie A. Akl, Marlisa Bianchi, Andrew Mente, Reem Mustafa, et al., "Effects of Higher-versus Lower-Protein Diets on Health Outcomes: A Systematic Review and Meta-Analysis," *European Journal of Clinical Nutrition* 66 (2012): 780–788, https://doi.org/10.1038/ejcn.2012.37.

6. Anne Raben Skov, Søren Toubro, Birgitte Rønn, Lars Holm, and Arne Astrup, "Randomized Trial on Protein vs. Carbohydrate in Ad Libitum Fat-Reduced Diet for the Treatment of Obesity," *International Journal of Obesity and Related Metabolic Disorders* 23 (1999): 528–536, https://doi.org/10.1038/sj.ijo.0800867.

7. Margriet S. Westerterp-Plantenga, Manuela P. Lejeune, Ineke Nijs, Margriet van Ooijen, and Eva M. Kovacs, "High Protein Intake Sustains Weight Maintenance After Body Weight Loss in Humans," *International Journal of Obesity and Related Metabolic Disorders* 28 (2004): 57–64, https://doi.org/10.1038/sj.ijo.0802461.

8. Susanna H. Holt, J. C. Miller, P. Petocz, and E. Farmakalidis, "A Satiety Index of Common Foods," *European Journal of Clinical Nutrition* 49 (1995): 675–690.

9. Judith Bowen, Manny Noakes, and Peter M. Clifton, "Appetite Regulatory Hormone Responses to Various Dietary Proteins Differ by Body Mass Index Status Despite Similar Reductions in ad Libitum Energy Intake," *Journal of Clinical Endocrinology & Metabolism* 91 (2006): 2913–2919, https://doi.org/10.1210/jc.2006-0609.

10. Anders Belza, Christian Ritz, Mette Q. Sørensen, Jens J. Holst, Jens F. Rehfeld, et al., "Contribution of Gastroenteropancreatic Appetite Hormones to Protein-Induced Satiety," *American Journal of Clinical Nutrition* 97 (2013): 980–989, https://doi.org/10.3945/ajcn.112.047563.

11. Olga Davidenko, Nicolas Darcel, Gilles Fromentin, and Didier Tomé, "Control of Protein and Energy Intake: Brain Mechanisms," *European Journal of Clinical Nutrition* 67 (2013): 455–461, https://doi.org/10.1038/ejcn.2013.73.

12. Marlon Calcagno, Hana Kahleova, Jasmol Alwarith, Natasha N. Burgess, Rosie A. Flores, et al., "The Thermic Effect of Food: A Review," *Journal of the American College of Nutrition* 38, no. 6 (2019): 547–551, https://doi.org/10.1080/07315724.2018.1552544.

13. Kevin J. Acheson, "Influence of Autonomic Nervous System on Nutrient-Induced Thermogenesis in Humans," *Nutrition* 9 (1993): 373–380.

14. Klaas R. Westerterp, "Diet Induced Thermogenesis," *Nutrition & Metabolism* (London) 1 (2004): 5, https://doi.org/10.1186/1743-7075-1-5.

15. Dalila Azzout-Marniche, Claire Gaudichon, Claire Blouet, Claire Bos, Véronique Mathé, et al., "Liver Glyconeogenesis: A Pathway to Cope with Postprandial Amino Acid Excess in High-Protein Fed Rats?" *American Journal of Physiology: Regulatory, Integrative and Comparative Physiology* 292 (2007): R1400–R1407, https://doi.org/10.1152/ajpregu.00566.2006.

16. Mark F. McCarty, "Promotion of Hepatic Lipid Oxidation and Gluconeogenesis as a Strategy for Appetite Control," *Medical Hypotheses* 42 (1994): 215–225, https://doi.org/10.1016/0306-9877(94)90120-1.

INDEX

C

G

H

I

N

O

P

Q–R

S

T

V

W

X–Y

Z